Harmful to Minors

The Perils
of Protecting
Children from Sex

Judith Levine

Foreword by Dr. Joycelyn M. Elders

Thunder's Mouth Press
New York

HARMFUL TO MINORS: THE PERILS OF PROTECTING CHILDREN FROM SEX

Passage from *Weetzie Bat* text copyright 1989 Francesca Lia Block; used by permission of HarperCollins Publishing. "Brown Penny" by W.B. Yeats, from *The Collected Works of W.B. Yeats, Volume 1: The Poems, Revised*, edited by Richard J. Finneran (New York: Scribner, 1997); reprinted with permission of Scribner, a division of Simon & Schuster, Inc. Fragment from *Sappho: A New Translation*, by Mary Barnard (Berkeley: University of California Press, 1958); copyright 1958 by the Regents of the University of California, renewed 1986 by Mary Barnard; used by permission of the University of California Press.

Published by
Thunder's Mouth Press
An Imprint of Avalon Publishing Group Incorporated
161 William Street, 16th Floor
New York, NY 10038

Originally Published by
University of Minnesota Press
111 Third Ave. South, Suite 290
Minneapolis, MN 55401

First Thunder's Mouth Press edition 2003

Library of Congress Cataloging-in-Publication Data is available.

ISBN 1-56025-516-1

9 8 7 6 5 4 3 2 1

Printed in the United States of America
Distributed by Publishers Group West

Praise for *Harmful to Minors*

"In the best tradition of social criticism, *Harmful to Minors* offers a cogent and passionate critique of the war against young people's sexuality. An uncompromising humanist and feminist, Judith Levine exposes the moral panic behind such politics as "abstinence-only" sex education and insists on adults' responsibility to give affirmative support to children's and teenagers' sexual develop-ments. . . . Levine and her publisher deserve the highest praise for launching a necessary, overdue debate on one of the most stubborn taboos of our era."

—From the judges of the 2002 *Los Angeles Times Book Awards*

"A sane, provocative, and well-researched effort to make readers think critically about what acts are, exactly, harmful to minors; what we should, and should not, be trying to protect our children from; and how we can separate legitimate worries from irrational panics, and real dangers from false alarms."

—*Times Literary Supplement* (London)

"Judith Levine is one of a rare species—she's an independent scholar and journalist who, unlike many in the academy, writes clearly and with great force. . . . *Harmful to Minors* is a carefully researched ex-amination of the myriad ways American culture attempts to control, monitor, suppress, and even eradicate children's access to informa-tion about sexuality, sexual health, and reproduction—all in the name of protection—and how it pathologizes and criminalizes chil-dren's and teens' sexual expression. . . . Levine argues strongly, thoughtfully, and persuasively that children are far more harmed by these misguided attempts at "protection" than they would be by having full access to honest information about sexuality. . . ."

—Michael Bronski, *The Boston Phoenix*

"[Levine's] research offers a potent challenge to the conventional wisdom about sex, sexuality, and sex education. Written with verve, humor, and wit, [*Harmful to Minors*] is a trenchant look at America's failure to extol the erotic, and an insightful observation of our preoccupation with pedophilia, deviance, illness, and mis-conduct."

—*The Progressive*

"*Harmful to Minors* is one of the most respectful and compassionate books I've read in a long time. It's thoroughly documented and brilliantly argued, often angry for good reason and often painful, because Levine holds up a stunning, eye-opening, shake-your-head-and-clear-the-cobwebs-away mirror to what she rightly calls a continuing national panic." —Pat Holt, *Uncensored*

"Likely to be on of the most significant books of the season...convincingly arguing that socially conservative beliefs and policies are largely to blame for the problems they purport to address." —The San Francisco Examiner

"*Harmful to Minors* is a sage, intelligent, industriously reported and eminently sane book...dedicated to recounting how the right wing, through sham social science, media sensationalism and self-righteous congressional inquiries, convinced the mainstream that sex is by nature dangerous to children." —*In These Times*

". . . A blistering critique of the current American approach to teaching children about sex . . . [Levine's] brand of sexual libertarianism is injected with a healthy dose of contemporary feminism and multicultural sensitivity, and tempered by an acknowledgment of the new dangers attending sex today. This engaging book takes as its premise the still shocking notion that even children are entitled to basic sexual freedom, privacy, and pleasure." —*Yale Review of Books*

"What Levine does argue, quite effectively, is that a lot of what teenagers are taught about sex these days makes it seem like a dangerous, dirty business. . . . The most disturbing thing about the reaction to Levine's book is the assumption that the subjects she discusses should not be discussed at all, because there is only one thing to be said about them." —*The New York Times Magazine*

"The greatest virtue in Levine's book is its hope that children might learn to find joy in the realm of the senses, the world of ideas and souls, so that when sex disappoints and love fails, as they will, a teenager, a grown-up, still has herself, and a universe of small delights and strong hearts to fall back on." —*The Nation*

To Paul

Contents

II. Sense and Sexuality

Foreword

Dr. Joycelyn M. Elders

In America we are in the midst of a sexual crisis. We lead the Western world in virtually every sexual problem: teenage pregnancy, abortion, rape, incest, child abuse, sexually transmitted disease, HIV/AIDS, and many more.[1] Yet when the Surgeon General issues a call to action on sexual health urging comprehensive sex education, abstinence, and other measures to promote responsible sexual behavior, and advocates that we break our "conspiracy of silence about sexuality," we want to fire the Surgeon General. Sexually transmitted diseases, ranging from the serious to the fatal, are a fact of life in high schools and neighborhoods across the country. Misinformation and scare tactics about common sexual practices like masturbation are rampant. Despite these facts, and despite parents' overwhelming desire for their children to receive detailed sex education at school as well as at home,[2] our society remains unwilling to make sexuality part of a comprehensive health education program in the schools and anxious to the point of hysteria about young people and sex. Our public health policy concerning sexuality education appears to be ideologically motivated rather than empirically driven. Yet no matter how widespread, politically viable, or popular a program may be, efficacy in preventing and modifying behavior associated with this sexual crisis must remain the primary criterion by which programs are changed.[3]

Ironically, for someone who has come to be closely associated with forthrightness about sexuality, I was raised in an environment in which sex was never discussed. During my life I have moved from complete, community-imposed silence about sex to dealing professionally almost every day with some of the toughest issues about sexuality. I know firsthand what it was like to be ignorant, and I also know how vital it is to be informed. I have talked with parents who have just learned that their newborn baby was born with sexually ambiguous genitals and with parents whose child isn't advancing toward puberty. I have spent large parts of my professional life trying to educate people and develop social policies to address problems that are eating away at the very fabric of our society—teenage pregnancy and its frequent result, inescapable poverty, ignorance and enslavement, HIV, AIDS, and other sexually transmitted diseases. The day-in, day-out nature of this work leads me to be impatient with people who object to Surgeons General, teachers, parents, and others advocating the use of condoms, for instance. As Ira Reiss states so eloquently in his book *Solving America's Sexual Crisis,* "the vows of abstinence break far more easily than do latex condoms."[4] Hysteria about sex has hindered attempts to address these pressing concerns, and the people hurt most are those who most need the information—our young people, the poor, and the uninformed. Ignorance is not bliss.

All of this makes *Harmful to Minors* such a vitally important book, one that brings an essential new perspective to this crucial set of issues. Drawing together stories in the media (as well as those that are less known), interviews with young people and their parents, and astute analysis, Judith Levine passionately argues for honesty and forthrightness in talking to children about sex. She lays bare the conservative political agenda that underlies many supposed "child protection" efforts. Perhaps what is most valuable about this book is the way it outlines the dominant, and often hidden, fact of discussions about sexuality in this country: the influence of the religious right (or what I have been known to call the "very religious non-Christian right"). I have spoken and written many times about my disgust with people who have a love affair with the fetus but won't take care of children once they are born. *Harmful to Minors* not only makes explicit the crucial importance of frank and accurate information about sexuality being widely available to people of all ages, it lays out a sensible, positive, and possible program to do so.

Treating sex as dangerous is dangerous in itself. We need to be matter-of-fact about what is, after all, a fact of life. Judith Levine argues convincingly that there is an intimate connection between the values we display in our sexual lives and the values we display as a society. She is right—sex is a moral issue, but not in the way the Christian right claims. Children must be taught sexual ethics and responsibility, inside and outside the home, just as they are taught how to behave in any number of public and private arenas. Teaching children to have self-respect, to feel good about themselves, to make good decisions: to me, that is sexuality education.

Author's Note

Most of the research for this book, including interviews, was conducted between 1996 and early 2000, and pertinent statistics were updated in 2001. The names of all nonprofessionals have been fictionalized, along with some identifying characteristics.

Acknowledgments

Among the most pleasurable tasks of writing a book is thanking the people who helped you. Of course, that includes everyone who has fed you a meal, suggested an idea, or cheered you up when the going got rough, during all the years you worked on the project. Because this book's going was frequently rough and the years were many, I was the recipient of many meals and many ideas—and an inordinate amount of much-needed cheering. So I begin by asking forgiveness from those I have not named; and to those I have, I extend the usual disclaimer: you are held harmless in any breach, infringement, violation, or stupidity herein committed.

Thanks to my writers' group—Allan Bérubé, Jeffrey Escoffier, Amber Hollibaugh, Jonathan Ned Katz, and Carole Vance—for their monthly infusions of loyalty, wisdom, and pasta. Members of the group, as well as Bill Finnegan, James Kincaid, Harry Maurer, Vanalyne Green, Peggy Brick, Leonore Tiefer, and Sharon Lamb read all or part of the manuscript (sometimes more than once!) and commented with acuity and generosity. At *Mother Jones,* Sarah Pollock provided excellent and endlessly patient editorial guidance to what is now chapter 3, and Jeanne Brokaw saved my skin with her meticulous fact-checking. Steve Fraser first acquired this book when others shied away and gave it learned and encouraging editorial guidance before he left commercial publishing. The industry is much diminished by the loss of his erudition, seriousness, and courage. I feel fortunate to have ended up with Carrie Mullen at the University of Minnesota Press, who has proven her commitment to unpopular ideas and her enthusiasm for scholarship without disciplinary borders. Great thanks too to the press's outside readers, who put their fingers directly on the book's weaknesses. Where I've cooperated, they greatly improved my arguments.

For much of its writing this book has felt like a battle. As time passed, both the political and commercial climate seemed to grow more hostile to its ideas—and, more important, to children's sexual happiness—and that has often rendered me lonely and discouraged. Those who stand by the ideals to which the book is committed, therefore, have risen even higher in my esteem. In my closest circle, Debbie Nathan, Bob Chatelle, and Jim D'Entremont earn my admiration for continuing to labor on behalf of those unjustly accused during the child abuse panics, when almost everyone else has forgotten them. Leanne Katz, the late executive director of the National Coalition Against Censorship, was prescient in recognizing the cultural calamity inherent in censoring sex and was never afraid to put herself on the line for all varieties of human expression. Her successor, Joan Bertin, is doing an impressive job filling her shoes. Among sex therapists, Leonore Tiefer doesn't always win friends, but she always influences the people in her profession and elsewhere with her tough, sane, pro-sex, antisexist thinking and activism.

In these pages, I hoist some javelins in the direction of the comprehensive sex-education community. But without organizations like Planned Parenthood, the Sex Information and Education Council of the United States (SIECUS), the Network for Family Life Education, and Advocates for Youth and without progressive educators like Peggy Brick, Susie Wilson, Pamela Wilson, Deborah Roffman, Konnie McCaffree, Elizabeth Casparian, and Leslie Kantor, there would be no decent sex education in this country at all. Even when my criticism is sharp, it is meant humbly.

Several libraries and their librarians were invaluable: SIECUS, Political Research Associates, the University of Vermont, and the New York Public Library. The Goldensohn Fund provided needed funds for much of the research in chapter 2.

One of the ongoing themes of my intellectual life is the insufficiency of most commonly accepted categories—Man, Woman, Child, Normal, Deviant—to capture the meanings of what they purport to describe. Most of what interests me falls into the wide-open noncategory of Other. So, under the honorable heading of Other Contributors, in alphabetical order only, I thank: Ann Agee,

Bill Andriette, Lynn Mikel Brown, Julius Levine Cillo, Diane Cleaver, the staff and youth at District 202 in Minneapolis, Emily Feinstein, Roger Fox, Debra Haffner, Marjorie Heins, Jenni Hoffman, Carol Hopkins, Janet Jacobs and family, Philip Kaushall, Marty Klein, Steve Knox, the Levines, Russell Miller, the National Writers Union, Paul Okami, Ursula Owen, the Passover group, Flavio Pompetti, Linda and Kevin Reed, Susan Richman, Joan and Steve Rappaport, Martha and Marty Roth, Ciro Scotti and the *Business Week* copy desk, the Sex and Censorship committee of the National Coalition Against Censorship, Jonathan Silin, Ann Snitow, Lisa Springer, Carolyn Stack, Larry Stanley, Sharon Thompson, Denise Trudeau, George and Betsy Whitehead, Elizabeth Wilson, and David Wolowitz. My deepest gratitude goes to every one of the hundreds of sources with whom I talked, and sometimes badgered relentlessly, but in particular to the many parents and kids who taught me much of what I needed to learn but whose names I promised to hold in confidence.

Joy Harris is the best agent a person could ask for and a lot more than that. Her talented associate Stephanie Abou stepped into the breach and found this book a home when I'd pretty much lost hope.

I met Janice Irvine not long after I started *Harmful to Minors,* and more than any other single person she has been its midwife. Opening her mind, heart, home, and vast knowledge of the subject to me, although she was working on a competing project, Janice became my chief intellectual sounding board and, just as important, a dear friend.

Finally, I dedicate these pages to Paul Cillo, whose constancy to all the right things inspires me, and whose love and humor in the face of all the wrong things are among the best reasons I have for getting up in the morning.

Introduction

Peril and Pleasure, Parenting and Childhood

Again, there is danger, the mother of morality—great danger—but this time displaced onto the individual, onto the nearest and dearest, onto the street, onto one's own child, one's own heart, one's own innermost secret recesses of wish and will.
—Nietzsche, *Beyond Good and Evil* (1886)

In America today, it is nearly impossible to publish a book that says children and teenagers can have sexual pleasure and be safe too.

Perhaps I should have gotten the hint five years ago, when my agent started sending around the proposal to commercial publishers. House after house declined. "Levine is an engaging writer, and her argument is strong and provocative," said one typical rejection. "But we don't see how this point of view will find the broad readership that would justify our commitment." They all closed with some version of the perennial editorial valediction "Good luck." I now hear that phrase as a snort of sarcasm.

When one of the most serious editors in commercial publishing did acquire the book, and I wrote a first draft, his comments were encouraging but sober. "It's a courageous book," he wrote me, "for which, as these chapters make abundantly and depressingly clear, the timing probably couldn't be worse." As it turned out, the timing could not have been worse, for him or for me. He was fired (not because of my book) and moved on to other enterprises, and my manuscript was passed to another senior editor. When she demurred (as the mother of a thirteen-year-old girl, she told me diplomatically, "I'm just not able to address some of the issues with enough objectivity to serve as your guide"), a new recruit at the house took the orphan in. That woman inaugurated a yearlong process by which the book would be rendered, as she put it, "more palatable to parents," who were now presumed to be the only interested readers. She asked for "comforting messages," mottled the manuscript with advisories, which begged for deletions: "This sentence will offend parents." "Many parents will find this hard to swallow." She suggested, in deference to parental anxiety, that I remove the word *pleasure* from the introduction.

In the end, the manuscript was not parent-friendly enough. It left that house and went to others, where it was also found commercially unviable. One editorial board called it "radioactive." The week I got that Geiger count, a full-page ad for John Gray's *Children Are from Heaven* ran in the *New York Times*. Its text seemed to promise parents that if they just read the book, their kids would become healthy, happy, obedient, and successful. The chubby cherubs floating around the margins implied that they might sprout wings, too.

To predict which books will sell, publishers try to keep their fingers on the collective pulse; they like to think their lists constitute a kind of EKG of the mainstream culture. The sensors through which this intelligence is derived are of two kinds: sales figures of similar books or the author's other books, and something less concrete—the acquiring editors' feelings, known in the trade as instinct.

Now, it is easy for writers to make excuses for rejection, and if I am doing so, well, kindly excuse me. But also allow me to offer this as explanation for what happened to *Harmful to Minors*: history happened. The "instinct" that moved those editors, who felt both as parents and as proxies for their imagined parent-readers, was shaped by particular cultural, economic, and political forces and events in the past and the present. The forces and feelings that almost ate *Harmful to Minors* are precisely what *Harmful to Minors* is about.

This book, at bottom, is about fear. America's fears about child sexuality are both peculiarly contemporary (I am certain I would not have had the same troubles twenty-five years ago) and forged deep in history. *Harmful to Minors* recounts how that fear got its claws into America in the late twentieth century and how, abetted by a sentimental, sometimes cynical, politics of child protectionism, it now dominates the ways we think and act about children's sexuality. The book investigates the policies and practices that affect children's and teens' quotidian sexual lives—censorship, psychology, sex education, family, criminal, and reproductive law, and the journalism and parenting advice that begs for "solutions" while exciting more terror, like those trick birthday candles that reignite each time you blow them out.

The architects and practitioners of all the above use the term *child protection* for what they do. But, as the stories of real children and families in this book show, they often accomplish the opposite. Indeed, the sexual politics of fear is harmful to minors.

Private Life

If parents at the turn of the twenty-first century are fearful, there are many reasons they should be. As the economy globalizes, its newly created wealth provides only a provisional and selective security. Census Bureau data released in early 2000 revealed that the U.S. poverty rate has stuck stubbornly around 12 percent for a quarter of a century, and the income and assets of the lowest fifth of wage earners have actually fallen. Even for the boom's beneficiaries, the sense of giddy potential can turn fast to the vertigo of instability[1]— exactly what many began to feel when the Nasdaq index of technology stocks started sliding in the spring of 2000, and layoffs began to come down the chute shortly thereafter. The latter was a nauseating reminder of the 1980s, when not even top executives were spared as their companies merged and shuttered, and the new broom of economic "flexibility" swept out job security as an anachronistic impediment to profit making.

The ticker-tape hieroglyphs of Wall Street, once of interest only to the rich and their brokers, have come to spell out everybody's fortunes, not only because more people own stock than ever before, but also because, increasingly, the private sector is all people have to count on. While cutting the taxes of the wealthiest Americans, politicians of both parties have whittled public support for the institutions that help and unite all citizens, such as schools and universities, libraries, mass transit, day care, and hospitals; the government has even gotten out of the "business" of running its own prisons. The resulting "surpluses," President George W. Bush declared as he signed a historically huge tax cut into law, should be returned in the form of more tax cuts to "the people," or at least the richest percentile thereof.

The social correlate of economic privatization is "family values"—the idea, as cultural theorist Lauren Berlant put it, that citizenship is a matter of intimate life, reserved "only for members of families."[2] Aside from disenfranchising everyone who is not a card-carrying family member (singles, gays and lesbians, runaway youths, the neglected elderly) this new declaration of the United Families of America, coupled with the demand for economic self-sufficiency, has a paradoxical effect. It leaves the vaunted Family to tread water on its own.

Beleaguered parents have only the media and the marketplace as sources of advice and help. The parenting magazines indict a hazard of the month, providing fretful mothers and fathers with a ready list of names for their vaguest fears: television radiation, chlorine, medicine droppers, iron pills, automatic garage door openers, latex balloons, trampolines, drawstring sweatshirts. The newsweeklies chime in with perils of a less concrete, more moral nature. "How Can We Keep Our Children Safe?" asked the cover of *Life* magazine in the mid-1990s, ringing the vulnerable face of a blond-haired, blue-eyed girl with a boldfaced wreath of horribles: "SEXUAL ABUSE, ABDUCTION, TELEVISION, ACCIDENTS, NEGLECT, VIOLENCE, DRUGS, VULGARITY, ALIENATION." The article, like the pieces on chlorine and sweatshirts, offered few solutions that were not purchasable, and private.

Parenting has become an escalating trial of tougher standards for success and surer penalties for failure, *personal* failure. In the late 1990s, a nineteen-year-old single mother, rebuffed and delayed in her efforts to get infant care from Medicaid, diligently kept up breast feeding, unaware her milk was insufficient. The baby wasted away, and the mother was convicted of starving him to death. Meanwhile, in the suburbs, middle-class parents are scrambling to meet the requirements of molding hardier, healthier, more computer-literate, "emotionally intelligent," and, since the Columbine High School shootings in Littleton, Colorado, nonhomicidal children. "As Chelsea gets ready to leave for college, Bill and I can't help reviewing the last 17 years," wrote the former First Mom in *Newsweek* when her nest was about to empty. "We wonder if we've made the most of every minute to prepare her for the challenges of adulthood."[3] That's *every minute,* mind you.

Panic

As the sense of social and economic precariousness has escalated in the last two decades, a panic about children's sexuality has mounted with it. The currency of anxiety in America is frequently the sexual; sex is viewed as both the sine qua non of personal fulfillment and the experience with the potential for wreaking the greatest personal and societal devastation. And popular sexual fears cluster around the most vulnerable: women and children.

The political articulation of these fears in the late twentieth century came from two disparate sources. On one side were feminists, whose movement exposed widespread rape and domestic sexual violence against women and children and initiated a new body of law that would punish the perpetrator and cease to blame the victim. From the other side, the religious Right brought to sexual politics the belief that women and children need special protection because they are "naturally" averse to sex of any kind.

As we will see in these pages, the two streams came together in uneasy, though not historically unprecedented, alliances. Feminist sexual conservatives redefined explicit erotica as violence against women; the Right, gathered in a sort of summit with those feminists at the Meese commission on pornography in 1986, seized on their theory to legitimate a wholesale crackdown on adult porn and, eventually, on an alleged proliferation of "child pornography." The satanic-abuse witch-hunts (which dovetailed the pornography scare and later became a more general panic over child abuse) also alchemized feminist and right-wing fears. Feminist worries about children's vulnerability to adult sexual desire gradually reified in a therapy industry that taught itself to uncover abuse in every female patient's past. Religious conservatives, mostly middle-class women who felt their "traditional" families threatened by the social-sexual upheavals of the time, translated that concern into the language of their own apprehension. They saw profanity—in the form of abortion, divorce, homosexuality, premarital teen sex, and sex education—everywhere encroaching on sanctity. To them, it made sense that adults, with Satan as chief gangbanger, were conspiring in "rings" to rape innocent children.

Throughout the quarter century, in a complex social chemistry of deliberate political strategy, professional opportunism, and popular suspension of disbelief, sexual discomfort heated to alarm, which boiled to widespread panic; hysteria edged out rational discourse, even in the pressrooms of established news organizations and the chambers of the highest courts. The media reported that children faced sexual dangers more terrible than anything their parents had ever known. Along with lust-crazed Satanists, there were Internet tricksters, scout-leader pornographers, predatory priests—an army of sexual malefactors peopling the news, allegedly more wily and numerous than ever before. "'Don't talk to strangers' isn't good enough anymore," read the back cover of Carol Soret Cope's 1997 advice book, *Stranger Danger*. "What worked when we were children just isn't sufficient in today's world." Cops were brought in to instruct kindergartners in "good touch and bad touch," teachers catechized elementary school kids on sexual harassment, colleges rushed freshmen through date-rape seminars the first week they arrived on campus. And from the first sex-ed class on, children were drilled in the rigors of abstinence, the "refusal skills" to defend themselves against their peers' pressing desires, and their own.

The story behind these stories—one that was more plausible and therefore perhaps more frightening to baby boomer parents than tales of baby-rapists in black robes—was that of more teen sex, starting earlier and becoming more sophisticated sooner, with more dire consequences. In one sense, this is true. Earlier physical maturation coupled with later marriage meant that fifteen to twenty years elapse between physical sexual readiness and official sexual legitimacy.[4] It is hardly surprising that 90 percent of heterosexual Americans have intercourse before they wed, if they wed at all, and most do so before they exit the teen years. One in four of these adolescents contracts a sexually transmitted disease each year, with genital herpes, gonorrhea, and chlamydia leading the list.

On the other hand, the fear that children are having intercourse in middle school is largely unfounded: only two in ten girls and three in ten boys do so by the age of fifteen, with African American teens more likely to do so than Hispanics, and Hispanics more likely than European Americans.[5]

But looking at teens' sex lives in the 1990s and comparing them with their parents' in the 1970s and their grandparents' in the 1950s, we can see that rates of youthful activity are not galloping upward. At midcentury, 40 percent of teenagers reported having premarital sex, 25 percent of girls. During the 1970s those numbers increased substantially. But as Barbara Ehrenreich, Gloria Jacobs, and Deirdre English have pointed out, the "sexual revolution" was really a revolution for women only, who began to feel the license to behave more like men had always behaved; male sexual behavior didn't change much. By 1984, the proportion of sexually active unmarried fifteen- to nineteen-year-old women was just under half.[6] Since then, increases in teen sex have been smaller, with a bit of a drop-off in the last few years. In 1990, 55 percent of girls fifteen to nineteen years old were sexually active. And by 1995, the percentage was back to 50 percent. Today it remains at 50 percent—right where it was in 1984.[7] As for young teens, in the mid-1950s only three in one hundred girls had had sex before the age of fifteen; by the mid-1970s, one in ten had; today, that number is two in ten.[8] Another factor: In the 1950s, plenty of teens had sex, but it wasn't considered troublesome because it wasn't premarital: in that decade, America had the highest rate of teen marriage in the Western world.[9]

Furthermore, no matter how *many* teens are counted as "sexually active," meaning they've had intercourse at least once, that activity is various and, for a substantial number of kids, scant. In one typical study of sexually active boys ages fifteen to nineteen in the 1990s, more than half admitted they'd done it fewer than ten times in the previous year, and 10 percent had not had "sex," however they defined it, at all.[10] As one public-health researcher told me, "Most sexually active teens are not very sexually active."

Despite the less-than-electrifying facts, almost every major report on teen sexuality is pitched with the staples of sensationalism—the shock of what the story will reveal and the reproachful dismay that the readers don't know it already. "Everything your kids already know about sex* (*bet you're afraid to ask)," shuddered a *Time* magazine cover in the mid-1990s. "Dozens of interviews with middle-school kids reveal a shocking world parents would prefer not to confront," promised a *Talk* blurb of an account by Lucinda Frank about sex and drugs among a handful of privileged New York youngsters. The article, which managed within two paragraphs both to brood that the kids were too young to deal with the emotional complications of sex and to object to their having sex without enough emotional investment, was hyperbolically and typically headlined "The Sex Lives of Your Children."[11]

In almost every article or broadcast, experts are called in to catalogue the reasons that teens have sex, all of them bad: Their peers pressure them or pedophiles manipulate them; they drink or drug too much, listen to rap, or download porn; they are under too much pressure or aren't challenged enough; they are abused or abusive or feel immortal or suicidal; they're rich and spoiled or poor and demoralized, raised too strictly or too permissively; they are ignorant or oversophisticated.

Actually, these pundits are, for the most part, guessing. Demographers have run scores of sociological and biological developmental factors through their computers, thousands of times: race and ethnicity, urban or rural residency, family structure and closeness to mothers, drug taking, school performance, and immigration status, along with "outcomes" such as age and frequency of intercourse, type and frequency of contraception, abortions and live births, age difference between partners, number of partners, and, recently but still rarely, incidence of anal and oral sex. Still, the things these social scientists study cover a small corner of the territory of sexual experience. Conservative legislators have effectively shut down government-funded research on adults' sexual behavior, motives, or feelings. As for surveying minors about the same subjects, this is practically illegal.[12] How do children and teens feel about sex? What do they actually do? Only a handful of researchers are asking, and few are likely to soon.[13]

Squeamish or ignorant about the facts, parents appear willing to accept the pundits' worst conjectures about their children's sexual motives. It's as if they cannot imagine that their kids seek sex for the same reasons they do: They like or love the person they are having it with. It gives them a sense of beauty, worthiness, happiness, or power. And it feels good.

AIDS shadows these fears and exaggerations, and it feeds the fear mongers. It has become the symbol of all that is hidden and unknowable about sex—a fact exacerbated by public-health officials' and educators' reluctance to disseminate terror-quelling data and proven methods of containment to teens. Preventable, the disease has come to stand for the uncontrollable, which is the soul of terror. And if sex is the carrier of calamity, discussion of pleasure is unseemly, even rash.

Today, there's evidence that teens are learning to handle the dangers while enjoying the pleasures of sex (by the 1990s they were more consistent condom users than their elders),[14] yet teen sex is still viewed as the most uncontrollable, the most calamitous. Commonly in the professional literature, sex among young people is referred to as a "risk factor," along with binge drinking and gun play, and the loss of virginity as the "onset" of intercourse, as if it were a disease. One of the journals that frequently reports on teen sexual behavior is called *Morbidity and Mortality*.

The Birth of the Child

The wish to protect a child, while not natural or inevitable,[15] is almost poignantly understandable to anyone who has ever known one. "It comes down to this," said Janet Jake, a forty-six-year-old San Francisco mother, as we watched her twelve-year-old son careen down the steep sidewalk on his skateboard and fly over a jury-rigged obstacle course of crates and planks. "You don't want your babies hurt." Mostly, Janet has given her kids a lot of room (she cringed, but did not prohibit, the skateboard daredevilry). But about sex, she's found herself "turning into an ironclad conservative." Like many parents, Janet regards her sexual protectiveness as the way of all flesh.

But the idea that sex is the thing that can hurt your babies most of all is hardly the way of all flesh, not now and not in the past. Indeed, the concept that sex poses an almost existential peril to children, that it robs them of their very childhood, was born only about 150 years ago.

According to the influential French historian Philippe Ariès, European societies before the eighteenth century did not recognize what we now call childhood, defined as a long period of dependency and protection lasting into physical and social maturity. Until the mid-1700s, he wrote, not long after weaning, people "went straight into the great community of men, sharing in the work and play of their companies, old and young alike."[16] At seven, a person might be sent off to become a scullery maid or a shoemaker's apprentice; by fourteen, he could be a soldier or a king, a spouse and a parent; by forty, more than likely, he'd be dead.[17]

Ariès's invention-of-childhood theory has undergone furious debate and significant revision since he advanced it in 1960 (he can be thanked in large part for inaugurating the rich and active discipline of childhood history). While many historians accept his basic notion that the young moved more fluidly among their elders in centuries past, that they did not enjoy the special protections now extended them, and because of high early mortality adults did not become emotionally attached to them as quickly as they do today, there is general agreement that adults and children in the past did recognize a category of person, the Child. L. A. Pollack, for instance, studied 415 primary sources from 1500 to 1600 and concluded that Ariès's argument is "indefensible. . . . Even if children were regarded differently in the past, this does not mean that they were not regarded as children."[18]

Concerning sexuality and its role in worldly corruption, however, children were regarded quite differently before the eighteenth century from how they are today: they were not necessarily "good," nor adults "bad," merely by virtue of the length of their tenure on earth. In Puritan America, in fact, the opposite was true. Infants were conceived and born in sin, but they were considered perfectible through religious guidance and socialization, which happened as they got older. Early colonial toys and children's furniture, wrote Karin Calvert in her marvelous history of the material culture of childhood in America, "pushed the child forward into contact with adults and the adult world. The sharing of beds with grown-ups, the use of leading strings and go-carts to place children in the midst of adult activities, and other practices all derived from a world view that saw development from the imperfect infant to the civilized adult as a natural and desirable progression."[19]

In the mid-eighteenth century, first in Europe, ideologies about this "progression" reversed. As the cultural critic James Kincaid has shown, the English and French philosophers of the Romantic Era conjured the Child as a radically distinct creature, endowed with purity and "innocence"—Rousseau's unspoiled nature boy, Locke's clean slate. This being, born outside history,[20] was spoiled by entering it: the child's innocence was threatened by the very act of growing up in the world, which entailed partaking in adult rationality and politics. In the late nineteenth century, that innocence came to be figured as we see it today: the child was clean not just of adult political or social corruption, but ignorant specifically of sexual knowledge and desire.[21] Ironically, as children's plight as workers worsened, adults sought to save them from sex.

European American ideas about the transition from prepubescence to adulthood have also undergone momentous transfiguration in recent decades. For most of recorded European history, there existed a vague period called youth, roughly consistent with what we call adolescence, but defined socially more than biologically. In colonial America as in its European home countries, young men (not women) gained economic independence gradually, in the form of inherited property, familial financial responsibility, and political rights. When their elders deemed them prepared to support a household, youth married and officially became adults.[22]

Sexual knowledge came gradually too, and neither the sacredness of female virginity nor the prohibition on premarital sex was universal. On the American continent during the colonial period, among slaves from West Africa "marriage sanctioned motherhood, not sexual intercourse," and a woman usually married the father of her first child, after the fact.[23] In the Chesapeake Bay Colony, because women and girls were scarce, they enjoyed a certain sexual liberty, as well as suffering considerable sexual exploitation. In Maryland, women wed as young as twelve, and extramarital sex, both wanted and unwanted, was common: before 1750 one in five maidservants gave birth to a bastard child, often the issue of rape by the master. As for the Puritans, their real lives did not always evince the stiff-backed moralism with which their name has become synonymous. Premarital intercourse, though interdicted, could be redeemed by marriage, and as many as a third of New England's brides were pregnant at the altar.[24]

Back in Europe, as the curtains opened on the twentieth century and Queen Victoria lay on her deathbed, the idealized child met a radical challenger: Freud. His *Interpretation of Dreams* posited a sexual "instinct" born in the child, incubated in the oedipal passions of family life, and eventually transformed into adult desire, ambition, and creativity, or, if inadequately worked through, into neurotic suffering. A few years later, the man who brought Freud to U.S. shores for the first time defined, and added an enduringly hellish reputation to, a chapter of Freudian sexual development whose biggest hurdle had been feminine: the transfer of clitoral eroticism to the vagina. In a huge eponymous tome, child psychologist G. Stanley Hall coined the term *adolescence*—the state of becoming adult—and it tested all comers. Adolescence was a "long viatacum of ascent," resembling nothing more than one of the hairy scenes from an Indiana Jones movie. "Because his environment is to be far more complex, there is more danger that the youth in his upward progress . . .

will backslide," he wrote. "New dangers threaten all sides. It is the most critical stage of life, because failure to mount almost always means retrogression, degeneracy, or fall."[25] Greatest among those dangers was sexual desire.

Freud's theory of the sexually roiling unconscious was a critique of Enlightenment rationality, but he also endorsed a certain rationality as the road to maturity and social order. In their embrace of sexuality as part of human relations at all stages of life, Freud and Hall were renegade Victorians. But they were still Victorians. The father of psychoanalysis normalized youthful sexuality, but he tucked it out of sight during most of the troubling neither-here-nor-there years of prepubescence, in "latency."[26] And Hall, even more than Freud, painted "awakened" adolescent desire as inevitably a source of trouble and pain.

All this history lives on in us: zeitgeists do not displace each other like weather systems on a computerized map. We still invest the child with Romantic innocence: witness John Gray's cherub-bedecked *Children Are from Heaven*. The Victorian fear of the poisonous knowledge of worldly sexuality is still with us; lately it's reemerged in the demonic power we invest in the Internet. Hall's image of teen sexuality as a normal pathology informs child psychology, pedagogy, and parenting: think of "risk behaviors" and "raging hormones."

Since Freud, the sexuality of children and adolescents is officially "natural" and "normal," yet the meanings of these terms are ever in dispute, and the expert advice dispensed in self-help books and parenting columns serves only to lubricate anxiety: Is the child engaging in sex too soon, too much? Is it sex of the wrong kind, with the wrong person, the wrong meaning? Children and teens continue to live out their diverse heritages—African slave, Chesapeake Bay colonist, errant-but-forgiven Puritan. And the modern family is vexed by its Victorian-Freudian inheritance: the self-canceling task of inducting the child into the social world of sexuality and at the same time protecting her from it.

And just as the grimy, glittery realities of young people's lives in the industrialized cities of the nineteenth century clashed with the ideology of cloistered, innocent childhood and its enforcement, events in the twentieth century have tended to pull children and their sexuality in two directions at once. Beginning with the child-protectionist reforms of the Progressive Era, law and ideology have laid stone upon stone in the official wall between childhood and adulthood. At the same time, the century's cultural, political, and economic developments have been bashing away at that wall, most violently at its weakest point, the in-between stage of adolescence. The Depression and World War II pushed teens into the workforce, out on the road, to the battlefront, and into freer sexual arrangements. In the postwar years, the automobile gave them mobility; their newly flush parents and a booming economy gave them spending money. And the mass media gave them knowledge.

By the end of the twentieth century, the traditional landmarks of adult enfranchisement had been scattered into disorder. Marriage can now follow the establishment of a household, a career, and a credit history; the birth of a child can predate all of these. Preteens enroll in college; adults return to school at midlife; young surrogate mothers gestate babies for women who want to start families after their reproductive years are past. Many grown-ups live single and childless all their lives.

As the plots of late-modern life read more like postmodernist "texts" than like nineteenth-century novels, the characters of Child and Adult become harder to distinguish from one another. While remaining utterly dependent in many ways, children worldwide share in every aspect of the work and play of the great communities of adults—labor and commerce, entertainment, crime, warfare, marriage, and sex.

Though we locate them in a separate political category, a medical and psychological speciality, a social subculture, and a market niche, children in the twenty-first century may be more like adults than they have been since the seventeenth century.

Is Sex Harmful?

The child is father to the man; the man, to the child. Our ambivalence about children and about our role in their lives is old and deep. "Christianity worships its god as a baby in a manger, but the Christian moral tradition also held, simultaneously, the inherent sinfulness of children," writes Marina Warner in her eloquent "Little Angels, Little Monsters."[27]

Modern efforts to protect the idealized child while squashing the sinner, all to produce a decent adult, resemble in their solicitude and their cruelty the footbinder's techniques of enhancing the beauty of the woman by stunting the graceful foot of the girl. Current youth policy and parenting advice teeter between high-anxiety child protection and high-anger child punishment. It would appear that children are fragilely innocent until the moment they step over some line, at which point they become instantly, irredeemably wicked. One striking pair of contradictory trends: as we raise the age of consent for sex, we lower the age at which a wrongdoing child may be tried and sentenced as an adult criminal. Both, needless to say, are "in the best interests" of the child and society.

What are the best interests of the child? Politician and public-health doctor, pastor and pundit disagree on the practical strategies and tactics of ensuring those interests, because Americans disagree vastly at the question's heart: what is good, in its broadest definition, not only for children but for everyone? Childhood, as we've seen, is historical and cultural, which makes it ideological too: it is, in addition to being a physical phenomenon, an idea constructed on the spine of moral beliefs. Childhood is historical, cultural, and moral, just like sex. And so the questions of child sexuality are moral questions.

What questions regarding child and teen sex have preoccupied Americans over the past two centuries? Mainly, *whether* and *when.* And what are the answers? *No* and *later,* when they are married or at least "mature." The manifest popular support for abstinence masks discord below the pollsters' radars, though: even when the answers are similar, the moral underpinnings may not be. Most adults want to save young people the pain and possible harms of sex. But some feel that the risks outstrip almost all young people's abilities to contend with them; and others just think sex is wrong unless the person is of legal majority, heterosexual, and married.

In any case, *whether* and *when* are not the questions that this book engages, except insofar as it explores the meaning of Americans' obsession with these questions and the ways in which they delimit our understanding of sexuality and children's relationship to it. Lest you consider my approach peculiar or irresponsible, I remind you that in Western Europe *whether* and *when* aren't the burning questions either. Sex education in those countries begins with the assumption that young people will carry on a number of sexual relationships during their teen years and initiate sex play short of intercourse long before that (which they do) and that sexual expression is a healthy and happy part of growing up. The goal of sex ed, which grows out of a generally more relaxed attitude toward sexuality, is to make sure that this sexual expression is healthy and happy, by teaching children and teens the values of responsibility and the techniques of safety and even of pleasure. Abstinence is not emphasized in European classrooms, if it's discussed at all.[28]

I don't mean to imply that if adults would just quit trying to suppress youthful sex, everything would be hunky-dory in American teens' bedrooms and automobile backseats. Homophobia and misogyny are as robust in the suburban middle-school hallway as in Jesse Helms's office or a gangsta' rap studio; dating violence is rampant.[29] In part because of this youthful bigotry, anecdotal evidence indicates that many kids, especially girls, are having sex they don't want or do not enjoy. Four million teenagers are infected with sexually transmitted diseases each year,[30] and half of the forty thousand new HIV infections a year are in people under twenty-five.[31] And while AIDS deaths are dropping in general in the United States,[32] since 1993 the disease has been the leading cause of death among people twenty-five to forty-four.[33] Sex among America's youths, like sex among its adults, is too often neither gender-egalitarian, nor pleasurable, nor safe. This book will argue that current psychological, legal, and educational practices exacerbate rather than mitigate this depressing state of affairs.

Harmful to Minors says sex is not in itself harmful to minors. Rather, the real potential for harm lies in the circumstances under which some children and teens have sex, circumstances that predispose them to what the public-health people call "negative outcomes," such as unwanted pregnancy and sexually transmitted diseases, not to mention what I'd also consider an unwanted outcome: plain old bad sex.

Not surprisingly, these are the same conditions that set children up to suffer many other miseries. Some, such as the denial or degradation of female and gay desire, may express themselves differently in different economic classes and social locations, but they strike everywhere. Others are unequal-opportunity afflictors. More than 80 percent of teen mothers come from poor homes.[34] A hugely disproportionate number of youngsters with AIDS are African Americans and Hispanics: Although these two groups make up only about a quarter of the general U.S. population, they account for 56 percent of adolescent males with the disease and 82 percent of females.[35] And nearly a third of black, gay urban men in their twenties are HIV-positive.[36] Even incest is correlated with poverty and the family chaos that is woven closely with it: a child whose parents bring in less than fifteen thousand dollars a year is eighteen times more likely to be sexually abused at home than one from a family with an income above thirty thousand dollars.

It is these unhappy conditions, and not the desire for physical intimacy, not child pornographers or abortions, not even the monstrous human immunodeficiency virus, that leave a young person with her defenses down, loitering in harm's way. Poor people aren't less moral than rich people. But poverty, like sex, is a phenomenon rooted in moral priorities, a result of deliberate fiscal and social policies that obstruct the fair distribution of health, education, and wealth in a wealthy country. The result, often, is an unfair distribution of sexual health and happiness, too.

Sex is a moral issue. But it is neither a different nor a greater moral issue than many other aspects of human interaction. Sex is not a separate category of life; it should not be regarded as a separate category of art, education, politics, or commerce, or of emotional harm or benefit. Child or teen sex can be moral or immoral. And so can our treatment of the children and teens who desire it and act on that desire.

Harmful to Minors launches from two negatives: sex is not ipso facto harmful to minors; and America's drive to protect kids from sex is protecting them from nothing. Instead, often it is harming them.

But the book aspires to the positive too. It is based on the premise that sex, meaning touching and talking and fantasizing for bodily pleasure, is a valuable and crucial part of growing up, from earliest childhood on. I'd even submit that the goodness of pleasure is an all-American value. Let's face it, a country that produced rock 'n' roll music and the double-fudge brownie is a pleasure-loving place. *Life, liberty, and the pursuit of happiness*: the founding fathers considered happiness so important, they made it a principle of Americanism. Part of that happiness is sexual happiness. Even Christian fundamentalists, who often seem intent on pooping everybody else's party, have produced a large, lively literature of sexual—or, as they call it, marital—advice.

For better or worse, American culture places a lot of value on sex—*a lot*. But if sexual expertise is expected of adults, the rudiments must be taught to children. If educators want to be credible about sexual responsibility, they have to be forthright about sexual joy. If parents want their kids to be happy now and later, it is their duty, and should be their delight, to help them learn to love well, which is to say respectfully of others and themselves, skillfully in body and heart, morally as lovers, friends, and citizens.

For our part, adults owe children not only protection and a schooling in safety but also the entitlement to pleasure.

I

Harmful Protection

1. Censorship

The Sexual Media and the Ambivalence of Knowing

The twin concepts of innocence and ignorance are vehicles for adult double standards. A child is ignorant if she doesn't know what adults want her to know, but innocent if she doesn't know what adults don't want her to know.
—Jenny Kitzinger, "Children, Power, and the Struggle against Sexual Abuse"

At the turn of the twenty-first century, America is being inundated by censorship in the name of protecting "children" from "sex," both terms capaciously defined. In the 1990s among the most frequent targets were Judy Blume's young-adult novel *Deenie,* in which a teenage girl likes to touch her "special place," and Maurice Sendak's classic *In the Night Kitchen,* because its main character, a boy of about five named Max, tumbles through his dream with his genitals bare. The student editor of the University of Southern Louisiana yearbook was dismissed because she published a picture of a young woman feeding spaghetti to a young man. Both were shirtless.[1] The New York State Liquor Authority denied a license to Bad Frog Beer. According to the authority, the label—a cartoon frog with his middle finger raised and the legend "An Amphibian with Attitude"—was "harmful to minors." Paul Zaloom, the star of the children's television science program *Dr. Beekman's Universe,* was forbidden by his producers to answer his viewers' most-asked question: What is a fart?[2] Even sex educators are not allowed to speak about sex. In 1996, when author Robie Harris went on the radio in Oklahoma to promote her children's book *It's Perfectly Normal: Changing Bodies, Growing Up, Sex and Sexual Health,* the host requested that she not mention the S-word. Harris was obliged to refer to sex as "the birds and the bees."[3]

The cultural historian Michel Foucault said that sex is policed not by silence but by endless speech, by the "deployment" of more and more "discourses" of social regulation—psychology, medicine, pedagogy. But our era, while producing plenty of regulatory chatter from on high, has also seen an explosion of unofficial, anarchic, and much more exciting discourses down below. When the sexual revolution collided with the boom in media technologies, media sex mushroomed. We started collecting statistics to prove it: 6.6 sexual incidents per hour on top-rated soap operas (half that number ten years before); fourteen thousand sexual references and innuendos on television annually (compared with almost none when Ozzie and Harriet slept in twin beds); movies most popular with teenagers "contain[ing] as many as fifteen instances of sexual intercourse in less than two hours"[4] (*Gone with the Wind* had one, off-screen).

Sexual imagery proliferated like dirty laundry: the minute you washed it and put it away, there was more. In Times Square, whose streets were transformed into a Disney-Warner "family-friendly" mall, the neon signs from shut-down peep shows were put on exhibit in a sort of museum of the smutty past at the back of the tourist information office. Meanwhile, looming over the heads of camera-toting tour groups from Iowa, half-block-long billboards advertised Calvin Klein underwear, inside of whose painted shadows lurked penises as large as redwood logs.

As the ability to segregate audiences by age, sex, class, or geography shrinks, we have arrived at a global capitalist economy that, despite all our tsk-tsking, finds sex exceedingly marketable and in which children and teens serve as both sexual commodities (JonBenét Ramsey, Thai child prostitutes) and consumers of sexual commodities (Barbie dolls, Britney Spears). All this inspires a campaign with wide political support to return to reticence,[5] especially when the kids are around.

History refutes the notion that we live today in a world of sexual speech but did not, say, three centuries ago. A child could witness plenty of dirty song-singing and breast- and buttock-grabbing in any sixteenth-century public house. Yet there *is* reason for concern about the world of unfiltered, unfettered sexual knowledge that is particular to the past several decades: pictures and words have attained unprecedented cultural influence in our time. Our marketplace produces few actual widgets; we make almost nothing but digitized ideas and the media to distribute them. As the economy moves from the Steel Belt to Silicon Valley, the boundary between the symbolic and the real is disappearing. Representation is no longer just a facsimile of a thing: it is the thing itself.

Nobody lives more in the "hypermediated" environment than the young.[6] The critic Ronald Jones, writing about two young artists in the 1990s, distinguished them from the now-middle-aged postmodernists of the 1980s, who stressed that "the way the media represented the world was a constructed fabrication." Younger artists, the critic said, work from an assumption of "inauthenticity as a normal course of life."[7] At the end of the twentieth century, a quarter of kids had their own televisions by the time they were five years old.[8] It was no use telling them to go outside and get a "real" life. Why play sandlot baseball when you can pitch to Sammy Sosa from a virtual mound? Even technologized sexual speech no longer just stands for sex; it *is* sex. Sherry Turkle, a social analyst of computer communication at the Massachusetts Institute of Technology, described the on-screen erotic exchanges that Netizens call "tinysex": "A 13-year-old informs me that she prefers to do her sexual experimentation online. Her partners are usually the boys in her class at school. In person, she says, it is 'mostly grope-y.' Online, 'they need to talk more.'"[9]

Where do you learn about sex? a television interviewer asked a fifteen-year-old from a small rural town. "We have 82 channels," the girl replied.

Oversophisticated

The chat on any contemporary sitcom might make Alice Kramden blush. But public steaminess was around long before the Summer of Love, and for centuries there were Tipper Gores and Dan Quayles at hand to decry it. "It is impossible to prevent every thing that is capable of sullying the imagination," lamented the anonymous author of *Onania, or the Heinous Sin of Self-Pollution, and All Its Frightful Consequences, in Both Sexes Consider'd, &c,* a best-selling antimasturbation treatise, published in England around 1700 and exported to America soon after. "*Dogs* in the Streets and *Bulls* in the

Fields may do mischief to Debauch's Fancy's, and it is possible that either Sex may be put in mind of Lascivious Thoughts, by their own *Poultry.*"[10]

In the late 1800s Anthony Comstock, head of the New York Society for the Suppression of Vice, pored over the innumerable moral "traps for the young" set right inside the bourgeois household, in half-dime novels, "story papers," and the plain old daily newspaper. The New York Society for the Prevention of Cruelty to Children "kept a watchful eye upon the so-called Museums of the City," whose advertisements were "like magnets to curious children." According to one of the society's reports, a play featuring "depravity, stabbing, shooting, and blood-shedding" so traumatized a ten-year-old girl that she was found "wander[ing] aimlessly along Eighth Avenue as if incapable of ridding herself of the dread impressions that had filled her young mind."[11]

By 1914, Agnes Repellier, a popular conservative essayist, was inveighing against a film and publishing industry "coining money" by creating a generation hypersophisticated in sin. "[Children's] sources of knowledge are manifold, and astoundingly explicit," she wrote in the *Atlantic*. Repellier may have been the first to propose a movie-rating system, asking "the authorities" to bar children "from all shows dealing with prostitution."[12]

The media-abetted breakdown of morality was news again in 1934. "Think of [the adolescent's] world of electric lights, lurid movies, automobiles, speed, jazz and nightclubs, literature tinged with pornography, and the theater presenting problems of perversion, the many cheap magazines with fabricated tales of true love, the growing cults of nudism and open confessions, the prevalence of economic uncertainty," Dr. Ira S. Wile wrote, discoursing on "The Sexual Problems of Adolescence" in the journal published by the American Social Hygiene Association. "Society is in a state of heated flux," Wile opined, indicting feminism, atheism, science, and even capitalism for the moral and sexual drift of the young.[13] Sound familiar?

Against such invective has always stood a kind of faute de mieux realism, which articulates the same sad tale but sees the outcome as inevitable. In 1997, a Disney executive explained how media and changes in the family created the sophisticated child, who created the media, which changed the family, who created the child . . . and the beast chased its tail faster and faster until it turned into butter (and went rancid). "Today's eight-year-olds are yesterday's twelve-year-olds. They watch some very edgy programs on television. There isn't this innocence of childhood among many children, what with broken homes and violence. We can't treat children as if they're all living in tract homes of the 1950s and everyone is happy. That is ridiculous."[14]

On kids' sophistication, the evidence is with him. In a survey of thirty-two hundred urban and suburban elementary school kids in the 1970s (before MTV!), "the most productive responses were elicited with the instructions, 'Why children shouldn't be allowed to see R and X rated movies'; or 'What is in R and X rated movies that children are too young to know about?' Here, the children proceeded with aplomb to tell all that they knew but were not supposed to know." Samuel Janus and Barbara Bess, the psychologists who conducted the study, concluded: "One learns that what the adult world has established is an adult psychic censor that will not admit of children's growth and experience. Selective perception may becloud and avoid awareness of childhood sexuality, but it does not eliminate [that sexuality]."[15]

Curious

Centuries of censorship notwithstanding, we are hardly unambivalent about knowing. On the one hand, Prometheus did his time in chains for delivering science to man. The Bible tells us that to stir curiosity, as the Serpent did, is to corrupt. Eve lusted for interdicted knowledge; this, not sex, was the first sin.[16] But we are also heirs of the Enlightenment, who for three centuries have insisted that to know is a human right, democracy's foundation, and the gift of our heroes. Knowledge is protector, healer, and liberator.[17]

In young children, we regard curiosity as a virtue, and by the mid-twentieth century curiosity about body parts and the making of babies was considered normal and nice. In fact, curiosity is a reassuring explanation of what otherwise might look like the quest for bodily pleasure. "In a child's mind, this investigation [of the body] is much the same as, say, tinkering with toys to see how they operate or watching birds build a nest," Toni Cavanagh Johnson, a self-styled expert on what she calls children's "touching problems," told a women's magazine advice columnist.[18] This explanation washes when Junior is reaching into his training pants, but it is harder to countenance when he's unzipping his baggy men's-sized

Tommy Hilfigers; now, it is a "risk behavior." If curiosity is cute in the kitten, we suspect it could kill the cat.

Our crudest and oldest fear about letting out too much sexual information is that it will lead kids to "try this at home" as soon as they are able—a sort of user's manual, or propaganda, model of sexual knowledge.

The relationship between seeing and doing is, to say the least, exceedingly complex. On one hand, it is intuitively clear and affirmed by social science that learning about sex affects what a person does and feels about it. "The body has a history and a social context that shape meanings and lived experience," wrote University of Massachusetts sociologist Janice Irvine.[19] Sex is cultural. In the United States kissing is step one of sex. In Burma, making love does not include kissing, which is considered unsanitary and disgusting.[20] Sex is historical. Awareness of the erotic utility of silk may date back millennia, but a rubber fetish could not possibly predate 1823, when the first process was developed for rolling rubber into sheets. Even the idea that people have "sexual identities" is less than a hundred years old, as gay historian Jonathan Ned Katz has shown. Before that a man who engaged in genital acts with another man was simply a man engaging in acts; he was not a particular kind of person, a "homosexual."[21] Sex is influenced by books, art, movies, television, advertising, and what your friends say. How many women in the 1970s figured out how to have orgasms by reading other women's techniques in *The Hite Report on Women's Sexuality*?

But learning about a sex act doesn't toggle the desire switch to "on" or the body switch to "go." Rather, one reacts to an image or idea according to her own experiences and all the scripts she's learned. For a child, those experiences might include an incident of incest, a thrilling experience of mutual masturbation with another child, a course in good touch and bad touch, or a joke heard on the playground. The relationship between learning about sex and doing sex is "more like the world weather system than a chemical reaction," University of Hawaii early childhood educator Joseph Tobin told me. "It's a chaos model we need: one cause can have various effects or different effects than we expected."

Still, the dark suspicion of a direct link between knowing and doing created from the start a conundrum that has endured for sex educators: how to inform youth about the facts of sex without inflaming their lust. Educators, like parents, worry that if the right adults ("us") do not tell kids the right things about sex (disease and reproduction) in the right way (clinically), the wrong ones will tell them the wrong things. Put another way, sex education, like obscenity law, was founded on the notion that you can separate clean sex from dirty sex.

For the purposes of edification, clean sex is the sex that occurs in committed, preferably legally sanctioned, age-of-majority, heterosexual, reproductive relationships; and it includes responsible precoital conversation, safer-sex devices, and postcoital cuddling. Clean sex is "scientific." For little kids it is still often explicated in narratives that begin with a pistil and a stamen or a "lady fish and a gentleman fish," as the child in *Auntie Mame* described them, and proceeds gingerly to the making of babies. (These "birds and bees" stories can misfire on account of young children's literal-mindedness. In the 1980s, psychologist Anne Bernstein asked a four-year-old, "How would a lady get a baby to grow inside her?" The child, who had studied the sex-ed picture books, began, "Um, first you get a duck.")[22] Older kids' clean sex is carried on in anatomically correct language and explicated in two-dimensional renderings of pelvises sliced in half to reveal fallopian tubes and vas deferens, without pictures of fleshly, hairy genitals as they might be encountered in life. Dirty sex is all the rest: the sex of the servants' quarters, the street, the schoolyard, of *Penthouse Letters, Baywatch,* 1-900-923-SUCK, and Hotbutts.com. It comes in willy-nilly, festooned with advertising.

But the enterprise of sanitizing sex is always quixotic. For one thing, clean sex doesn't capture the attention of the young. "When schools teach you about sex, it's just a big blah," one high school girl told a CBS reporter. "This is a penis, this is a vagina," a male classmate elaborated. At the same time, even what we consider the highest-minded texts and images, the Bible or Shakespeare or ancient Indian miniatures, can be as filthy as a barnyard. Frank McCourt, in *Angela's Ashes,* remembers opening the morally improving pages of Butler's *Lives of the Saints* as a boy and discovering "stories about virgins, martyrs, [and] virgin martyrs . . . worse than any horror film at the Lyric Cinema." The anthropologist Mary Douglas tells us that dirt is "matter out of place," but to the child who is forbidden it, all sexual knowledge is knowledge out of place and therefore dirty. Ask the child who has thrilled at uncovering a little cache of penis-related words, right there in the dictionary between *peninsulate* and *penitence,* and she will agree with Douglas: "Dirt is in the eyes of the beholder." A resigned father summed it up in answering a *New York Times* survey about media and children: "Kids are always going to want to watch what we don't want them to."[23]

In part, they want to do so because we don't want them to. Confessing the schoolboy misdemeanor of stealing forbidden fruit, Saint Augustine, one of the fathers of Western sexual anxiety, put it this way: "My pleasure was not in those pears. It was in the offense itself."

Harmed

The idea that young minds (and female minds and feeble minds) are vulnerable to bad thoughts, which might lead to bad acts, may be considered the founding principle of obscenity law. In 1868, an English anticlerical pamphlet called *The Confessional Unmasked* was deemed punishably obscene because its text might "suggest to the minds of the young of either sex, and even to persons of more advanced years, thoughts of a most impure and libidinous character."[24]

The legal definition of obscenity is "variable," according to First Amendment lawyer Marjorie Heins. The "compelling" public interest constitutionally required to justify restraint of the First Amendment is considered more compelling if the presumed viewer is a minor. For adults, a ruling of obscenity depends on the work passing the three-pronged "Miller" test, named for the 1973 Supreme Court case *Miller v. California*: it must be "patently offensive" and appeal to the "prurient interest"; it must meet the above criteria under local "community standards" (so a book considered okay in California might be banned in Oklahoma); and it must lack "serious legal, artistic, political, or scientific value." Together these raise a deliberately high bar, which has significantly cut down the number of obscenity prosecutions. The "harmful to minors" standard, established in the 1968 Supreme Court case *Ginsberg v. New York,* is the obscenity standard applied to minors. The same criteria must be met, only less so. Still, both before and since *Miller,* the courts have upheld restrictions on children's access to a wide swath of less-than-legally-obscene, not-quite-pornographic stuff judged "indecent" and thus conceivably harmful to minors. As is true of every obscenity charge, the nature of the harm is not physical or even measurable, but metaphysical: the content may cause bad thoughts.

As the broadcast media matured, they posed a far greater challenge to would-be censors than books and magazines did. Individual printed items can presumably be kept out of the hands of underage readers simply by placing them out of reach in the shop or newsstand. But you can't direct a radio wave or television image to adult ears and eyes only, so the courts have upheld laws restricting programming with sexual content and putatively offensive speech to "safe harbor" hours, supposedly after the children (whether they're preschoolers or high schoolers) are in bed.[25]

When the Internet erased both space and time, efforts arose to penalize creators and distributors of "indecency" if their material was accessed by minors at all. In 1996, as part of an omnibus telecommunications law, Congress passed the Communications Decency Act (CDA), which would have imposed a fine of $250,000 or a sentence of two years in jail on anyone who might "display" materials deemed "indecent, lewd, lascivious, or filthy" on the Internet in such a way that young Net surfers might see them.

The U.S. Supreme Court, in *Reno v. ACLU* (1997), struck down the CDA, because it decided the Internet was more like a telephone system than a television network: it was too vast and much of it too private to police. To keep children "safe," every one of the millions of daily online communications and the then-estimated 320 million separate Web pages would have to be reduced to a level of speech appropriate on *Mr. Rogers' Neighborhood*,[26] a restriction akin to what former Supreme Court justice Felix Frankfurter, in another case, called "burn[ing] the house to roast the pig."[27] Though bloodied, conservatives were unbowed. In many states legislators continued to propose bills restricting minors' access to everything from Web sites to rock concerts but substituted "indecency" with the better-defined, though still vague, "harmful to minors."

In 1998, the 105th Congress passed the Child Online Protection Act (COPA), which was substantially the same as the CDA but was more narrowly aimed at commercial "adult" sites, ordering them to take steps to foil minors' access, such as requiring a credit card number for entry. Under COPA, as under the CDA, a prosecutor anywhere could indict a Web owner whose site originated anywhere else. Penalties included fines up to $150,000 per day of violation, as well as six months' prison time. In 1999, enjoining enforcement of COPA, Judge Lowell A. Reed of the Philadelphia U.S. District Court evinced the time-honored objection that the law would chill adult free speech, with a technological twist: a site would be unable to verify the age of the visitor, so its owner might unknowingly break the law.

The government appealed, and when the U.S. Third Circuit Court upheld the preliminary injunction in June 2000, its ruling went beyond the trial court's and struck in a new and potentially profound way at the basis of obscenity law. Troubled by the possibility of a small-town prosecutor in Louisiana attempting to shut down a Web site originating in San Francisco—in effect, restricting the Californians' speech to the standards of the most conservative burb in America—Judge Leonard I. Garth argued that the very notion of community standards had become obsolete in an age of global communications among people of vastly varying cultures and moralities.[28]

Evidence of the harm of exposure to sexually explicit images or words in childhood is inconclusive, even nonexistent. The 1970 U.S. Commission on Obscenity and Pornography, the "Lockhart commission," uncovered no link between adult exposure to pornography and bad behavior and called for dismantling legal restrictions on erotica. Not only did the panelists fail to find harm to children in viewing erotica, moreover, they went so far as to suggest it could "facilitate much needed communication between parent and child over sexual matters."[29] The 1985 Commission on Pornography (the Meese commission), chaired by Reagan's attorney general Edwin Meese and assembled specifically to overturn the 1970 findings, could not establish factual links between sexually explicit materials and antisocial behavior either. Indeed, researchers have found more evidence that the opposite is true. Interviews of sex criminals including child molesters reveal that the children who eventually became rapists were usually exposed to pornography less than other kids;[30] if they'd seen the same amount, the exposure had not occurred earlier in life than the other children's.[31] According to Johns Hopkins University's John Money, one of the world's foremost authorities on sexual abnormalities, "the majority of patients with paraphilias"—deviant sexual fantasies and behaviors—"described a strict anti-sexual upbringing in which sex was either never mentioned or was actively repressed or defiled."[32]

But such data were, in a sense, politically irrelevant. Heins, former head of the ACLU's Arts Censorship Project, found that such laws were routinely passed and upheld without recourse to any evidence whatsoever.[33] The moral wisdom of shielding minors from sexy materials is seen as self-evident. In spite of its findings to the contrary, and in spite of its historical moment at the height of the sexual revolution, even the liberal-dominated Lockhart commission deferred to popular sentiment and refrained from recommending that restrictions be lifted on minors' access to sexual materials.[34]

By the time the Meese commission sat, the presumed harm to minors of dirty pictures, and thus the good of keeping such pictures from them, was even more "evident." The Right was in ascendancy, and a rump caucus of feminists had singled out pornography not only as the cause of sexual violence to women but as a species of sexual violence in itself. The commission was convened by conservative attorney general Edwin Meese and stacked with fundamentalist preachers, Republican prosecutors, vice cops, and antiporn activists. And while the lion's share of the testimony it heard concerned adult materials and consumers (and found no solid evidence of harm), the commission pitched its pro-restriction recommendations to popular fears about children: "For children to be taught by these materials that sex is public, that sex is commercial, and that sex can be divorced from any degree of affection, love, commitment, or marriage," the report read, "is for us the wrong message at the wrong time."[35]

The Meese commission lent new legitimacy to the idea that pornography causes harm, especially to children, and since its hearings that notion has mushroomed, morphing into the suspicion that exposing children to *any* explicit sexual information can hurt them. In recent years, whether the target was nude photos in museum exhibitions, contraceptive information videotapes, or (according to one Florida pastor) the satanic Barney the Purple Dinosaur, censorship proponents have advertised nearly every assault on speech as a defense of children. Critics suspect that the Right's true agenda is a radically conservative one: to scrub the public space clean of sexuality entirely. Artists and civil libertarians have resisted, but what was once controversial has become commonsensical. By the 1990s, commercial media all posted "harmful to minors" warnings before programs containing sexual language or images, and—a practice unheard of even a decade before and still considered ludicrous in

Europe—American public art spaces routinely post similar advisories that an exhibition might be "inappropriate" for children. Many such exhibits display nothing more than paintings or sculptures of nudes. And, as we will see in the next chapter, the most sacrosanct subject of all is the representation of children's own bodies.

The story of one sex-ed curriculum demonstrates this change in attitude over a third of a century. Just around the time the Lockhart commission was convened, the national Unitarian Universalist Church was devising a sex-education program called "About Your Sexuality" for preteen and teenage church members. In some "AYS" sessions, educators showed filmstrips featuring naturalistic, explicit drawings of people engaged in sexual activities from masturbation to two men kissing. For decades, the program received praise and gratitude and no objections from parents in the church, which embraces liberal politics. Indeed, graduates were glad to enroll their own children in the program.

Then, in 1997, two parents in Concord, Massachusetts, protested. Someone informed CBS's right-wing libertarian commentator Bryant Gumble, who rushed in to expose the shocking truth. "Guess who's showing sexually explicit films to children? The church!" blared the segment's teaser. One of the aggrieved mothers was filmed in tears, and a child-abuse "expert" intoned, "It could be disturbing to some kids—and even harmful."[36] The hour wound up with an instant poll of viewers: 74 percent said it is "never okay to show graphic sexual visuals to teenagers in the context of sex education."[37]

Shortly thereafter, the church introduced a new sex-ed curriculum, "Our Whole Lives," which had been in development for several years. According to the church's curriculum director, Judith Frediani, "OWL" was not more conservative than "About Your Sexuality" but in fact "far more inclusive and pro-active" in its "positive message about sexuality." For instance, the discussion of transsexuality is extensive and "sympathetic" within its section on gender and sexual identity, and while it explores abstinence, "we don't tell [youngsters] what decision to make" about their sexual activity, said Frediani. "Nor do we take the position that it is our right to tell them." Nevertheless, the explicit visuals (filmstrips for junior high school students and videos including stills of sexual activity for high schoolers) were removed from the new program and repackaged, along with Unitarian-specific religious instruction, as an optional supplement called "Sexuality and Our Faith." Only

Unitarian Universalist–affiliated congregations may purchase the supplement, only specially trained instructors may teach it, and only children whose parents have previewed the visuals and given written permission may participate in it.

Did sexually explicit images suddenly become more dangerous? The new arrangement "puts our stuff most squarely under the protection of the First Amendment," said Frediani, "and our congregations are a little more protected in their communities, particularly the more conservative, Bible Belt communities." Did the pictures suddenly become harmful to minors? As we've seen, current conventional wisdom says yes, and, Frediani said, even liberal Unitarian Universalist members are not immune to popular persuasion: "Like everyone else, our folks are more cautious, more conservative." In writing the curriculum, her committee talked with many parents, teachers, and child-development experts. Of the last group, she told me, "No one was willing to say [the pictures] were helpful or necessary or even appropriate. And the truth is, we have no data to demonstrate their value, or even their harmlessness, beyond anecdotal reports." Still, anecdote adds up. Although thirty years of preteens and teens have cycled through "About Your Sexuality," a sufficient subject pool in any social scientist's estimation, the psychological literature contains no reference to a disproportionate number of Unitarians among sexual deviants.

Filtered

When the U.S. Supreme Court rejected the Communications Decency Act, civil libertarians sighed relief for the First Amendment rights of adults and rose en masse, along with the parenting magazines and cyber columnists, to salute a fleet of new software packages that would guard the borders by "filtering" Net-borne filth from kids. The software came with names evoking caregivers (Net Nanny, CyberSitter) and cops (Cyber Patrol). The telecommunications bill, to which the CDA would have been an amendment, was also the first to propose the V-chip, a device to be installed in televisions that could screen out programs according to ratings coded for sex, vulgar language, violence, and so forth. Around that time, a *New Yorker* cartoon showed a computer scientist at her workstation, telling a colleague, "I have in mind a V-chip to be implanted directly in children."

As the joke suggests, these people's relief was misplaced. Sure, parents had a hand in deciding what movies their kids saw, what books they read, and what Web sites they visited. But they could not filter out all the "dirty" sex, even if they wanted to. And technology was not going to solve the problem, no matter how smart the programmers made it. For one thing, computer-savvy kids were smarter. One enterprising twelve-year-old A student programmed the computer to record his father's keystrokes as he set up the filter, then deleted them, downloaded some porn, and sold it to his friends.[38]

Moreover, this artificial intelligence was about as discriminating as Senator James Exon, the Nebraska Democrat who sponsored the CDA. CyberSitter couldn't tell the difference between the dirty word *penis* and the clean one any better than a person could. So the programs, and the people employed to scroll through the names of Web sites looking for potential offenders, erred on the far side of caution. America Online blocked the word *breast* until cancer patients complained they couldn't get to their support groups and information sites. Cyber Patrol's top-secret CyberNOT list banned Planned Parenthood's sites, feminist, youth, and gay sites, as well as free speech and Second Amendment sites and such "violent" information as that posted by the city of Hiroshima about its peace memorial.[39] CyberSitter blocked the site of the National Organization for Women. The poet Anne Sexton and the Sussex County Fair were universally banned because of the spelling of their names, as were Christian sites advertising videos about sexuality.[40] Even the allegedly more sensitive PICS (Platform for Internet Content Selection), software that employs a site-rating system and was recommended for schools and public libraries as well as homes, could leave kids "confined to a research world smaller than their school library," attorney Heins pointed out, "because after all, the *Encyclopedia Britannica* has an entry on 'contraception,'" a word that would give it the equivalent of an R or X rating. Nevertheless, by 1999, almost a third of online households had installed a filtering device on their computers.[41] And in December 2000, unnoticed during the prolonged presidential postelections, Bill Clinton signed the Child Internet Protection Act (CIPA), requiring public libraries to filter their computers or lose federal funding; upon his assumption of the presidency, George W. Bush affirmed his commitment to Internet censorship. At this writing, the American Library Association and the ACLU have brought suit challenging CIPA's constitutionality.

Opponents of government regulation of the Net usually maintain that parents, and not the state, should decide what their children see and read. But there are some adults who believe kids can make their own decisions. In *Wired* magazine, journalist Jon Katz argued that by accepting technological surrogates for government censorship under the Communications Decency Act, liberals had sold out their kids' free-speech rights. Katz said he and his wife were concerned for their fourteen-year-old daughter's safety, but they had also schooled her in media literacy and instilled moral intelligence, also known as conscience. In short, they trusted her. So the girl surfed the Net unsupervised, discussing what she found there just as she'd discuss a movie or an event at school. If an uncomfortable or threatening situation arose, she was instructed to employ the tactic she learned in preschool: "Use your words." The appropriate phrase for Internet creeps, said Katz, is "Get lost."[42]

Premature

It is hard to say what children are "taught" by porn or any other sexual imagery or by words they encounter in the media. However, as testimony before the Lockhart commission suggested, many sexologists suspect that sexual information gleaned before a person can understand it either bores or escapes or possibly disgusts him or her but doesn't hurt.[43] The New Jersey mother of a ten-year-old told me her son asked out of the blue what a "rim job" was. When she answered him explicitly, she said, "He looked at me like, 'Are you kidding?' and then he said, 'Oh,' and got out of the car and went to play soccer. He seemed fine after that."

Like Katz's daughter, a child who has been allowed to leaf through the coveted contraband and offered adult guidance may be able to critique or even reject sexual images that he's not ready for. Craig Long, a father I met in Chicago, had carried on a frank and continual conversation with his son, Henry, about sex since earliest childhood. Then, on his eleventh birthday, the boy asked shyly for a *Playboy* magazine. After discussing the matter with Henry's mother, Craig gave him the magazine, accompanied by a small lecture. "I told him real women do not look like the models in *Playboy*, and they're not generally splayed out for immediate consumption." After a few weeks, Craig checked in with his son. Had he been looking at the magazine? "Hmm, not so much." Was he enjoying it?

"Hmm, not so much." Why not? "I don't know, Dad," the boy finally said. "I guess I'm too young for this stuff."

Given the gradual and idiosyncratic nature of children's maturation and learning, the timing mechanism of sex education probably resembles a sundial more than the IBM Olympic stopwatch. Yet timing, or "age-appropriateness," is usually represented as a determination of high sensitivity, with miscalculations carrying grave, possibly irreversible, consequences. "Although secrecy makes for dangerous ignorance, too much openness can turn on what is meant to stay turned off until later," child-raising adviser Penelope Leach ominously warned the readers of *Redbook*.[44]

In the 1990s, concerns about timing inspired two strategies of restriction. Movie producers, and later their colleagues in television, sliced the young viewing public into precise age categories: this film was appropriate for thirteen-year-olds but not twelve-year-olds, that one for seventeen-year-olds accompanied by an adult (who could be eighteen) but not without one. The Communications Decency Act took the other tack: its "minor" status covered a territory as wide as Siberia. For the law's purposes, those who were considered vulnerable to the trauma of seeing a picture of a penis entering a vagina included both the seventeen-year-old sexually active high school senior and the three-year-old preschooler who pronounced the word "bagina."

All this classification reveals deep anxieties about what childhood is and about the waning ability to separate the boys and girls from the men and women. The liberal educator Neil Postman dated the "disappearance of childhood" to the invention of the telegraph in the mid-1800s, which eventually spurred a mass media that availed all people at all ages of all sexual secrets. And "without secrets," he wrote, "there is no such thing as childhood."[45] Although it was based on geography, not age, Judge Garth's ruling against the Child Online Protection Act in 2000 suggested something similar about age. The courts had long determined which bricks in the legal wall between statutorily defined minors and the adult sexual world would unduly restrict the comings and goings of adults. Now, the judge might have been admitting that the wall was irreparably blasted down, and the vandals were not pornographers or online pedophiles but technology itself. Just as global capitalism and modern warfare dictate that many of the world's children partake in the activities long considered exclusively adult—commerce and crime, mothering and soldiering—the modern mass media avail even "sheltered" children of knowledge of those formerly adult realms. Ten-year-olds in the twenty-first century know about interest rates and dot-com IPOs, about police brutality and the hole in the ozone layer. And they know about adult sexuality, from abortion to sadomasochism.

It is unlikely the air will get less dense with information or with sex. No law, no Internet filter, no vigilant parent will be able to keep tabs on every page and pixel that passes before a child's eyes beyond about the age of two. In that exquisite teenage tone of sarcastic pity, high school freshman Laura Megivern addressed parents who imagined they should and could "protect" their children in this way. "I have something else you might be interested in," she wrote in her local Vermont newspaper. "A closet with a lock"—to put the kids in and keep them there.[46]

Adults may have more influence over their kids' media consumption than Laura thinks. But she is right that censorship is not protection. Rather, to give children a fighting chance in navigating the sexual world, adults need to saturate it with accurate, realistic information and abundant, varied images and narratives of love and sex.[47]

2. Manhunt

The Pedophile Panic

All children should be told in simple words that there are some grown-up men who are "slightly ill and not quite right in the head" and who would rather embrace and kiss little girls than grown-up women. They should be told that there are only a few such men, but that they should avoid them. After such a warning the child has a more or less realistic appraisal of the situation: on the one hand it knows of the possibility of such sexual approaches; on the other hand it does not suspect sex-maniacs behind every bush. An explanatory warning not only lessens the likelihood of contact between girls and male adults, it also reduces to a minimum the emotional and psychological effects should contacts take place.

—Paul H. Beghard, Jan Raboch, and Hans Giese, *The Sexuality of Women* (1970)

Obviously, our children should always stay outside a molester's zone of control. Once a child comes under the control of an abductor/molester, the child will almost certainly be molested, and may even be kidnapped or killed. You probably don't need to put the fear of death in your child, however. Most children are naturally fearful of being separated from their families. The possibility of being abducted or kidnapped is sufficiently frightening without adding the specter of cold-blooded murder.

—Carol Soret Cope, *Stranger Danger* (1997)

"MONSTROUS" shouted the banner of the *Boston Herald* on October 4, 1997. For once, the paper's notoriously hyperbolic headline writers had struck the right tone.[1] Three days earlier, ten-year-old Jeffrey Curley of Cambridge had disappeared in the middle of the afternoon while washing his dog outside his grandmother's house. Now he was dead.

Jeffrey's neighbor Salvatore Sicari, twenty-one, and Charles Jaynes, twenty-two, of Brockton, had reportedly lured the child into Jaynes's Cadillac with the promise of a new bike. Sicari, according to his own confession, drove the car while Jaynes wrestled with Jeffrey in the back seat, trying to force him to have sex. For many minutes, the 80-pound boy fought off the 250-plus-pound man; finally, Jeffrey succumbed to the burning suffocation of the gasoline-soaked rag held over his face.

The men loaded the body into the trunk and made their way to a Manchester, New Hampshire, apartment that Jaynes had rented and decorated with children's posters. In the early hours of the morning, again according to Sicari, Jaynes laid the corpse on the kitchen floor and raped and sodomized it. After that, the men mixed cement in a fifty-gallon storage container, stuffed Jeffrey's body into it, sprinkled lime on his face to speed decomposition, and traveled north to a bridge in South Berwick, Maine, where they hefted the plastic coffin into the river.

In separate murder trials a year later, each man blamed the other. Sicari was convicted of kidnapping and first-degree murder, for which he received a sentence of life without parole. Jaynes was found guilty of second-degree murder, because the jury could not positively place him at the crime scene. No sex charges were brought. Jaynes protested his innocence to the end, even shouting out during the prosecutor's final arguments that he had not hurt Jeffrey. His first parole hearing would come after twenty-three years' incarceration.

The story was terrifying enough to inject freon into the veins of any parent. But terror begs for reason, and while the Curley family struggled to find spiritual lessons in their child's demise, other parents watched their own kids pedal down the street on their bikes and looked desperately to the authorities to do, to say . . . something. Everyone wanted to understand how two men could commit such an atrocity against the affable, gap-toothed little guy in a Little League cap who smiled from the front page every day.

Sicari, according to his neighbors, was a menacing punk. He'd been picked up loitering near a schoolyard with cocaine on him, allegedly to sell, and been convicted of punching and kicking the twenty-year-old mother of his then one-year-old son. One of his favorite means of scaring up cash was to steal little kids' bicycles. Jaynes, who, unlike his accomplice, was employed, nevertheless had a rap sheet and a trail of seventy-five unanswered warrants, mostly for passing bad checks and coaxing other people's money out of ATMs.

Yet these ordinary criminal pedigrees held no warning of the cruelty the men would inflict on Jeffrey. They surely failed to supply the *meaning* the Curley family and an increasingly restive community longed for. It did not seem sufficient to call Jeffrey's murder what it was: an event utterly without sense, a ghastly aberration of high psychopathology, a crime of such rarity as to be, statistically, almost nonexistent. This inexplicable tragedy needed an explanation.

No one needed to look far. Both the media and its audience were adept at fitting any happening—an election, a new food product, a child's murder—into some sociological "trend," and every mother and father in America had heard of this one. Experts were on hand to supply analyses, newspaper databases were searched for crimes and criminals similar, or similar enough, to this one. The monsters needed a name, and they got one, in the first phrase of the *Boston Herald*'s first article on the apprehension of the suspects: "A pair of sexual predators smothered a 10-year-old Cambridge boy. . . ."

How could such a vile event have occurred? It occurred because of the kind of people Salvatore Sicari and Charles Jaynes were: they were sexual predators, "pedophiles." From hundreds of other articles and television reports, readers already knew that kind of person and were sure these two were not alone in the world.[2] Indeed, the men's photographs, reproduced scores of times atop the hundreds of columns of newsprint the story would command over the next year, suggested a crowd of compatriots, an army of murderers compelled by perverse desire.

The Pedophile: The Myth

Hear the word *pedophile* and images and ideas flood to mind. Pedophiles are predatory and violent; the criminal codes call their acts sexual attacks and sexual assaults.[3] Pedophiles look like Everyman or any man—"a teacher, a doctor, a lawyer, a judge, a scout leader, a police officer, an athletic coach, a religious counselor"[4]—but their sexuality makes them different from the rest of us, sick: *pedophilia* is listed in the American Psychiatric Association's *Diagnostic and Statistical Manual of Mental Disorders,* the canon of psychopathology.[5] Pedophiles are insatiable and incurable. "Statistics show that 95% of the time, anyone who molests a child will likely do it again," declared an Indiana senator proposing community notification laws for former sex offenders.[6] "The only molesters who can be considered permanently cured are those who have been surgically castrated," Ann Landers once wrote.[7]

Pedophiles abduct and murder children, and people who abduct and murder children are likely to be pedophiles. "The pedophile who kidnapped Adam from a mall and killed him in 1981 . . ." began a feature on molesters by *Boston Herald* reporter J. M. Lawrence, following Jeffrey's killing. He was referring to the still-unsolved abduction-murder of six-year-old Adam Walsh, whose case helped spur the creation of the National Center for Missing and Exploited Children and (some say) the career of his father, John, now the host of *The FBI's Most Wanted.* Even if a child survives a liaison with a pedophile, we believe, he will inevitably suffer great harm. "The predatory pedophile is as dangerous as cancer. He works as quietly, and his presence becomes known only by the horrendous damage he leaves," stated the children's lawyer and sex-thriller writer Andrew Vachss.

And pedophiles are legion, well-organized, and cunning in eluding detection. "I believe that we're dealing with a conspiracy, an organized operation of child predators designed to prevent detection," Kee MacFarlane, director of the Children's Institute International in Los Angeles and a premier architect of the satanic-ritual-abuse scare of the 1980s, told Congress in 1984.[8] "If such an operation involves child pornography or the selling of children, as is frequently alleged, it may have greater financial, legal, and community resources at its disposal than those attempting to expose it."[9] Ten years later, after a far-reaching national network of state and federal agents had been put in place to track them down, pedophiles were still strangely invisible. "There really aren't any figures. It's a hidden offense that often doesn't come to the surface," said Debra Whitcomb, director of Massachusetts' Educational Development Center Inc. in 1994, referring to the "child sexual exploitation" on the Net that her organization had just received a $250,000 government grant to combat.[10]

Perhaps it is no wonder that in a Mayo Clinic study of anxieties reported to pediatricians, three-quarters of parents were afraid their children would be abducted; a third said it was a "frequent worry," more frequent than fretting over sports injuries, car accidents, or drugs.[11] And no wonder Jeffrey Curley's murder, the crest of a wave of highly publicized criminal brutality, revived the crusade for capital punishment in Massachusetts, or that it was in this movement, as a spokesman for state-administered revenge, that his father, a firehouse mechanic named Bob, briefly found voice for his unutterable grief.[12]

The Facts

The problem with all this information about pedophiles is that most of it is not true or is so qualified as to be useless as generalization. First of all, the streets and computer chat rooms are not crawling with child molesters, kidnappers, and murderers. According to police files, 95 percent of allegedly abducted children turn out to be "runaways and throwaways" from home or kids snatched by one of their own parents in divorce custody disputes.[13] Studies commissioned under the Missing Children's Assistance Act of 1984 estimate that between 52 and 158 children will be abducted and murdered by nonfamily members each year.[14] Extrapolating from other FBI statistics, those odds come out between 1 in 364,000 and fewer than 1 in 1 million.[15] A child's risk of dying in a car accident is twenty-five to seventy-five times greater.

Fortunately, pedophilic butcheries are even rarer than abduction-murders. For instance, in 1992, the year a paroled New Jersey sex offender raped and killed Megan Kanka, the seven-year-old after whom community-notification statutes were named, nine children under age twelve were the victims of similar crimes, out of over forty-five million in that age group.[16] As for Adam Walsh, invoked by the *Boston Herald* as the Ur-victim of molestation murder, no defendant was ever indicted in his disappearance. According to detectives in Hollywood, Florida, where the crime occurred, Adam's father spread the rumor that the abductor was a pedophile, most prominently in a much-quoted book about child molesters, although there was neither suspicion nor evidence of sex in the case.[17]

Molestations, abductions, and murders of children by strangers are rare. And, say the FBI and social scientists, such crimes are not on the rise.[18] Some researchers even believe that some forms of molestation, such as exhibitionism, might be declining.[19]

There are, moreover, few so-called pedophiles in the population, though it is hard to say how few. "I write '1, 5, 21, 50' on the board and ask my students, 'Which is the percentage of pedophiles in the country?'" said Paul Okami, in the University of California at Los Angeles psychology department, who has analyzed the data on pedophilia in America. "The answer is all of them." That's because a "pedophile," depending on the legal statute, the perception of the psychologist, or the biases of the journalist, can be anything from a college freshman who has once masturbated with a fantasy of a twelve-year-old in mind to an adult who has had sexual contact with an infant.[20]

As for the "pure" clinical species, Okami believes that the proportion of Americans whose primary erotic focus is prepubescent children hovers around 1 percent. Estimating from lists of so-called pedophile rings, arrest records, and his own experience, David Techter, the former editor of the Chicago-based pedophile newsletter *Wonderland*, put the number at "maybe 100,000."[21] Criminal records do not indicate there are large or growing numbers of pedophiles. Even as the age of consent has risen and arrests for lower-level sex crimes have increased dramatically,[22] arrests for rape and other sex offenses, including those against children, still constituted only about 1 percent of all arrests in 1993.[23]

Pedophiles are not generally violent, unless you are using the term *sexual violence* against children in a moral, rather than a literal, way. Its perpetrators very rarely use force or cause physical injury in a youngster.[24] In fact, what most pedophiles do with children could not be further from Charles Jaynes's alleged necrophilic abominations. Bringing themselves down to the maturity level of children rather than trying to drag the child up toward an adult level, many men who engage in sex with children tend toward kissing, mutual masturbation, or "hands-off" encounters such as voyeurism and exhibitionism.[25]

Indeed, say some psychologists, there may be no such thing as a "typical" pedophile, if there is such a thing as a pedophile at all. Qualities by which social scientists and the police have marked him, such as his purported shyness or childhood sexual trauma, do not bear out with statistical significance.[26] More important, sexual contact with a child does not a pedophile make. "The majority of reported acts of sexual abuse of children are not committed by pedophiles," but by men in relationships with adult women and men, said John Money, of Johns Hopkins, a preeminent expert on sexual abnormalities.[27] They are men like Charles Jaynes, who wrote in his journal about a fast crush on a "beautiful boy" with "a lovely tan and crystal-blue eyes" and in whose car police found literature from the North American Man/Boy Love Association (NAMBLA) but who had an adult girlfriend and was rumored to be lovers with Sicari, who also had a girlfriend.[28]

In other words, there may be nothing fundamental about a person that makes him a "pedophile." So-called pedophiles do not have some genetic, or incurable, disease. Men who desire children can change their behavior to conform with the norms of a society that reviles it. Pedophilia can be renounced; in the medical language we now use to describe this sexual proclivity, it can be "cured." Indeed, contrary to politicians' claims, the recidivism rates of child sex offenders are among the lowest in the criminal population. Analyses of thousands of subjects in hundreds of studies in the United States and Canada have found that about 13 percent of sex offenders are rearrested, compared with 74 percent of all prisoners.[29] With treatment, the numbers are even better. The state of Vermont, for example, reported in 1995 that its reoffense rates after treatment were only 7 percent for pedophiles, 3 percent for incest perpetrators, and 3 percent for those who had committed "hands-off" crimes such as exhibitionism.[30]

The Enemy Is Us

All this rational talk may mean nothing to a parent. Nine in forty-five million children are raped and murdered: slim odds, sure, but if it happens to your baby, who cares about the statistics? Still, most parents manage to put irrational fears in perspective. Why, in spite of all information to the contrary, do Americans insist on believing that pedophiles are a major peril to their children? What do people fear so formidably?

Our culture fears the pedophile, say some social critics, not because he is a deviant, but because he is ordinary. And I don't mean because he is the ice-cream man or Father Patrick. No, we fear him because he is us. In his elegant study of "the culture of child-molesting," the literary critic James Kincaid traced this terror back to the middle of the nineteenth century. Then, he said, Anglo-American culture conjured childhood innocence, defining it as a desireless subjectivity, at the same time as it constructed a new ideal of the sexually desirable object. The two had identical attributes—softness, cuteness, docility, passivity—and this simultaneous cultural invention has presented us with a wicked psychosocial problem ever since. We relish our erotic attraction to children, says Kincaid (witness the child beauty pageants in which JonBenét Ramsey was entered). But we also find that attraction abhorrent (witness the public shock and disgust at JonBenét's "sexualization" in those pageants). So we project that eroticized desire outward, creating a monster to hate, hunt down, and punish.[31]

In her classic 1981 study, *Father-Daughter Incest*, feminist-psychologist Judith Lewis Herman suggested another source of self-revulsion that might lead us to project outward. Child abuse, she said, is close to home, built into the structure of the "normal," "traditional" family. Take the family's paternal authority enforced through violence, along with its feminine and child submission, its prohibitions against sexual talk and touch, and its privacy sanctified and inviolable, she said. Add repressed desire, and the potential of incest festers, waiting to happen.[32]

Herman's work was at the front edge of a horrifying suspicion, the truth of which is now firmly established. Even if child-sex crimes against strangers are rare, incest is not. Like pedophilia, it's hard to say how common it is, since incest figures are almost as muddied as those of adult-child sex outside the family. On one hand, child abuse statistics are notoriously unreliable; for example, of the 319,000 reports of sexual abuse of children in 1993, two-thirds were unsubstantiated.[33] The expansion of the definitions of family members, the ages of people considered children, and the types of interactions labeled abuse have jacked up incest figures. So has the popular suspicion of incest as an invisible source of later psychological distress, especially among women. Since the 1980s, self-help authors have claimed that you don't even have to remember a sexual event to know it occurred. "If you think you were abused and your life shows the symptoms, then you were," wrote Ellen Bass in *The Courage to Heal*.[34] The symptoms of past molestation listed in such books range from asthma to neglect of one's teeth.[35]

On the other hand, professionals under the influence of Freud have denied the existence of incest for decades, interpreting children's reports of real seductions as oedipal fantasies, and still may count only cases involving physical coercion, discounting the inestimable pressures on children to yield to a parent's sexual advances out of dependency, fear, loyalty, or love.

At any rate, reliable sources show that more than half, and some say almost all, of sexual abuse is visited upon children by their own family members or parental substitutes.[36] The federal government recorded over 217,000 cases in 1993 (fewer than the media hysteria would indicate, but still plenty).[37] Research confirms what is intuitively clear: that the worst devastation is wrought not by sex per se but by the betrayal of the child's fundamental trust. And the closer the relation, the more forced or intimate the sex acts, and the longer and later in a child's life they persist, the more hurtful is the immediate trauma and longer-lasting the harm of incest. Incest is a qualitatively different experience from sex with a nonfamily adult; almost inevitably, the former is a lot worse.[38]

Even those who don't buy Kincaid's claim that the cultural "we" are drooling over the prepubescent Macaulay Culkin cavorting through *Home Alone* in his underpants or Herman's metaphor of the family as incest incubator might be surprised to find that their own secret yearnings could be illegal. The vast majority of so-called pedophiles do not go out and ravage small children. So-called criminals are most often caught not touching but looking at something called child pornography (which I will get to in a moment). And their desired objects are not "children" but adolescents, about the age of the model Kate Moss at the start of her modeling career.[39] "The clients are usually white, suburban, married businessmen who want a blow job from a teenage boy but don't consider themselves gay, and heterosexual men who seek out young girls," said Edith Springer, who worked for many years with teenage prostitutes in New York's Times Square. "I have never in all my years of therapy and counseling come across what the media advertise as a 'pedophile.'"

Psychologists and law enforcers call the man who loves teenagers a hebophile. That's a psychiatric term, denoting pathological sexual deviance. But if we were to diagnose every American man for whom Miss (or Mr.) Teenage America was the optimal sex object, we'd have to call ourselves a nation of perverts. If the teenage body were not the culture's ideal of sexiness, junior high school girls probably would not start starving themselves as soon as they notice a secondary sex characteristic, and the leading lady (on-screen or in life) would not customarily be twenty to forty years younger than the leading man. I asked Meg Kaplan, a widely respected clinician who treats sex offenders at the New York State Psychiatric Institute's Sexual Behavior Clinic, about the medicalization and criminalization of the taste for adolescent flesh. "Show me a heterosexual male who's not attracted to teenagers," she snorted. "Puh-leeze."

Rather than indict our Monday night football buddies, rather than indict the family, though, we circle the wagons and project danger outward. "Screen out anyone who might be damaging to your child. Whenever possible, assume childcare responsibilities," the FBI's Kenneth Lanning advised the readers of *Life*. "Tell your kids that if an adult seems too good to be true, maybe he is."[40]

Genealogy of a Monster

Days after Jeffrey Curley's murder, the *Boston Herald* was fulfilling its public duty to provide sound-bite cultural analysis. "[S]exually oriented Internet chat rooms, the proliferation of sexual situations on TV, and easy access to hard-core pornography are creating more damaged children and possibly the next generation of pedophiles," opined one "expert." Another blamed welfare reform, which sent single mothers to work, leaving their kids to fend on their own. "And there are always child molesters looking for these kids."[41]

As we saw in chapter 1, dire assessments of a morally anarchic world are not new. But they tend to crop up in times of social transformation, when the economy trembles or when social institutions crumble and many people feel they're losing control of their jobs, their futures, or their children's lives. At times like these, the child-molesting monster can be counted on to creep from the rubble.

He first showed his grizzly face in modern Anglo-American history at the height of industrialization, in the late nineteenth century. In the cities and mill towns, poor and working-class children and adolescents left their homes and went out to work, where they met with new opportunities for sexual pleasure and new sources of sexual and economic pain. The young working girl's pleasures— to dance, flirt, or engage in casual prostitution to augment her meager wages—offended Victorian and religious morals. Her pains— exploitation and harassment in the factories, rape, disease, and

unwed motherhood—outraged feminists and socioeconomic re-
formers. The English writer Henry Worsley called the factory a
"school of iniquity" producing in the child an unseemly "precoci-
ty" about "the adult world and its pleasures."[42] The press, eager to
heat up these simmering sensitivities, "discovered" in the gutters a
marketplace in which venal capitalism fornicated with sexual license. This commerce was called white slavery.

In 1885, the popular tabloid *Pall Mall Gazette* introduced London's readers to the "white slaver." Its sensationalist series "The
Maiden Tribute of Modern Babylon," one of the most successful
"exposés" in journalistic history, told of a black market in which
virgin girls were sold by their hapless mothers to wicked neighborhood procuresses, who in turn prostituted them to eager, amoral
"gentlemen." The articles ignited one of the greatest moral panics
in modern British history.[43]

When a similar panic took hold in America a decade or so later,
it had literally a different complexion. Waves of immigrants from
China, southern Europe, and Ireland, as well as blacks from the
South, were pouring into the cities. And while African chattel slavery had been abolished, racism was hardly dead. "White slavery"
was so named to denote that its alleged victims were of northern
European descent (the institutionalized rape of African slaves would
not be acknowledged until a century later). Meanwhile, the sexual
salesmen described in almost all accounts of "white slavery" were
swarthy—sinister almost by definition—Jews, Italians, and Greeks.[44]

Although adult prostitution did flourish in the new industrial
cities, the trade in children on either side of the Atlantic was virtually an invention.[45] The *Gazette*'s editor, it turned out, had engineered
the abduction of the "five-pound virgin" (referring to her price, not
her weight) around whom his exposé was built;[46] "the throngs
of child prostitutes" claimed by London's anti-white-slavery campaigners were "imaginary products of sensational journalism intended to capture the attention of a prurient Victorian public," according to the historian Judith Walkowitz.[47] Rates of American
prostitution were also hugely inflated: one figure reported in the
New York suffragist press was multiplied tenfold from probable reality.[48] Nevertheless, both moral campaigns led to a spate of sex-
restrictive legislation. Following the "Maiden Tribute" articles, the
British age of consent rose from thirteen to sixteen.[49] In America,
between 1886 and 1895, twenty-nine states raised theirs from as
low as seven to as high as eighteen.[50] Some of the laws, like the Brit-

ish criminalization of homosexuality, stayed on the books into the late twentieth century.

As the twentieth century progressed, the sex monster went into hibernation. He was briefly roused during the Depression, when widespread financial failure threatened an epidemic of foundering masculine confidence and sparked suspicions of a compensatory "hypermasculinity" that would burst out in pathological desires for young bodies.[51] The child molester slumbered again, however, when World War II gave America a real enemy, and plenty of debauchery was tolerated both stateside, between the women and high schoolers left to run the factories, and near the front, where single and married fighting men took sexual R&R with the residents of the war's scarred cities.[52]

When the war ended, however, it was time to get gender and the family back to "normal." Men had to resume the breadwinning and women the bread baking. The homosexual culture that had seen its first sparks in the barracks and soldiers' bars had to be extinguished.[53] And teenagers, who had enjoyed a taste of adult wage earning and adult sexual license during the wars and the Depression, had to be dispatched back to childhood. Lingering resistance required an antidote: a social menace to make the renewed old order more attractive. And before FBI director J. Edgar Hoover and Senator Joseph McCarthy began painting that menace red, they set their sites on pink: the first targets of their inquests were homosexuals in the State Department. The hounded homosexuals in high places stood as a public example of (and to) perverts allegedly on the loose everywhere. The photomontage running beside Hoover's famous 1947 article "How Safe Is Your Daughter?" announced the return of the sex monster: three white girls in fluffy dresses and ankle socks fleeing from a huge, hovering masculine hand. "The nation's women and children will never be secure," the caption read, inserting a heart-stopping ellipsis ". . . so long as degenerates run wild."[54]

During this time, psychology was establishing itself as a profession, the apex of a centuries-long process by which the management of social deviance shifted from the purview of preachers to that of clinicians. Modern case books gave the monster a new name: the "sexual psychopath," compelled to molest children by "uncontrolled and uncontrollable desires."[55] By the mid-1950s, prewar anxieties about masculinity had zeroed in on sex between men, and in both the academy and the public imagination the psychopath took on the stereotypic characteristics of the homosexual, and vice versa. Boys were alerted never to enter public toilets alone. And after every grisly crime against a child, the gay bars were sure to be raided.[56] As they had a half century earlier, the headlines rang out alarms of a crime wave against children: "Kindergarten Girl Accosted by Man," "9 Charges against Molester of Girls," "What Shall We Do about Sex Offenders?"[57] But also like the panic of that earlier era, this one reflected no actual increase in violent sex crimes against children. Nevertheless, commissions were empaneled, new laws were passed, and arrests increased. Whereas most of these, like most arrests today, were for minor offenses such as flashing or consensual homosexual sex,[58] a few highly publicized violent crimes drew a clangor of public demand for dragnets, vigilante squads, life imprisonment, indefinite incarceration in mental institutions, castration, and execution of the psycho killers,[59] all of which were revived in the 1980s and 1990s.

During the 1960s and 1970s, sex panic gave way to sexual liberation, including, for a brief moment, the notion that children had a right to sexual expression. "Sex is a natural appetite," wrote Heidi Handman and Peter Brennan in 1974, in *Sex Handbook: Information and Help for Minors*. "If you're old enough to want to have sex, you're old enough to have it."[60] But as women's and children's sexual options were proclaimed, their experiences of coercion were also thrown into relief. Feminists started speaking out against sexual violence under the cloak of family and romantic intimacy; suspicion grew that child sexual abuse was epidemic. An industry of therapists specializing in unearthing past abuse and curing its purported effects began to prosper.

The cold war was melting into detente; for the first time in living memory, Americans were bereft of national enemies and native subversives. The new political-therapeutic alliance unearthed the same old nemesis to children's sexual innocence and safety. But, in the age of media, the old white slaver–child molester wore a modern hat. Now, besides kidnapping and ravishing children, he was taking their pictures and selling them for profit. The pedophile had taken up a sideline as a pornographer.

The Modern Monster

The child pornographer, when he first came to public light in 1976, was a feeble beast and an even worse businessman. In fact, he was almost bankrupt. Raids aimed at cleaning up Times Square for the Democratic Convention uncovered only a minuscule cache of kiddie porn.[61] But those few stacks of dusty, decades-old black-and-white rags, already illegal, were enough to launch a crusade. It was led by a team that would epitomize the anti-child-porn forces: a child psychiatrist, Judianne Densen-Gerber, who founded the drug-rehabilitation empire Odyssey House in New York, and a vice cop, Sergeant Lloyd Martin, of the Los Angeles Police Department.

The two careened from sea to sea, stoking outsized claims. Before a congressional committee in 1977, Densen-Gerber estimated that 1.2 million children were victims of child prostitution and pornography, including "snuff" films in which they were killed for viewers' titillation.[62] Martin traveled the country orating speeches of evangelical fervor, warning America on one Christian television show, for instance, that "pedophiles actually wait for babies to be born so that, just minutes after birth, they can grab the post-fetuses and sexually victimize them."[63] At that 1977 congressional committee, he declared that the sexual exploitation of children was "worse than homicide."[64]

Within a few years, police testified that child porn had never been more than a boutique business even in its modest heyday in the late 1960s. The first law wiped out what little kiddie porn remained on the street, and by the early 1980s, the head of the New York Police Department's Public Morals Division proclaimed the stuff "as rare as the Dead Sea Scrolls."[65] The 1.2 million figure, which Densen-Gerber subsequently doubled,[66] was revealed to be the arbitrarily quadrupled estimate of an unsubstantiated number one author said he'd "thrown out" to get a reaction from the law enforcement community.[67] Densen-Gerber would soon slip from the public eye under suspicions of embezzling public monies and employing coercive and humiliating methods at Odyssey House.[68] Martin would later be removed from his post at the LAPD for harassing witnesses and falsifying evidence.[69]

But their work had been accomplished. The press continued to broadcast their bogus statistics. And hardly a year after Densen-Gerber's first press conference, Congress passed the Protection of Children against Sexual Exploitation Act of 1977, prohibiting the production and commercial distribution of obscene depictions of children younger than sixteen. One of the first casualties was *Show Me!*, a sex education book for prepubescent children featuring explicit photographs of children, from around six to their early teens, engaged in sex play. When it was published in 1970, the book was showered with awards. Under the new restrictions on "child pornography," it became illegal to publish, distribute, and, eventually, even to own anywhere in the United States.

Then, in 1979, a six-year-old middle-class white boy named Etan Patz turned the corner on his way to school in lower Manhattan and was never seen again. Two years later, six-year-old Adam Walsh's head was found floating in a Florida canal. Federal and private money began funneling toward a newly named victim, the Missing and Exploited Child. Soon, hundreds of "missing children" were beseeching would-be rescuers from the containers of that quintessentially maternal food, milk. Local police departments set up child-finding units, which distributed pamphlets and dispatched trainers and speakers. Parents and teachers were getting the message: the molester-kidnapper was everywhere.

Most frightening, he was lurking where the most vulnerable children were sent for nurture and safekeeping: nursery school. And he had joined up with an omnipotent ally: none other than Satan. In 1984, the media started following breathlessly as the trial unfolded in southern California of Peggy Buckey, the elderly proprietor of the McMartin Preschool, and her son Ray, a beloved teacher. The two had been accused by three-year-olds of bizarre tortures—anal rape with knives and pencils, animal mutilation, oral sex performed on clowns—"satanic ritual abuse" allegedly carried out in broad daylight in open-door classrooms, where parents and other teachers could walk in at any time.

No child had volunteered any such story until being interviewed by Kee MacFarlane and her team of social workers at the Children's Institute International in Los Angeles, and the videotapes of these interviews revealed bewildered and resistant babies being hectored into assenting to the narratives fed them by their interrogators. Indeed, by the end of the longest and most expensive criminal trial in U.S. history, it was the tapes themselves that exonerated the Buckeys. But eerily identical tales began to surface in schools across the nation.[70] In 1994, the U.S. government's National Center on Child Abuse and Neglect reported on its five-year survey of eleven thousand psychiatric and police workers nationwide, covering the more than twelve thousand accusations of satanic ritual abuse. The investigation found "not a single case where there was clear corroborating evidence," not a single snapshot or negative of the alleged rolls and rolls of child pornography produced by the deviants.[71] But new accusations, all unsupported, kept coming. The latest were in Wenatchee, Washington, in 1995, where forty-three people were accused of some twenty-nine thousand counts of sexual abuse involving sixty children, all without a shred of evidence.[72] At the beginning of the new millennium, many innocents are still behind bars.[73]

Debbie Nathan and Michael Snedeker argued in *Satan's Silence* that the day-care abuse scares tapped popular anxieties about women working outside the home and leaving their children with others. But these fears were given shape and heft by a certain world view, which was attached to a certain political agenda. It was that of the religious Right (who believed that Satan literally walked the earth), with the cautious endorsement of feminist sexual conservatives—the same bedfellows who would lie down together in the 1986 Meese commission.

As anthropologist Carole S. Vance pointed out, the Meese commission was not inclined to recommend any policies that feminists would champion, such as aid to women who wanted to leave abusive men or legal protections of sex workers from violence and economic exploitation. Rather, it erected a broad federal network to chase and prosecute symbolic assaults on its own ideas of morality, that is, on smut peddlers. But its offensive against adult pornography failed to generate heartfelt support in the heartland. Several municipal antipornography ordinances crafted by the influential feminist theorists Catharine MacKinnon and Andrea Dworkin, had already fallen to constitutional challenge. Prosecutors backed off bringing obscenity cases against "adult" material, which were almost impossible to win.

Right-wing organizations that had long fought for censorship of erotica were determined to stay the course. Shrewdly, they abandoned their old maiden in distress, "decency," and took up the cause of "families and children." Citizens for Decency Through Law (founded in 1957 by that paragon of decency through law, savings-and-loan swindler Charles Keating) became the Children's Legal Foundation, which metamorphosed into the National Family Legal Foundation. Reverend Donald Wildmon's National Federation for Decency became the American Family Association, and the National Coalition Against Pornography (N-CAP) spun off the

National Law Center for Children and Families. The Justice Department's National Obscenity Enforcement Unit, set up after the Meese commission, was rechristened the Child Exploitation and Obscenity Section. The wide, fat enemy "pornography" began to fade from view. Now both antiporn feminist and conservative propaganda aimed at the sleaker "hard-core," the scarier "child pornography."

And where was this new pornographer? Densen-Gerber and Martin had been unable to run him down on the urban streets. He'd eluded capture in the suburban childcare centers. Now, said his pursuers, the fugitive had found his way to everywhere and nowhere. He was on the Internet, where he had joined a vast club that zipped pictures of copulating kids among them, sidled up to children in chat rooms, and enticed them into real-world motels and malls. With the family room connected by a mere modem to the wild open cyberspaces, even the home was no longer safe. As the cover of one "family-values" magazine blared, "CYBERPORN STEALS HOME."

Snared in the Web

In spite of proud FBI claims, many lawyers and journalists, including me, suspect that the child pornographer is the same penny-ante presence online as he was in Times Square. Bruce Selcraig, a government investigator of child pornography during the 1980s who went online in 1996 as a journalist to review the situation, concluded the same. In the cyberspeech debate, he said, the dissemination of child porn amounted to "a tuna-sized red herring."[74]

Aficionados and vice cops concede that practically all the sexually explicit images of children circulating cybernetically are the same stack of yellowing pages found at the back of those X-rated shops, only digitized. These pictures tend to be twenty to fifty years old, made overseas, badly re-reproduced, and for the most part pretty chaste. That may be why federal agents almost never show journalists the contraband. But when I got a peek at a stash downloaded by Don Huycke, the national program manager for child pornography at the U.S. Customs Service, in 1995, I was underwhelmed. Losing count after fifty photos, I'd put aside three that could be called pornographic: a couple of shots of adolescents masturbating and one half-dressed twelve-year-old spreading her legs in a position more like a gymnast's split than split beaver. The rest tended to be like the fifteen-year-old with a 1950s bob and an Ipana grin, sitting up straight, naked but demure, or the two towheaded six-year-olds in underpants, astride their bikes.

So when these old pictures show up on the Net, who's putting them there? Attorney Lawrence Stanley, who published in the *Benjamin A. Cardozo Law Review* what is widely considered the most thorough research of child pornography in the 1980s, concluded that the pornographers were almost exclusively cops. In 1990 at a southern California police seminar, the LAPD's R. P. "Toby" Tyler proudly announced as much. The government had shellacked the competition, he said; now law enforcement agencies were the sole reproducers and distributors of child pornography.[75] Virtually all advertising, distribution, and sales to people considered potential lawbreakers were done by the federal government, in sting operations against people who have demonstrated (through, for instance, membership in NAMBLA) what agents regard as a predisposition to commit a crime. These solicitations were usually numerous and did not cease until the recipient took the bait. "In other words, there was no crime until the government seduced people into committing one," Stanley wrote.[76]

If, as police claim, looking at child porn inspires molesters to go out and seduce living children, why were the feds doing the equivalent of distributing matches to arsonists? Their answer is: to stop the molesters before they strike again. Newspaper reports of arrests uniformly follow the same pattern: a federal agent poses as a minor online, hints at a desired meeting or agrees to one should the mark suggest it, and then arrests the would-be molester when he shows up.[77] But another logical answer to the almost exclusive use of stings to arrest would-be criminals is that the government, frustrated with the paucity of the crime they claim is epidemic and around which huge networks of enforcement operations have been built, have to stir the action to justify their jobs.

The same logic can explain why the volume of anti-child-porn legislation has increased annually. From a relatively simple criminalization of production and distribution, the law eventually went after possession and then even viewing of child-erotic images at somebody else's house. It raised the age of a "child" from sixteen to eighteen and defined as pornography pictures in which the subject is neither naked, nor doing anything sexual, nor, under the 1996 Child Pornography Prevention Act, is even an actual child. Legislation that was first

justified as a protection of real children evolved to statutes criminalizing the sexual depiction of anyone *intended to look like a minor,* including "virtual" computer-generated children. In 2002 the Supreme
Court struck down the CPPA. It found the government's claimed link
between looking at images and child abuse "contingent and indirect.
The harm does not necessarily follow the speech, but depends upon
some unquantified potential for subsequent criminal acts.[78]

Such bills have almost invariably been sponsored by conservative
Republicans with support from right-wing and fundamentalist Christian organizations and antipornography feminists. And even while
some legislators privately express doubts that they protect children,
these proposals are unstoppable. "When the Senate votes on child issues, they're all on one side," Patrick Trueman, a lobbyist for the
American Family Association and former head of Justice Department's National Obscenity Enforcement Unit, told me in 1989. "We
got the toughest law in 1988"—the Child Protection and Enforcement Act—"because it had the words *child exploitation* in it, though
most of it was directed to adult pornography." So, have the government's efforts worked to round up dangerous pedophiles?

In 1995, the FBI launched its child-pornography task force Innocent Images, which trains special agents under a congressional grant
of ten million dollars to rout out pedophiles on the Net. From 1996
to 2000, the unit initiated 2,609 cases. But barely 20 percent of
those generated indictments, with just 17 percent resulting in convictions.[79] The FBI's Peter Gullotta told James Kincaid that Innocent Images had achieved 439 convictions since 1995. How were
these criminals found? "It's like fishing in a pond full of hungry
fish," Gullotta told Kincaid. "Every time you put a line with live bait
in there, you're going to get one."[80] This might sound like induce-
ment (especially to journalists like myself, who have talked to the
fish)—the same tactics that Stanley described in the 1980s, only updated from snail mail to e-mail.[81]

The federal government's biggest success to date concluded in
August 2001, with the arrest of the two owners of Landslide Pro-
ductions, Inc., and one hundred of their customers in Fort Worth,
Texas. Landslide maintained a profitable pornography Web site
that offered, in addition to adult porn, links to foreign sites that
contain images considered child pornography under U.S. law. The
two owners were arrested for possession and distribution, not production, of child pornography, and the subscribers were arrested

for possession. While one of these customers was identified as a "registered child sex offender" and another as having been convicted of four "sex crimes" in the past, none arrested in this operation was indicted for abuse of an actual child. To draw out the child-porn aficionados from among the site's 250,000 mostly law-abiding subscribers, the government advertised sales of child-pornographic tapes and CD-ROMs under the name of the company, which it had seized in 1999. When a person placed an order, a package was sent and the buyer arrested on its delivery.

Although the shutdown of one site and the arrest of one hundred customers took four years and engaged unnumbered Justice Department agents, as well as thirty federally financed local task forces nationwide, U.S. Postal Service Inspector General Kenneth Weaver claimed that Landslide was "the tip of the iceberg" in what the *New York Times* paraphrased as "a growing market for child pornography via the Internet."[82] The story was front-page news in every market I checked, and the *Times* ran it in the spot reserved for the day's most important story, the top right-hand column.

Were these customers predisposed to crime, besides the illegal act of looking at images of minors who might or might not be engaging in sex? According to the FBI's Gullotta when he spoke to Kincaid, the typical catch has no previous criminal record. Almost no such case goes to trial; the defendants plead guilty. The government calls this more evidence of guilt.[83] But, again, closer examination of such cases (in fact, of most child abuse charges) reveals that pleas are often taken under advice of counsel to eliminate the chance of a long prison sentence and also to limit the personal destruction that publicity wreaks even if the accused is exonerated.[84]

Unfortunately, plea bargains, because they lack the details of depositions, interrogations at trial, and the defense's version of events, make it almost impossible to tell what the person is accused of doing, much less whether he did it. Federal statistics aren't much help. According to Kincaid, neither the FBI nor the National Center for Missing and Exploited Children now keeps track of how many children are actually lured to danger after online assignations, the feared eventuality that motivates these operations. Journalists are frustrated by more than insufficient data, though. In 1995, while I covered the story of the first man convicted for possession of "lascivious" videotapes of minors who were neither naked nor doing anything sexual, I arrived at the Justice Department in Washington,

D.C., only to learn that my scheduled viewing of the evidence had been canceled because, well, the tapes were illegal. Exposing the models to my eyes, an agent told me, would criminally harm them (I later learned that portions of the tapes had aired on Court TV). I drove six hours to western Pennsylvania, where the court clerk set me up with a VCR, and I yawned through hours of badly filmed images no racier than a Bahamas tourism commercial. Similar restrictions were placed on reportage of the Landslide investigation. According to the *Times,* "the authorities did not release the addresses of the actual [foreign] sites" allegedly offering child-pornographic images, and the only models described were two British siblings, a girl and a boy, ages eight and six.[85] But agents did not reveal whether these children were photographed engaging in sexual activity, and journalists were obviously unable to inspect the images themselves. In 1999, thirty-two-year veteran radio journalist Larry Matthews was sentenced to eighteen months in federal prison for receiving and transmitting a child-pornographic image in the process of reporting a story on child-porn chat rooms. In fact, prosecutors were alerted to his activities when he reported what he called "terrible things"—the posting by a mother apparently offering up her children for sex with adults.[86]

Statistics that I got from the National Center for Missing and Exploited Children in 1996 indicated that the feared eventuality that motivates all this activity had rarely come to pass. Only twenty-three minors were enticed to malls and hotel rooms by their adult suitors between 1994 and 1996, none of these "children" was under thirteen, and most were at least a couple of years older than that. A 2001 survey conducted by the University of New Hampshire found that almost a fifth of ten- to seventeen-year-olds who went online received sexual solicitations from "strangers," an unspecified number of whom may have been adults. However, it would be hard to impute widespread harm to these experiences. Three-quarters of the youth said they were not distressed by the posts. And, wrote the researchers, "no youth in the sample was actually sexually assaulted as a result of contacts made over the Internet."[87] As for pedophiles caught in the act, as far as I can gather only one such case has occurred: the infamous Orchid Club, whose members took turns having sex with a child in front of videocams that broadcast their doings to their compatriots in real time.[88] This act of sexual violence was already a crime before child porn law and remains so, as it should.

Meanwhile, local authorities have dived enthusiastically into the broadening legal definitions of smut, with the result that more and more citizens are finding themselves entangled with the law for making and keeping truly innocent images. In the early 1990s, the Nebraska attorney general ordered a local policeman to burn nine thousand slides, each of an individual naked child, assembled by psychologist William Farrall to be used with the penile plethysmograph, an instrument that measures sexual arousal. Psychologists employed the pictures along with the device to assess the progress of thousands of sex offenders in treatment nationwide.[89] After the passage of the Child Pornography Prevention Act of 1996, Oklahoma police seized a copy of the film of Günter Grass's Nobel Prize–winning *The Tin Drum* from a video rental store because of an inexplicit scene in the movie in which a man who refuses to grow out of his child's body (to avoid participating in fascism) performs what some construed as oral sex on an adult woman. And in the 1990s, cases proliferated in which clerks in photo-developing shops, instructed to alert the police of any "suspicious" pictures, flagged such classic "bear rug" shots as moms in the tub with their babies, which led to the arrests of the photographers, and worse.[90] In New York, Fotomat employees reported nude shots of a six-year-old son taken by a photography student. The father was handcuffed and taken from his home, while his children were rushed out in their pajamas to be examined for sexual abuse. No evidence of abuse was found, and the man was not brought to trial. But he was barred from his home for two months and forbidden to see his youngest daughter. Cynthia Stewart, an Oberlin, Ohio, mother, was nabbed when a photograph of her eight-year-old daughter in the bath was fingered as "pornographic" by a photo-shop clerk. Stewart escaped prosecution (and potential imprisonment) only after agreeing to state publicly that two of her pictures could be interpreted as "sexually oriented" and allowing prosecutors to destroy them; she also consented to participate in six months of anti-abuse counseling. Although she found the smarmy implications of these measures abhorrent, she complied in order to save her daughter the trauma of a trial.[91]

False Security

Civil libertarians have called these laws unconstitutionally vague: a reasonable person can't know in advance if he is breaking them. They've diverted millions of taxpayer dollars from real child welfare and created an atmosphere of puritanical surveillance over all U.S. citizens in the dubious name of catching a small number of people who, if left alone, might do nothing more harmful to minors than sit around and masturbate to pictures of ten-year-olds in bathing suits.

But the legislative legacy of the child-abuse panic has done more than abridge the First Amendment. For Americans convicted of any sex crime, legislation passed in the 1990s arguably constitutes cruel and unusual, and perpetual, punishment. By 1999, according to the Center for Missing and Exploited Children, all fifty states had enacted "Megan's laws," requiring paroled sex offender registration and community notification; more stringent laws win states more federal crime-fighting funds.[92] In many states, parolees are required to register regardless of the nature of their crime. In 2001, a judge in Corpus Christi, Texas, ordered twenty-one registered offenders to post "DANGER: Registered Sex Offender" notices on their homes and cars.[93]

Sweeping over individual differences, politicians routinely refer to the former convicts as sexual predators, a phrase connoting insatiable appetite and sharp teeth. But as the rhetoric mounted during the 1990s, even *predator* wasn't scary enough. Following Kansas's lead in 1994, "sexually violent predator" laws spread across the states, which allowed the indefinite incarceration in psychiatric facilities of sex criminals who had completed prison sentences but were deemed likely to commit another crime.[94] To qualify as a sexually violent predator, the convict had to manifest a "mental abnormality" or "personality disorder," diagnoses about as exact as "a real fruitcake" and as common as compulsive eating. They were also remarkably reminiscent of the "uncontrollable desires" of the 1950s.[95]

Those who work with sex offenders have warned that such policies might do no good and even could do harm. For one thing, former sex offenders are at far lower risk of committing new crimes than those released from prison after serving time for other crimes.[96] Nevertheless, rage against sex criminals is often far greater, and community notification laws serve to focus that rage. Since their inception, such programs have fueled harassment and vigilantism,[97] which further isolate and unnerve the parolee, leading to the exact opposite of the law's intended effect. "You ban somebody from the community, he has no friends, he feels bad about himself, and you reinforce the very problems that contribute to the sex abuse behavior in the first place," Robert Freeman-Longo, former director of the Safer Society Program and president of the Association for the Treatment of Sexual Abusers, told me. "You make him a better sex offender."

Some criminal-justice practices, moreover, seem to have no other intent but to keep the public on the edge of its seats. During the summer of 1997, California's Justice Department set up a sort of side-show booth at state fairs featuring an LED screen that endlessly scrolled the names of the state's registered sex offenders, along with their addresses—sixty-four thousand in all. What the shocked viewers did not know was that because registration in that state covered crimes committed as far back as the 1940s, many of the "predators" on the list had been arrested for victimless misdemeanors like soliciting a prostitute or cruising a man in a gay bar.[98] Tom Masters, program director of correctional treatment services at Oregon State Hospital, described such policymaking succinctly: "A lot of crime legislation is a function of politics, and not of rehabilitation or community safety."

Nor, I would add, is it a function of community sanity. In 1984, at the beginning of the sex-lawmaking frenzy, the authors of the final report on U.S. Senator William V. Roth's Child Pornography and Pedophilia hearings noted what they called a paradox. "Good laws often lead to more arrests," they wrote, "thus making it appear that more new laws are needed to curb what the public perceives as an increase in crime."[99] Nevertheless, the commissioners recommended more laws, which led to more bureaucracy, more agents, more investigations, and more arrests. And that, said Eric Lotke of the National Center for Institutions and Alternatives, created another paradox: the public felt falsely safer and also more fearful.

Lynn Johnston, in the comic strip "For Better or For Worse," described the sadness and bafflement that can accompany these contradictory feelings. In a strip at the end of the 1990s, John, the father, amiably chats with a five-year-old at the supermarket. Her panicked mother swoops down the aisle. "VANXXESSA!!!" she cries. "Don't talk to that man . . . we don't know who he is!!!" Back at home, John's wife comforts him as he holds his own toddler in his lap. "She was just protecting her child, honey," says Elly. "I know," John answers. "It's just that now and then I hate the world we're living in." The reader was left to infer what about the world this archetypal baby boomer hated, the pedophiles or the paranoia.

Vanessa's mother was doing the "right thing," according to the local police who would have spoken at her daughter's school. But for the child's sake, it was the wrong thing. Panic about adult-child sex, like panic about anything, prompts fewer right decisions than wrong ones, and the wrong ones can be breathtakingly wrong. Attorney General Janet Reno's decision to lay siege to the Branch Davidian compound in Waco, Texas, was based in part on rumors of child abuse going on inside.[100] In the ensuing conflagration, eighty people died, including twenty-four children.[101]

Trying to fortify the nuclear family by fomenting suspicion of strangers fractures the community of adults and children; it can leave children defenseless in abusive homes. Projecting sexual menace onto a cardboard monster and pouring money and energy into vanquishing him distract adults from teaching children the subtle skills of loving with both trust and discrimination. Ultimately, children are rendered more vulnerable both at home and in the world.

3. Therapy

"Children Who Molest" and the Tyranny of the Normal

> Although this type of behavior is perfectly normal, it is socially inappropriate.
> —Dr. Lawrence Kutner, on "playing doctor," *Parents Magazine* (1994)

When I met him at the end of 1996, Tony Diamond was an unhappy boy. Charming and tractable one minute, he might be flailing in rage or brooding in despair the next. Tony's schoolwork was outstanding; he read widely and wrote winningly. (He proudly showed me his report on Napoleon, whom he quoted as uttering, "Able was I 'ere I saw Elba." Not coincidentally, he was a fan of palindromes.) Yet Tony had trouble at school—he got into fights and disobeyed teachers—and in his short life had attended several. Like other boys his age, twelve at the time, Tony liked *Star Wars*, baseball, and animals. At home, there was a small menagerie: a hamster named Fidget, fish, a rabbit, and a garrulous cockatiel.

Tony could be mean to his sister, Jessica, one year his junior, blond and plump where he is dark and slender, slow in class where he excelled. Their relationship, it seemed, was fierce—fiercely affectionate and fiercely antagonistic. One evening, they sat touching, playing quietly. Another time, she climbed into the car and he slapped her, unprovoked.

In November 1993, the San Diego County Child Protective Services pronounced Tony Diamond a grave danger to his sister. Jessica told someone at school that her brother had "touched her front and back." Mandated by the 1974 Child Abuse Prevention and Treatment Act to report any suspicion of child abuse, even *by* a child, the school called the Child Abuse Hotline. The social worker who did the family's intake interview elicited a record of Tony's earlier offenses: In elementary school, he used sexual language and looked under girls' skirts. At four, he lay on top of Jessie in the bath.

With only Jessica's testimony to go on, the juvenile court charged Tony with "sexual abuse" of "the minor" Jessica, "including, but not limited to touching her vaginal and anal areas . . . placing a pencil in her buttocks" (that is, he poked the flesh of her buttocks with a pencil), and threatening to hurt her if she "disclosed the molest." Jessica's story would change over the weeks and months, and none of what transpired between them is clear.

Nevertheless, the interviewer made this confident assessment: "It would appear from a review of the case that Tony is a budding sex offender." Tony was nine years old.[1]

Tony was to become one case in a new "epidemic," the "sexualization" of children; a new class of patient, "children with sexual behavior problems"; and a new category of sexual criminal perpetrator, "children who molest." Although some youngsters, particularly teen boys, do commit real sexual intrusions, even rape of other kids, "children who molest" are of another order. As young as two, they are diagnosed and treated, and sometimes prosecuted, for "inappropriate" behaviors like fondling, putting things inside genitals, or even flashing, mooning, or masturbating "compulsively." From the anecdotes I have gathered since reporting on Tony, it appears that sex play between siblings is considered the gravest, though ironically the commonest, species of a grave and not uncommon problem.

Children who molest are accused of coercion, though often the "victim" complies willingly, enjoys, or does not notice the "abuse." And while some such kids are aggressive in other ways, such as fighting, stealing, or setting fires, their doctors practice under the assumption that any sexual acting-out is of a wholly different, and worse, order of behavior. So, with little supportive evidence, a new group of self-styled experts has persuaded the child-protective systems that "sex-offense-specific" therapy is necessary for any minor with a "sexual behavior problem."

Although the events that befell Tony and his family may seem extreme, they are not unique. While in San Diego reporting on the

Diamonds for *Mother Jones Magazine,* I also met Brian Flynn, who at fourteen in 1993 had been charged with lewd and lascivious conduct and oral copulation with a minor, felonies punishable by three- and eight-year terms of incarceration, respectively. His crime, denied by both alleged participants, was asking—or, depending on who told the story and when, allowing—his ten-year-old sister to lick his penis. After much persuasion, Brian pled to the first count, for which he spent more than two years in the state's punitive custody. When he went AWOL from one of his placements, the county sent a SWAT team: half a dozen squad cars with loudspeakers warning neighbors to beware of "a dangerous sex offender" and a helicopter buzzing the scrubby backyards of his father's community. Brian scrambled up a hill; an officer took chase and pulled a gun. The fugitive jumped a fence into the night. His mother finally, reluctantly, turned him in. "I was scared he was going to get himself killed," she told me.[2]

After the *Mother Jones* story came out, I began reading more and more stories like Tony's and Brian's in the papers. In 1996, in Manchester, New Hampshire, a ten-year-old "touched [two girls] in a sexual manner" (he grabbed at them on the school playground) and was charged with two counts of rape.[3] In New Jersey, a neurologically impaired twelve-year-old who groped his eight-year-old stepbrother in the bath was compelled to register as a sex offender under Megan's Law,[4] a mark that could stigmatize him for life. In 1999, the newspapers briefly bristled with reports of a "child sex ring" in York Haven, Pennsylvania, in which "children as young as 7 . . . taught each other to have sex." An eleven-year-old girl was convicted of rape.[5]

My research has made me suspicious of these reports, and my doubts were heightened by the phone calls I was receiving from distraught parents and grandparents whose kids were being charged in similar situations. A single mother in Long Island, New York, tracked me down in 1999 to ask for help for her thirteen-year-old son, Adam, who had been accused of sexually rubbing against his eleven-year-old sister (she had boasted of her sexual experience to her friends, who were urged by her to report him to a school counselor). Adam was arrested, handcuffed, threatened with prosecution on adult felony charges, then placed in a youth sex offenders' program in an austere Catholic residence (he was Jewish), where he was paroled after a year on the condition that he undergo at least another year of outpatient treatment. A Michigan grandmother wept over the phone, recounting how a sex-offender institution refused to release her eleven-year-old grandson because he wouldn't confess to an offense he insisted he did not do. "They kept saying he was 'in denial' and the therapy wasn't taking. So they just kept keeping him locked up," she told me. After four years, in the mid-1990s, she said, the boy killed himself.

Equally important as the individual tragedies that have befallen these children is the effect the trend has on all children, including those who will never go near a child-protective agency or set foot in a juvenile detention facility. What Tony's story represents is the gradual pathologizing of *normative* children's sexuality, that is, behavior that most kids do.[6] This has consequence not just for the behavior deemed "deviant" but for all children's sexual behavior. Each time a new category of sexual deviance is identified—or, you might say, invented—the entire scale of so-called normal behavior is calibrated a few notches to the right. Professionals' and laypeople's idea of what is okay for children, teens, or families slides in a more conservative, more frightened, and more prohibitive direction, away from tolerance, humor, and trust.

Normal is not an exact scientific term. It can mean what most people do or what some people consider healthy, moral, regular, or natural, as opposed to sick, sinful, weird, or unnatural. It can mean what my mother, my priest, or the psychologist on *Oprah Winfrey* says is okay. Or it can mean what *I* think is okay.[7] Normal is enormously susceptible to swinging with the gusts of politics and history. Disguised as scientific and fixed, it is subjective and protean. That is why I used the word *normative* above, a term derived from statistics, simply meaning what most people do. It's why I do not resort anywhere in this book to the common liberal defense of kids' sexuality: that it is "normal and natural." Normal is problematic, because you can't have normal without abnormal. Acceptable behavior needs "unacceptable" (or "inappropriate") behavior to find its place in the world. To have an in-crowd, you have to have outcasts.

Tony's story is both a cause and a symptom of the conservative drift of "normal" in the past twenty-five years, a combination of the Right's influence in national sexual policy on one side and feminist concerns about abuse on the other. As a result, everybody in the everyday business of child raising at the turn of this century is on the qui vive for pathology. The eminent sex educator Peggy Brick, who spent decades traveling the country giving parent and teacher workshops on child sexuality, told me she was alarmed when such panels began to be dominated by "experts" on "sexual behavior problems," and when parents who were once confused, but also amused, by their kids' sexual pleasure-seeking were now worried that their kids were treading into danger. A psychologist friend recounted the events at an exclusive private school on Manhattan's Upper East Side, also in the late 1990s. In the kindergarten teacher's presentation to parents, she allowed that children in her class sometimes dressed in opposite-sex clothes when acting out fairy tales. It helped them literally to walk in the other person's shoes, she said. The parents flew into a frenzy. Were the children being prematurely "sexualized"? Could such play be harmful to their fragile gender identifications? A raft of meetings and panels followed, but the invited expert, a child psychologist, did not put the parents' minds to rest. Instead, he suggested that such play might mobilize "gender dysphoria," an extremely rare sense of being in the wrong-sexed body.

Parenting-advice columns in women's magazines, which for decades handed out reassurances that it's perfectly fine if kids touch each other, masturbate, and talk incessantly about penises, now anatomize how much might be too much or when is the wrong time. Where the avuncular Dr. Spock and the hip shrink Sol Gordon once sat on these magazines' daises of experts, now readers attend to a furrow-browed Toni Cavanagh Johnson, the guru of "sexual behavior problems," pointing at charts with the danger zones marked in red.

And if there is creeping pathology, adults have begun to fear, then there must also be more danger to the other, "healthy" children. Most people felt that the North Carolina school administration overreacted almost ludicrously when it censured the freckle-nosed first-grader Johnathan Prevette for kissing a classmate. But since then, "zero-tolerance" rules on student flirtation have become more extreme in some places. For instance, in 2001 the eight-year-old daughter of a Vermont acquaintance had the charge of "sexual harassment" entered in her elementary school record. Her crime: sending a note to a classmate asking if he wanted to be her boyfriend.

These school policies do not fall far outside the norm. The principals were acting inside a growing consensus: that physical demonstrations of affection between children are "sex" and that sex between children is always traumatic.

Unsuspecting

When Diane Diamond invited a caseworker into her house, cluttered with angels and Buddhas, kids' trophies, and plants, she had a naive faith in the helping professions. The small, quick woman had undergone plenty of healing herself, of both the traditional and the New Age varieties, and she poured out her family's history in sentences studded with psychologisms. She told the caseworker that she'd fled, pregnant with Jessica, from a husband who beat and raped her and choked one-year-old Tony; she said she'd been "drug and alcohol free" for fifteen years; she reported that a man had exposed himself to Jessica in the park when she was little, and she'd brought charges against him. Diane told Child Protective Services (CPS) she was concerned about her son's volatility and depression; she thought he might be suicidal and was hoping they'd help find him therapy.

But this story of self-improvement, courage, and concern for her children only seemed to condemn her; of it, her interrogators built a case of family pathology. A psychologist wrote that Tony had "witnessed" his mother's rape, though he was only months old; thus, he had a history of abuse. Jessica's unwanted glimpse of a penis was added to her list of victimizations. One evaluator wondered whether Diane had a propensity for substance abuse. And because at the time Diane was more worried about Tony than about Jessica, who seemed okay, CPS decided Diane was "minimizing" the "molest" and judged her incapable of protecting her daughter. Tony was made a ward of the dependency court and removed from his mother's custody.

What Diane hadn't realized was that panic over child abuse sprouted from the desert soil of San Diego as abundantly as the neon-fuchsia succulents and deep-red bougainvillea. The county had been the scene of a string of highly publicized false allegations of abuse, including satanic ritual abuse, going back to the 1980s. In 1992, a major grand jury investigation found the county's child welfare agencies and juvenile courts to be "a system out of control," so keen on protecting children from abuse that it took hundreds from their parents on what turned out to be unfounded charges. When Tony's case came into the system, many of the same people indicted in that report were still working in the agencies, courts, and police department.[8]

Diane didn't know that southern California was also the epicenter of a national movement. *San Diego Times Union* reporter Mark Sauer had seen the hysteria coming. In the early 1990s, he watched psychologist Toni Cavanagh Johnson and social worker Kee MacFarlane presenting their work on children who molest at a sex-abuse conference in the city. He was astonished. "First they state that there is no research, that we really don't know anything about normal children's sexual behavior," he recalled in a 1996 interview. "Then out come the pie charts and graphs, and they go on for an hour defining this new abnormality. And everybody is madly taking notes."

MacFarlane was practiced at routing out abuse that might not have happened. At Children's Institute International in Los Angeles, where she still worked, MacFarlane headed the team that interrogated 400 children for the prosecution of the infamous McMartin Preschool trials and found 369 to have been victimized in bizarre rituals of "satanic abuse," including anal rape, animal mutilation, and kidnapping through secret tunnels,[9] none of which was substantiated. Johnson first coined the term *children who molest* in 1988, while working with MacFarlane at the institute's Support Program for Abusive Reactive Kids, or SPARK,[10] which continues to treat juvenile "abusers."

As they did during that last plague, the prophets of this one claimed the problem was enormous, but that we didn't see it because we weren't looking. "[Children who molest] make all of us uncomfortable," wrote MacFarlane in *When Children Abuse,* "so uncomfortable we've had to deny their existence and/or minimize their behavior until now. We've called their behavior 'exploration' or 'curiosity' until they were old enough for us to comfortably call it what it is: sexual abuse of other children. Who are they?" she continued. "So far, relatively few have come to our attention."[11] One *LA Weekly* article said professionals in the field claimed that 80–90 percent of such crimes go unreported.[12] Neither the "professionals" nor the reporter cited any evidence of this allegation. Soon they'd have it, generated by the perpetual motion machine of expanded definitions of sexual abuse, which lead to changed criminal codes, which lead to increased arrests, which lead to more "proof" of epidemic sexual abuse. Although it is unlikely that juvenile sexual behavior had undergone a radical turn toward the violent over a decade's time, in 1994 the U.S. Department of Justice recorded ten thousand "Other Violent Sex Offenses" by juveniles (these exclude forcible rape), an increase of 65 percent from 1985.[13]

The discursive hyperbole—and invigorated police activity—was good for business. In the mid-1990s, catalogues of child-abuse literature devoted more and more pages to this young deviant,[14] much of it, like much of Johnson's, self-published, meaning it did not undergo the peer review of a university press or professional journal. Training tapes and symposia proliferated and were costly: in 1996, an audiotape sold for fifty dollars; today the bill for a two-day workshop is in the several hundreds.

In 1984, there were no treatment programs for such kids. MacFarlane's SPARK was founded in 1985. A dozen years later, Vermont's Safer Society Foundation database listed 50 residential and 394 nonresidential programs for kids under twelve with "sexual behavior problems" and over 800 programs for teens.[15] Asked why his ninety-year-old Massachusetts residence for troubled adolescents had recently initiated such a program, one exhibitor at a large conference on sex abuse told me that judges were less and less willing to refer delinquent kids for general rehabilitation, preferring to send them directly to jail. But, no doubt partly because of the hubbub being created by people like MacFarlane, the courts were willing to put young sex offenders into sex-treatment programs. "Frankly," the man said, "it was a business decision."

All this activity was based on a near vacuum of empirical data about what young children actually do sexually (I used the word *normative* above, but to be honest, given the paucity of real information, *normative* is almost as null a term as *normal*). The therapists relied heavily on a few studies, particularly one by psychologist William Friedrich of the Mayo Clinic in Rochester, Minnesota, who asked some 880 midwestern mothers what sexual behaviors they observed in their two- to twelve-year-old kids.[16] Paul Okami, a University of Southern California psychology postdoctoral fellow who wrote the first critiques of this diagnosis in the professional literature,[17] dryly noted that for information on children's sex, a less reliable source than mothers could hardly be found.[18] For the details of diagnosis, most of these new specialists turned to Johnson's checklist of child sexual behaviors, divided between those that are "natural," those that an observer should worry about, and those that require rushing the child to the doctor. For kindergarten to fourth-grade children, for instance, "looks at the genitals, buttocks, breasts of adults" was in the "Natural and Expected" column, but "*touches/stares* at the genitals, etc." was listed under "Of Concern," and "*sneakily or forcibly* touches genitals . . ." was under "Seek Professional Help."[19] These determinations, beyond being arbitrary, were based on conclusions reached from observations in the 1980s that were so tenuous and tautological that they might have been reported in Wonderland: "While norms do not presently exist for what is normal sexual behavior of children," wrote Johnson in 1988, "the behaviors exhibited . . . led us to label the behaviors as being outside the normal range of sexual activity for their age group."[20]

Nonetheless, as the diagnosis of "sexual behavior problems" gained currency in sex-abuse circles, it also was on its way to wider ratification, which in turn boosted media attention, funding, and business. A five-year study that provided and evaluated therapy for hundreds of "sexualized" children under age twelve in Oklahoma, Vermont, and Washington State was funded with two million dollars from the government's National Center on Child Abuse and Neglect, the largest and longest-running single appropriation on its rosters during that time.[21] And if this major financial endorsement did not serve to institutionalize the new deviance, some psychologists, frustrated that they could not officially diagnose a child who has sex with a younger child as a "pedophile," were promoting the inclusion of "sexual misconduct/abuser disorder" in the psychiatrists' bible, *The Diagnostic and Statistical Manual of Mental Disorders*.[22] Before the *DSM* made the move, the National Incidence Study of Child Abuse and Neglect, the U.S. government's official count of family-inflicted harm to children, in 1996 added a category of "other or unknown sexual abuse": "inadequate or inappropriate supervision of a child's voluntary sexual activities."[23] All children, in other words, need to be protected from their own errant sexuality. And parents who take a laissez-faire stance regarding sex play are, by their failure to intervene, "abusers."

"Sexualization"

The theory just discussed would be the undoing of Diane Diamond and her family. The minute her son came under investigation by the authorities, not only he, but she, was under suspicion as an abuser.

Jessie was identified as the victim from the start, although it will probably never be known how much of the sex play between the siblings was consensual. Later, a state-employed social worker would deem her unable to "differentiate between imagination and reality." Still, in May 1994, Jessie told the social worker that her mother had lain on top of her in bed. (She also said a social worker "wanted to molest" her, but this charge was not followed up.) Diane, whose criminal record consisted of one unpaid fine for a broken taillight, explained that she'd reached across her daughter to turn off the electric blanket. Nevertheless, a "true finding" of abuse was made, and Jessie was sent to a foster home inhabited by two disturbed teenage girls—an odd choice for a child at risk for "oversexualization." The foster mother ran a tight ship, complaining to the social worker that during family visits Diane touched her children's knees and necks, and put her arm around Jessica's waist.

Indeed, the records comprised, along with a narrative of the family's life under surveillance, what looked like an extended effort to justify the decision to separate Diane's children from her. In spite of frequent descriptions of smooth and happy visits and the family's mutual love and concern, Diane was called "defensive and histrionic," mistrustful and resistant, "sabotaging" the so-called reunification plan, ironically, by insisting that she be allowed to spend more time with her children. There was no suggestion that any of her maladies might have been iatrogenic, caused by the state's "cure" itself. Reading these several thousand pages, one finds it hard not to infer that the child-protective agents felt they knew what was going on in the Diamond family before looking into it.

What they had learned in their abuse training (if they'd had any; the chief parole officer for youthful sex offenders said the department provided none) was the main tenet of children-who-molest theory: that "age-inappropriate" behavior is a symptom that the perpetrator is himself a victim of abuse. Where else, the logic went, would a seven-year-old get the idea of putting a crayon, or a penis, into somebody's vagina? Hence, the terms *abuse-reactive* and *sexualized* are used almost universally when describing "molesting" kids under twelve.[24]

The first flaw in this theory is that the so-called cycle of abuse—that children who are abused go on to abuse others—has been widely questioned and substantially discredited. Even Toni Cavanagh Johnson averred that plenty of abused kids don't grow up to be abusers. In fact *most*—at least two-thirds—do not.[25] The second problem is the contention that prepubertal children who act out sexually are showing signs of abuse. But there is no identifiable set of "symptoms" of abuse that cannot be observed in other, similar-aged kids. Whether they've had traumatic experiences or not, most children seem to exhibit more or less the same sexual behaviors.[26]

Psychologists trying to ferret out the symptoms of abuse have pointed to these facts to demonstrate how hard diagnosis can be. But there would be another way of interpreting them: *a wide range of sexual behavior is normative in children.* In spite of a paucity of empirical data, we know that masturbation is ubiquitous from early on, more noticeably among little boys than little girls. So is "playing doctor," inserting fingers into orifices, and other such pastimes. In the so-called latency years, from about seven to eleven, children continue to masturbate, touch each other, and have crushes on their classmates and friends.[27] In fact, the disappearance of visible sexual behavior probably means only that children have gotten the message that adults don't want to see it. "It seems likely that sexual interest and probably some form of activity continue" in middle childhood, Friedrich wrote, "but that as children learn the cultural standards these interests are concealed."[28] Instead of recognizing this range of child-initiated sexual interest and behavior, however, the notion of a "sexualized" child assumes that it takes a pathological, traumatic event (probably a premature, coercive sexual engagement with an adult) to make a child act sexually or at least act sexually in certain ways.

The children-who-molest people argue that even if the kid is not being abused and even if he would not become a grownup abuser, "age-inappropriate" sex play is a sign of emotional distress. Of course, sometimes it is. But, on the other hand, who is to say that a sexual activity is a sign of distress if the child does not seem distressed either by the sex or otherwise? Toni Cavanagh Johnson offers a clue to the distress she and her colleagues are most concerned about: not children's. Her behavior chart alerts parents to seek professional help when children's eroticized play is "directed at adults who feel uncomfortable receiving" it, when the child "wants to be nude in public after the parents say 'No,'" or when he "touches the genitals of animals."[29]

What's wrong with these things? I asked University of Georgia social work professor Allie Kilpatrick, who conducted an in-depth study of women's childhood sexual experiences and their aftermath. "They make parents nervous," she answered.

Social workers, trained to sniff out abuse, are often even more nervous than parents. Judy Cole, clinical services director of San Diego's Center for Child Protection, told me in 1996 she was tired of "seeing parents minimize and deny the behavior of their children," as young as four. "What they don't understand is what their kids are doing is often molesting behavior that is not okay."

What would be okay? I asked.

"Occasional masturbation, as long as it's in private. Some sexualized play, questions about where babies come from. Same-age children will do 'you-show-me-yours-and-I'll-show-you-mine.'" She added hastily: "Not that it's appropriate or should be encouraged. But it's probably not traumatic."

So would "Look, don't touch," be a good watchword? I queried.

Cole smiled. "In an optimal world."

Cole is not unusual among child-protective professionals in suspecting that too much touching either by or of children is dangerous. In Virginia, for instance, the majority of mental-health and legal professionals in one survey said they believed that parents who hugged a ten-year-old frequently, kissed a child on the lips, or appeared naked before a five-year-old were candidates for "professional intervention."[30]

Values and Data

Adults are responsible for teaching children appropriate behavior. One does not let a child wear a bathing suit to a wedding or out in the snow. But if something is reasoned to be inappropriate because it might cause harm, how is harm determined—and correction undertaken—without asking the child if she feels hurt? I asked Barbara Bonner, who ran the largest component, in Oklahoma City, of the five-year study funded by the National Center on Child Abuse and Neglect, to explain the rationale for calling behavior inappropriate and harmful if it doesn't worry the child (or her parents). In short, why label a child a victim if she doesn't feel victimized?

Bonner, a helpful and well-meaning woman, thought a while. "I don't know if it's the degree of pleasantness or unpleasantness that ought to be the guideline that determines whether it is appropriate or not," she said at length. "The victim should be defined by somebody other than the child."

Why? "Well, if a kid is eating chocolate all day long, we stop them, whether they like it or not."

But eating chocolate all day is demonstrably harmful, I pressed. It gives them cavities and it has caffeine in it, which hypes them up and stunts their growth. Is unhurtful sex harmful?

Bonner laughed amicably at the chocolate analogy. Finally, she said: "As hopefully knowledgeable people, and as a society, we recommend what we consider to be appropriate and in the best interest of children." In "the best interests of the child," the program's Sexual Behavior Rules for six- to eleven-year-olds included "It's not OK to touch other people's private parts" and "It's not OK to show your private parts to other people"—acts that might be considered perfectly appropriate, normal, and even salutary in many families or communities.

Bonner admitted that her team's recommendations were not based in empirical study; it would be impossible to predict or measure the harm of certain sexual experiences, because replicating them in a clinical setting would pose obvious ethical problems. But, she conjectured, too much sex too early "might [cause children to] become oversexually stimulated and prefer sexual behavior to sports, dance, or other more appropriate activities. They might become promiscuous as adults." On the other hand, she added with midwestern frankness, "They may turn out to be normal. We don't really know. We don't have long-term outcomes."

In fact, we do have some "long-term outcomes" of childhood sex. At the University of California at Los Angeles, a thorough review of the literature and a major longitudinal study of families from a child's birth to its eighteenth year found that three-quarters of kids had engaged in masturbation or some kind of sex with other kids before the age of six. Was there a "pernicious influence" of such experiences, a "main effect" correlating early sex play with childhood distress or later maladjustment, as many psychologists hypothesize? "No such correlations were apparent," the California group concluded.[31]

Even incest between siblings (the most common behavior, as far as I can tell, in children-who-molest cases) is not ipso facto traumatic. A study of 526 New England undergraduates revealed "no differences . . . on a variety of adult sexual behavior and sexual adjustment measures" between those students who had had sexual experiences with brothers or sisters, those who'd had them with kids outside their families, and those who'd had none at all.[32] Sociologist Floyd Martinson, an éminence grise in the study of child sexuality, collected scores of reminiscences of happy consensual sex among kids under twelve, including play between siblings and kids five years or more apart in age, both crimson flags in the children-who-molest literature.[33]

Indeed, just about everything Toni Cavanagh Johnson considers worrisome is unremarkable someplace else in the world. Clellan Ford and Frank Beach in their classic *Patterns of Sexual Behavior* examined 191 of the world's peoples, including Americans. "As long as the adult members of a society permit them to do so," they discovered, "immature males and females engage in practically every type of sexual behavior found in grown men and women," including "oral-genital contact and attempted copulation."[34] Cunningham and MacFarlane, in their children-who-molest text, earmark the "reenactment of specific adult sexual activity" as "abnormal"[35]— a behavior so common around the globe that it has a well-worn name among anthropologists: "sexual rehearsal play."

But you don't have to study the Kickapoo to see that values differ. Dutch sexologists Theo Sandfort and Peggy Cohen-Kettensis replicated William Friedrich's influential survey in Holland and got wildly different results. A fifth of the Dutch mothers saw their daughters masturbating with objects, whereas fewer than 1 percent of American moms did; a fifth of Dutch mothers reported that their little boys undressed other people, but only 4.4 percent of Americans did. Sandfort and Cohen-Kettensis conjectured that maybe Little Hans was less inhibited about playing with himself with Mama in the room than Little Matthew was with Mommy or that Mama was less bashful about telling the survey-taker about it.[36] Friedrich's own 1998 retest found that "better-educated mothers with more liberal sexual attitudes reported more sexual behavior" in their children, perhaps because they felt "greater comfort" about the subject.[37]

These studies reveal something remarkable about values and research: a kind of Heisenberg Uncertainty Principle of social science that anthropologists talk about, in which the observer's presence and viewpoint affect her description—her measurement, so to speak—of the phenomenon she's studying. Seeing should not be believing, because values affect what is shown (children know what adults want to see, or not, and therefore choose what they reveal), and values also affect what we notice. Moral judgments, conscious and unconscious, affect not only the judgment of what is considered normal but even the "scientific" assessment of what is normative.

"The negative pairing of sex and aggression"

"For eight years, I have been talking about sex on a continuum," said Toni Cavanagh Johnson when I interviewed her in 1996 at her office in Pasadena, California. Perhaps suspecting I was among her detractors, she had canceled two interview appointments, which themselves took a dozen phone messages and several faxes each to set up, and when I arrived, spent the first twenty minutes of a scheduled hour-long session interrogating me on how I was going to represent her work. The woman who built a healthy business on extremity was now determined to be represented as a friend of moderation. "Normal, healthy sexuality is what we need in children," she insisted (not defining her terms). She added, "It's the negative pairing of sex with aggression that is a problem."

Of course, kids should be taught to stop sticking their fingers where others don't want them to be. Like Johnson, most observers on all sides of the sex debates (including me) are appalled by the "negative pairing" evinced by preteen boys who get their jollies assaulting girls in city pools and high school football players who gang-rape their classmates. Even the Supreme Court, in a 1999 ruling in favor of a girl who sued her school for failure to protect her from repeated hostile and unwanted sexual advances by male classmates, declared that sexual harassment should not be accepted as the normal course of events in adolescent life. Johnson is right to place the question of *consent* at the heart of her theories.

But where does the "pairing" of sex with aggression become "negative," and when is it "abnormal" enough to be treated as a disorder or a crime? Just like the word *abuse,* the word *consent* is subject to multiple meanings.[38] Negotiation is part of children's sex play. It may involve bribes and trickery, conflict, trade-offs, and power imbalances, like all other interactions between children. Older and bigger does not necessarily add up to more powerful, though. And a wide spectrum of behavior involving power differences between children seems to be normative (or if I've soured you on *normative,* then apparently harmless). Psychologists Sharon Lamb and Mary Coakley surveyed three hundred psychologically healthy Bryn Mawr students about their childhood sexual experiences. The young women wrote about thrilling games of porn star, prostitute, rape, and slave girl, all at ages in the single digits, indicating that the pairing of sex and aggression or sex and power differences, too, may be "normal."[39] Simone de Beauvoir described in her memoirs the titillation of enacting on her little sister the mortifications of the Catholic saints. And sexologist Leonore Tiefer suggested that even if coercion ought to be corrected, it shouldn't be pathologized. "Kids push and hit and demand, until they're socialized," she said. "Aggression is normal in children." Given contemporary American culture, it should surprise nobody that when a child acts out aggressively, he might use the lingua franca of sexuality to express himself.

Harm also exists on a continuum, and it can come from different sources. As we saw in the previous chapter, the trauma of youngsters' sex, with anyone, often comes not from the sex itself but from adults going bananas over it. As for "sexual behavior problems" the trauma inflicted by the "cure" may be far worse than the "disease" itself.

Heroic Intervention

In the summer of 1994, when psychologist Phillip Kaushall began supervising the Diamonds' family visits, he was shocked that the children were in foster care. He recognized troubles among mother and children, but nothing warranting separation. In September, he began recommending to the authorities that the kids go home.

Around that time, Jessie started attending Daughters & Sons United, a victims support group, where she reported learning about "good and bad guilt," the latter of which she understood as "when you tell on somebody about something and you feel bad about it." "She'd come out of those meetings angry and excited," recalls Diane. "And she'd go, 'I'm gonna report you, Mother,' every time she got mad."

Both the children's therapy continued with Kaushall, but what went on in his cozy office full of toys did not fulfill Tony's requirement to undergo "offender treatment." In October 1995, almost two years after the "offense," the court put him in a "sexually reactive children's" (SRC) group with social worker David McWhirter, an original and important researcher on gay couples who later became San Diego County's czar of juvenile offender treatment. Kaushall encouraged Tony and Diane to cooperate; he hoped it would be the last hoop the family had to jump through before they were reunited. But McWhirter, who described the SRC group work as "soft confrontation," wrote Kaushall to inform him that Tony was disruptive. The boy didn't want to call himself an offender, the first required step to "recovery," and was intimating that the other kids shouldn't either. It was clear to Kaushall and to Diane that Tony regarded the charge as inaccurate and unjust. "Mom," he reported one afternoon, "there's one kid in there for *mooning*!"

Privately, Kaushall felt McWhirter's approach might be a failure from the get-go. "There may be a need for therapy," said Kaushall, whose intervention in the family's case may have prevented the children from being put up for adoption. "But if you treat somebody specifically for a 'sex offense,' you are undercutting the treatment automatically, because you give them an identity as a sex offender, which is precisely what you don't want them to have."

Still, the doctor considered Tony lucky that he got off with "soft confrontation," because as hard as defense attorneys try to get their young clients into treatment instead of incarceration in tougher juvenile detention facilities, the distinction between punishment and treatment is becoming more difficult to discern. A great deal of what passes for sex-offender treatment (such as an increasing number of "emotional growth" and other behavior-modification programs for misbehaving and violent youths) has been challenged as dubiously therapeutic and even abusive in itself.[40] Moreover, unlike kids whose sentences are meted out by the juvenile justice system, those who become entangled in the mechanisms of "cure" are denied the legal protections afforded even adult perpetrators of the most heinous crimes.

When I visited it, the regime at McWhirter's STEPS, or Sexual Treatment Education Program and Services, in San Diego, was surely not the worst. But it was typical of youth sex-offender "therapy" today: steeped in conservative sexual values, behaviorist in approach, and employing classic good cop–bad cop manipulations by staff. Its stated intentions sounded like children's rights propaganda: promote self-esteem and empathy, consent and equality. But the practice was anything but consensual, and the rights of both children and parents were all but disregarded. The minute a child touched his neighbor's penis or buttocks, he had been assumed devoid of moral faculties; there was simply no debating whether what he did was wrong. A patient received no due process: as long as he protested his innocence, he was "in denial" (the psychotherapeutic equivalent of "in contempt") and could be dropped from the program that was a prerequisite of reunification with his family.

Or worse: His treatment, unlike a jail sentence, could go on for

years, during which he relinquished his own and his friends' rights
to privacy. Anything he said could be reported to the authorities,
and in many programs he was required to furnish the names of
everyone he'd had sex with.

"Stand up, Hector," barked STEPS assistant director Diane Barnett as she led me to her office past two early-teenage Mexican boys
slumping in the hallway. "Those boys are on in-house time out.
They've been able to slip by, manipulate, or do something under-
handed," she said. "They're good." She smiled and paused for effect. "But we're better."

On enrolling in STEPS, the boys and their parents signed a fifteen-
page contract, essentially giving over their liberty of thought and
action for what could amount to three or more years. The contract
read, in part:

> I understand that I am required to keep a daily written record in a
> journal . . . of my deviant sexual fantasies or other specific thoughts
> that are related to my sexually aggressive behavior. I will complete a
> written autobiography assignment during the first two months of my
> involvement at STEPS, that will include descriptions of: (a) my past
> sexual offenses, fantasies, and my state of mind during offenses.
> (b) Any sexual and/or physical abuse that has happened to me. (c) My
> history of sexual behavior other than outright offenses. (d) How I
> kept my problem a secret and avoided getting caught. This assign-
> ment will be completed with a minimum of six pages.[41]

Using a cognitive-behavioral approach common to many prison-
based sex-offender treatment programs, programs like STEPS aim
to change the boys' actions by teaching them to think differently.
As Barnett explained, the boys at STEPS were instructed to write
down a "cycle" of every thought, feeling, and sensation leading up
to, during, and after a sexual "offense." They then developed "back-
up plans"—thought processes free of "thinking errors"—to be used
to prevent "reoffending." When he started dreaming about sex
with a younger kid, for instance, a boy might substitute a picture of
himself behind bars. The inmates were required to report on their
masturbation in detail, confessing whatever fantasies were left in
their strip-searched imaginations. For eight hours a day, five days a
week, with about two hours off for schoolwork, they were under
surveillance, earning points for good behavior, losing them for, say,
uttering "fuck off." Touching, whether aggressive or affectionate,

by staff or inmates was prohibited, because, Barnett said, "these boys don't know their boundaries."

Even outside the building, STEPS was watching. The boys were not allowed contact with their "victims" without program permission or ever to be alone with anybody considered "victim age." They were required to submit to random drug tests, avoid being alone, and inform all potential romantic interests of licit age that they were sex offenders. "I will always lock the bathroom door whenever I am using the bathroom and when there is anyone else on the premises," read the contract.

"Once they've developed enough empathy," Barnett told me, "we start looking at atonement," which involves a twenty-step process from Exposing the Offense to Learning to Forgive Oneself, with Preventing Suicide and Finding Meaning in Life in between.

Step seven was Apologizing on the Knees to the victim, the victim's family, and the boy's own family. Such sessions tend to alarm and anger the inmate's family, Barnett told me. "Sometimes the parents will be saying, 'I will send you to court!' The mother is shouting, 'I'll kill you!' It's very emotional." She continued, her voice becoming smoother, "As soon as that kid's knees hit the floor, most often, he will be sobbing. To the parents, it will look like I am being mean. But I will tell them, '*When this is all over, you will have your own boy back.*'"[42]

Their own boy, obedient, broken, expiated of deviant fantasy. Or maybe of sexual fantasy altogether.

Does such treatment do any good? The ACLU Prison Project has sued a number of similar programs for adults, including one in Vermont, in which "drama therapy" compelled inmates to simulate anal rape while the therapist shouted obscenities at them.[43] Expert witnesses argued that such treatment was not only unproven as curative but likely to be psychologically damaging, and the court enjoined the prison to cease what the judge deemed to be cruel and unusual punishment disguised as treatment.[44] The program's director, William Pithers, was codirector of the Vermont component of Barbara Bonner's study on "sexual behavior problems," helping to devise treatment for children.[45] The methodology of McWhirter's and other such programs also strikingly resembles the "treatment" gays and lesbians were subjected to in the 1950s and 1960s to cure them of their attractions to others of their own sex. Those who underwent such cures usually attest to their dolorous effects on self-esteem and dignity and their utter failure to reroute erotic patterns of many years' standing. At least the "diagnosis" was on the mark, though; those people *were* homosexual. The kids in Toni Cavanagh Johnson's consulting room or in the building that housed David McWhirter's STEPS may not even have been afflicted by the disease of which they were being cured. They were not violent sex offenders (otherwise, they would be ineligible for the program); they may not even have been sexual aggressors. Many were kids who'd had sex that simply made adults nervous.[46]

I asked Vern Bullough, a sexologist who spent more than half a century studying childhood sexuality, what he thought of the "sexual behavior problem" theories and treatments. He sniffed in disgust. "This all reminds me of heroic gynecology [during the early twentieth century], which regarded the birth process itself as a pathological thing" and gave women drugs to make pregnancy more "normal." Said Bullough, "What we've got now is heroic intervention in childhood sexuality by people who don't know what they are talking about."

Cruel and Usual

In the state's eyes, Diane Diamond's increasing desperation as the months and years dragged on only proved the case that she was an unfit mother and damned her to longer separation. After she made a particularly angry call to one social worker's office, followed by a calmer, apologetic one, the worker recorded: "I have grave concerns about what just happened. I wonder if she is having some sort of breakdown."

Once the narrative was inscribed—crazy mother makes boy a molester, victimizes girl—no alternative story could be told. When Jessie confessed, almost immediately after her first testimony, that she had "told lies" about her mother, the child was presumed to be exhibiting "accommodation syndrome," that is, suffering the consequences of being removed from the life she knew and thus lying to put things back as they were. Only Kaushall and one case worker believed Jessie's retraction or evinced any sympathy for Diane. This worker chronicled excited gift-giving and calm vegetable-planting and endorsed the children's entreaties to go home. But her advice, which Kaushall echoed, was ignored, and she was inexplicably removed from the case. Near the end of 1994, Diane sold her car in order to hire a private lawyer to contest the court's dispositions. She spent Christmas without her children, waiting for the trial, which would be delayed eight months. In February 1995, she lost her appeal without comment.

Tony was at yet another foster home, losing weight and losing hope. "There are allegations that Ms. Diamond has been rude" to the foster mother, Child Protective Services reported in a court filing during this time. Kaushall wrote report after report to CPS that institutionalized life and separation from their mother were damaging the children.

After two years of holding a child in state custody, California law requires that the dependency court decide whether to place him in long-term foster care, terminate the parent's rights and refer him for adoption, or send him home. In what appears to be a combination of bureaucratic fatigue, a null case for adoption, and the knowledge that Diane would not give up her children without a savage fight, CPS made arrangements to move Tony and Jessica back home. The ragged family was reunited in early 1996.

"There is no doubt in my mind that what was done was a hundred times worse than any problem [the Diamonds] had to begin with," said an angry and disgusted Kaushall. "It was handled with a lethal combination of zealotry and incompetence." Jessica, he believed, "has learned that when she talks about sex, everyone will drop their forks and knives and listen. She knows sex is a powerful weapon." Tony suffered harshness and betrayal from adults; he remained depressed and mistrustful. For both kids, Kaushall said, "the developmental harm of breaking a bond with the parent is tremendous."

But when I visited them on a bright Sunday in March 1997, things seemed almost uneventful. Jessie went off to an "ugly-dog show" with a church volunteer, and the rest of us drove to La Jolla to wade in the tide pools. Tony hugged his mom frequently, demanded to be taken to McDonald's and moped when that didn't happen, all eminently normal behavior from my untrained perspective. "I'm a survivor," Diane told me, estimating that her ordeal had cost more than thirty thousand dollars. She chatted about "our plans" to move to Arizona, or maybe Oregon because "we love the beach." She used the first-person plural often, as if to repossess that fragile pronoun.

Tony and I peeled snails from a rock as Diane explained to him that I was writing about their family. His eyes became serious. "Are you writing about cruelty to children in California?" he asked.

From Badness to Illness

Over the past two centuries, the moral judges have moved from the pulpit to the clinic. As the medical historian Peter Conrad put it, "badness" has been rewritten as "illness." The process has not been thoroughgoing. Alcoholism, once a moral failure, is now treated as a disease, while drug addiction is still punished as a transgression, with harsh prison sentences mandated for anyone who even possesses illegal drugs, whether or not they've committed an act of violence to pay for them. The category of childhood "sexual behavior problems," with its healers' obsessive attention to excess and its dire predictions of future misery, is a reincarnation of the eighteenth- and nineteenth-century "disease" of masturbation insanity, crossed with the Progressive Era criminal designation "sexual precociousness" and the late-twentieth-century crime of sexual abuse, with a dollop of the popularly designated affliction "sex addiction" thrown in as well.

The cruel tactics deployed in disciplining deviants to the standards of normalcy are legendary in the annals of medicine. Water torture, drawing and quartering, castration, lobotomy—what went on at STEPS was like aromatherapy in comparison. Still, across America children are being harmed by being labeled as deviant, a stigma they may never live down.

The antidote to cruel or unusual treatment is not to argue that what is at any moment viewed as deviant is really "normal" or "natural." For normal is what a particular culture or historical era calls it: male homosexuality was regarded as normal in classical Greece; intergenerational sex has been normal as sexual initiation in many preindustrial societies;[47] even rape has historically been normal in wartime.[48] On a more local scale, we may look at subsequent editions of the *DSM* and find that the minute we stop diagnosing one psychopathology, there's something else to take its place (the year homosexuality was removed, after considerable pressure from the gay and lesbian rights movement, a new childhood syndrome, "gender dysphoria," or a profound discomfort with the biological sex one is born with, was entered). It is a real challenge to speak positively about children's sexuality without calling on the palliatives *natural* or *normal*; I find myself frequently turning to my battered *March's Thesaurus*. Instead of repairing to *normal,* with its assumption that anything that falls inside its purview is harmless and anything that falls outside is harmful, what's needed are some more neutral descriptions of actual experience and assessments of actual harm. Asking kids themselves is the best beginning. In the meantime, we might be as honest as Oklahoma's Barbara Bonner, who told me, "Until we are more informed about children's sexual development, our work will continue to be driven by values."

There are some values that parents and professionals, clerics and politicians would agree should be instilled in children: be kind, considerate, respectful of self and others, noncoercive in sex as in all things. But "normality" is a fickle and disputed virtue, and given its potential as a confederate in therapeutic abuse and social disenfranchisement, it is overrated.

4. Crimes of Passion

Statutory Rape and the Denial of Female Desire

I really don't think a crime has been commited [sic]. Two people loved each other & parents got in the way to stop it.
—Heather Kowalski, "victim," *United States v. Dylan Healy*

In April 1997, Robert Kowalski flew to New York from Pawtucket, Rhode Island, to appear on *The Maury Povich Show*. His wife, Pauline, was home waiting by the phone, over which Povich interviewed her. The Kowalskis were the parents of three teenagers. Their youngest child and only daughter, Heather, thirteen, had been missing for three weeks, in the company of her twenty-one-year-old boyfriend. "If Heather could call home, she would," insisted Rob, who, the newspapers reported, had been away on business when Heather took off.[1]

The Kowalskis said they did not allow Heather to date. A year earlier, when they learned she was talking to boys in an online chat room, Rob had discontinued the family's America Online subscription. But Heather soon was back in the room, using a friend's account, and in February she met a guy there named Dylan Healy. Dylan lived only ten minutes away, in an apartment in Providence. The two met five days later and Dylan began courting Heather devotedly, buying her jewelry and stuffed animals, calling her frequently at home. When the Kowalskis found out how old Dylan was, they later told the press, they forbade Heather to see him.

But passion likes obstacles, and the lovers persisted. Heather and her friends schemed ways of circumventing her parents' surveillance. "Next time you call my house and my dad asks who you are say you are Patrick from Huskies. OK? OK!" she wrote Dylan. When calling the house became impossible, he gave her a beeper and a cell phone. He called the Maple Street Junior High School, where she was an honors student, and impersonated her father so she could cut classes and go to his apartment. There, they talked, watched television, ate junk food, and made love.

The Kowalskis reported Dylan to the police, who charged him with interfering with the custody of a minor, a misdemeanor, and released him on bail with the order that he not see Heather. She showed up for his hearing, against her mother's injunction, and cried. They kept seeing each other. The Kowalskis, no doubt at their wits' end, got a restraining order. "I can't believe how bad all of this is getting," Heather wrote Dylan on March 23. "All we want is to be together. Is that so much to ask?! I ♥ U so much, I just don't want to lose you."

Two days later, Dylan picked Heather up at the school bus stop as usual. He did not threaten or coerce her, and later, in searching for them, the police considered her a runaway, not a kidnap victim. He, on the other hand, was a fugitive, violating bail and a restraining order. After the couple disappeared, the police charged him with eight counts of felonious sexual assault with a minor: statutory rape.

From March 25 to April 19, coincidentally a day after the *Maury Povich* broadcast, Heather and Dylan drove around Rhode Island, New Hampshire, and Massachusetts in his neon-green Jeep Wrangler. They stayed at a motel on the beach, rented videos, tasted exotic new cuisines (they especially liked Indian food), and when their funds dwindled, subsisted on biscuits and gravy at truck stops. They looked at the houses they passed and spun happily-ever-after fantasies of a wedding and children. On the last day, someone spotted a nervous young man at a bank near Pawtucket, trying to cash a check he'd stolen from his mother's bedroom. Outside, the witness spied a neon-green Jeep Wrangler with a teenage girl in it. He called the police. The last words Heather said to Dylan were, "The cops are coming."

It was no wonder the two were recognized. The story received almost daily coverage in the local newspapers and radio and television stations and in the Boston media. *USA Today* and newspapers across the country picked up the story. The FBI posted a

"Crime Alert/Missing" notice on its Web page featuring Heather's wide, white-toothed smile and flaxen hair, as well as one headlined "Wanted by the FBI" for Dylan, with the legend "Armed and Dangerous," though he was not the former, and there was little evidence that he was the latter, beyond the tautology that he was dangerous because the law said sex constitutes danger to a minor. His deep-set, dark eyes and pudgy face made him look younger than she, almost puppyish. The Guardian Angels put up their own Missing flyers throughout the Boston area transit system, and the civilian anticrime army's online platoon, CyberAngels, posted it on their Web site, with the impressive headline "CHRIST THE KING SPREADS PRAYER AND SEARCH FOR MISSING TEEN" (Christ the King was the Kowalskis' church). When the *Maury Povich* segment aired, false sightings of the couple were called in from as far away as Louisiana. The case was to be broadcast on *America's Most Wanted,* but Heather came home before the scheduled date.

Dylan was eventually sentenced to twelve to twenty-four years' imprisonment on state and federal charges. He was prohibited from speaking to Heather ever again.

Why so much attention to one girl, of the thousands of teenagers who run away from home every year? To the media and the townspeople, the prosecutors and police, to Heather's parents and the judges, two facts distinguished this couple from the rest: their ages—hers at the start of adolescence, his at the debut of adulthood—and the allegation that she was "lured off the Internet."

The latter made excellent copy. "Families who've been torn apart by the Internet!" Povich introduced the Kowalskis' segment of his show, giving the medium typically hyperbolic power. "I mean, it is out there, it is prevalent, it's—it's omnipresent!" For the prosecutors, who seemed bent on sending other online miscreants a message, Dylan provided an excellent example. "The problem with this case is the use of computers by sexual predators in the exploitation of children," said U.S. attorney Arnold Huftalen, speaking to reporters on the federal courthouse steps after Dylan's sentencing. "There's an epidemic of predators on the Internet." Dylan's lawyer stated repeatedly that if the youngsters had not met online, there would have been no publicity and his client would have gotten off with a much lighter sentence.

Danger Zone

"Just like you wouldn't let your child play alone in an urban park for three hours," one police sergeant warned the readers of a women's magazine, "you shouldn't let them play alone on the Internet."[2] But such warnings lose their utility, ironically, just when the child is old enough to know better. For if your "child" is thirteen or fourteen, he *is* likely to be playing alone in an urban park, quite possibly with friends you don't know and might not approve of. Adolescents, with money, wheels, and pressing desires, are ever on the move between the home and the street, childhood and adulthood. And "danger," wrote the anthropologist Mary Douglas, "lies in transitional states."[3]

Age-of-consent law, which dates to the late-thirteenth-century British Statutes of Westminster,[4] endeavors to bring safety to this danger zone by drawing a bright line between childhood and adulthood, and then by criminalizing, in statutory rape, an adult's trespass over it. The law conceives of the younger partner as categorically incompetent to say either yes or no to sex. Because she is by definition powerless both personally and legally to resist or to voluntarily relinquish her "virtue," the state, which sees its interest in guarding that virtue, resists for her.[5]

While we now presume such laws are based on the principle that minors have a differential right to protection, originally the protected object was not the child herself but her virginity, which was the property of her father. The victim was always female, and as late as 1981, the Supreme Court upheld the constitutionality of criminalizing sex with a female minor but not a male minor. The justices noted the greater risk of sex to a girl because of pregnancy but not the greater discrimination against a girl in assuming she never wanted sex.[6] A few years ago state statutes began to include boys as possible victims of statutory rape. But partly because it is so common for young women to have sex with men who are older than they by at least three years, and partly because statutory rape proceedings are often precipitated by a pregnancy, the vast majority of such cases still involve a male adult and a female minor.[7] These are followed in number by male adults in consensual homosexual liaisons with male youths,[8] who might be considered feminized in the eyes of the culture.

The law encodes an enduring sexist idea—that in sexual relations there is only one desiring partner, the man. In romantic language, we call him the seducer and her the debauched, or fallen, woman; in the contemporary cross between gothic metaphor and sociobiological jargon, he is the predator and she the prey; in legalese, he is the perpetrator and she the victim. In all, one person is guilty and the other innocent. Age, especially when the partners are close in age, often serves as a stand-in for other assumptions about gender. The man is allowed to desire, but he is also suspected of being sexually predatory by masculine nature, and thus morally indictable. That he's older makes him legally indictable.

Of course, young women do get raped: almost all rape victims are female, and more than half of the nation's rape victims are under eighteen, according to the Justice Department. The younger a girl and the wider the age difference between her and her older male sex partner, moreover, the likelier she is to feel coerced into having inter-course, at least the first time.[9]

But statutory rape is not about sex the victim says she did *not* want. It is about sex she *did* want but which adults believe she only thought she wanted because she wasn't old enough to know she did not want it. Still, teen girls persist in expressing their own desires. "If he's guilty, I'm guilty," one sixteen-year-old El Paso girl told me she had informed her parents when they threatened to report her twenty-year-old boyfriend to the police. Because a successful prose-cution needs a victim willing to testify against her lover, and few teens are, many prosecutors admit that the oxymoronic concept of consensual rape makes such cases hard to prosecute or win.

The "Internet Romeo" and a Juliet without Desire

The story of Dylan and Heather fit precisely the cultural codes writ-ten into the law and also the contradictions held therein. There was no doubt that Dylan committed a crime as an adult, but he acted like an adolescent: hungry, impetuous, irresponsible, desperate. Heather, in the eighth grade at the time, behaved just like a truculent young teen: she disobeyed her parents, cut school, and ran away. Yet with Dylan she collaborated in breaking the law. And she did what adults do: have sex.

Beyond this, and beyond his record and her family's descrip-tions, the media had little or no information about either Dylan or Heather. His family avoided the press, and her family revealed knowing virtually nothing about him. Absent facts, the media retold the melodrama, "Girl Lured Off the Internet," with the help of Heather's family. The police narrated a thriller, with good guys and bad guys and violence looming around every corner.

Usually, Dylan was referred to as Healy and Heather as Heather; he was called a man, and she a girl. Even when both were identified by their surnames, he was the actor, she the acted upon: "Healy persuaded Kowalski to meet him in person," wrote one reporter. The press dubbed Dylan the Internet Romeo. Rob Kowalski characterized him as a Svengali. "I think right now that Heather has been a victim of some psychological and emotional manipulation that happened over a very short period of time," the father said on *Maury Povich*. "So in—in my mind she may have left with this person willingly, but at some point her free will was lost and she may not even realize it." Pauline told the Associated Press that she believed Dylan had "brainwashed" her daughter.

The local papers hinted at Dylan's "dark" history, writing of his two children, then five and two, born "out of wedlock" and quoting the mothers, who accused him of controlling and abusive behavior. One of them, June Smith, had taken out a restraining order against him. He had also allegedly offered to pay two teenage girls to meet him at a motel room and have sex. When they refused, the police said, he called them and sent a threatening e-mail to one of the girls. He denied these latter charges.

These shady and disputed facts were used to cast suspicion on other facts that were incontrovertible. Once his record was revealed, the obviously shy computer nerd became a *"supposedly* shy computer nerd." The press consistently exaggerated by innuendo an already fairly hefty sheet of charges pending against him. "Healy also faces eight counts of rape in Providence and three counts of intervening with custody in Pawtucket," the papers reported at the end of a story about federal charges against him, making him sound like a serial rapist. What they neglected to say was that all those charges were related to his consensual relationship with one person, Heather Kowalski.

In inverse proportion to the evil and wiliness of the male character in "Girl Lured off the Internet" was the innocence and cluelessness of the female character. "She's still a little girl. She needs to be taken care of like a little girl," Rob Kowalski described Heather to Povich. "She went with him willingly," Heather's sixteen-year-old brother, Jason, told the *Boston Globe*. "Well, willingly in the sense of the five-year-old getting out of kindergarten and a grown man comes by in a van, offering her a lollipop."

To her elders, Heather's desire was a mistake, a misapprehension, and so was the love she told her friends she felt for Dylan. "I don't think a thirteen-year-old knows about love," said Pauline. "I think she's infatuated with him and is happy about the attention." Povich described Heather, along with a fourteen-year-old missing since Christmas with a twenty-two-year-old AWOL air force man, as "two children . . . manipulated and lured away from home by older men on the Internet." And the local press returned over and over to the tropes of Heather's childishness—the teddy bear Dylan gave her, the Beanie Baby one of her friends was "clutching" when they gathered to greet her on her return.

While she was gone, Rob and Pauline stressed how good and normal their daughter was. "She was always the most well behaved, always had the best grades, always the most polite. When the house needed to be cleaned, she would work with her mother," said her father, providing a sketch of ideal femininity and an unwitting glimpse of his own and his sons' roles (or lack thereof) in maintaining the household. Heather's tastes and interests were also "typical" of girls: she liked to shop, hang out with friends, and watch *Beverly Hills 90210,* said Mom. She also played trumpet in the band—not so typically feminine.

When she returned, care was taken to protect that image, and the family that had gone on national daytime television now took pains to guard their daughter's privacy. She appeared before the television cameras once, for a few minutes, flanked by her mother, her two brothers, and her best friend, Jennifer Bordeaux, who was fifteen. "I know what I did was wrong, and I don't want anyone else to do that, because I learned from my mistake," she recited distractedly, suppressing giggles. Asked what she and Dylan had done for twenty-two days, she replied, "We just watched TV and slept." If they had had sex, she did not mention it.

That was the last the press heard from Heather. At Dylan's sentencing, her family formed a phalanx around her. No phone number is listed for either of her parents. When I wrote to her, twice, she did not reply.

In the end, perhaps, her blankness served the melodrama better than if the public had been allowed to get to know her. In the tale of Girl Lured off the Internet, and in the law, the innocent child is defined by her very nullity, a template onto which others may inscribe passivity, naïveté, and desirelessness.

Real People

Anybody who investigated further would have immediately discovered Dylan and Heather as more complex and their story as far more ambiguous, less dramatic, and sadder than the press represented. Although nine years apart in chronological age, it seems the two young people were closer emotionally and intellectually. Dylan lived on his own, but his rent was paid by a trust fund left by his father, who had committed suicide. Dylan had dropped out of high school and could not hold a job because he was clinically agoraphobic (his doctor told him he had "social phobias"), as well as obsessive-compulsive and chronically depressed. Dylan, said his mother, Laura Barton, had always been "fragile." (He is now taking medication for his anxiety and obsessive disorder,[10] but when I saw him in prison he told me he was depressed and talked to almost no one. He seemed to have poured his obsessiveness into the blood-from-a-stone project of reaping a vegetarian diet from the cafeteria and junk-food machines. As a result he had lost a hundred pounds since his arrest.) His kamikaze notion of true love was concocted from television, the movies, and comic books. In the emotional and educational limitations he described in a lengthy statement, delivered at his sentencing by his lawyer, Dylan was like most other men who have relationships with younger teen girls, according to psychologists. In his honest love, according to prosecutors, he resembled other young-twenties men in such liaisons.[11] Like others of his confreres, Dylan's immaturity and lack of earning potential may have made him less attractive to adult women.[12] But he was glamorous and sophisticated to girls like Heather. At least he was equipped with a car, money, and the license to buy beer and cigarettes.

Possibly because of the psychological troubles he described in the eight-page courtroom *récitatif,* Dylan was not an eminently rational or responsible young man. But his crimes were not violent. And while his history is not one of tender or mature relationships, neither does it describe a "predator." Dylan is no "pedophile" by any stretch of the imagination. One of his former girlfriends was a year younger than he; one was older. As for Heather, "an important distinction was whether he ran away with a thirteen-year-old because he was attracted to young girls or because he was socially uncomfortable with his peers," commented Dylan's lawyer, saying that it was the latter. In his statement, Dylan confirmed that impression: "[Heather's] youth allowed me to overcome my fears," he wrote.

Nor was Heather the flat snapshot of a pure lamb on the cover of the newspaper. Most obviously, the polite, helpful, hardworking girl had also done everything she could to hoodwink her parents and defy their, and her school's, authority. Later, Pauline demurred to a reporter that Heather was perhaps "a little wild and rebellious," but, the reporter told me after the state sentencing, he did not report the comment in the paper. Ultimately, the girl cooperated in breaking a federal law to run away with her boyfriend, though it's likely she had little understanding of the consequences (it seemed to occur to neither kid that her parents might be looking for them, until one evening, drifting off to sleep in a motel room, they saw their faces on the eleven o'clock news). Still, at her press conference Heather showed no remorse or regret beyond the words she uttered. "She was very carefree about the stress she had put her mother through," a Providence reporter, who was present, told me. After her short statement, Heather skipped away arm in arm with her friend Jennifer, both of them laughing.

From her well-written letters to Dylan, it was clear Heather was an expressive girl, grown up for her age. And, though her parents and the judge would call it puppy love, she was plainly in love with Dylan. She was also silly, petulant, and moody. A progress chart of her side of the correspondence would plunge and spike with battles and reconciliations. At one point the newspaper reports of Dylan's other relationships and children apparently wounded her so much she was ready to break up with him, because he had kept a secret from her in spite of their "pact" to tell each other everything. "Were you going to wait until after we were married?" she demanded to know in a letter written after his arrest. But she also struggled to continue trusting him. "My heart tells me to forget about it. That was the past, it wasn't me, he really ♥s me. Then my brain tells me, are you fucking stupid, dump the asshole." By the next sentence, her reveries of romance outweighed her doubts. "I think that the best time I ever had being with you was when we were gone, I would watch you sleep & I would think about the wonderful life we would someday have. . . . I love you." She enclosed a little stone and a rose in the letter. Heather, it seems, was as taken with the romantic melodrama of her relationship as her media chroniclers were.

In most photos of her, Heather wore a heavy gold chain and a delicate crucifix around her neck, both gifts from Dylan. The combination sent an appropriately mixed message: she was tough and vulnerable, aggressive and feminine, "bad" and "good."

Parents' Rights, Parents' Responsibilities

The other hierarchy of power upheld by age-of-consent law is that of age in the family. By categorically abrogating a minor's right to consent, the law grants adults purview over her sexuality. In the thirteenth century, a father's right to his daughter's virginity was unquestioned. She (like her mother) was his chattel, and if he suspected somebody of trespassing on his property, he could haul the culprit before the magistrate like a horse thief. Today, in spite of prosecutors' preference for obtaining the girl's testimony against her boyfriend, it is not necessary to the case. The law makes a distinction between willingness to have sex and informed consent, and since a minor is statutorily "uninformed," if it can be proved that he or she and an adult partner had sex, a crime has been committed. Proceedings may be initiated by the people who are most aggrieved by the relationship: according to prosecutors, close to two-thirds of reports of illicit sex with minors come to the police from parents.[13] The law gives parents an inordinate amount of power: they can, effectively, put their daughter's boyfriend behind bars.

Of course, parents have a responsibility to guide their offspring toward safe relationships and away from unsafe ones, if they can, which for many means dissuading or forbidding them from romantic involvement with people who are much older than they. But families are different. One woman, now the mother of a teenager, told me she had a four-year relationship, starting at age sixteen, with a man a decade her senior. Her mother "went crazy" when she found out but eventually grew to love the boyfriend and welcome him into the family. Alternatively, parental care and counsel may be utterly absent at home, and that in itself may drive a girl into the arms of an older man, who may take on a quasi-parental role in her life. In the late 1990s, social psychologist Lynn M. Phillips talked with 127 New Jerseyites who were currently or had been in minor-adult sexual relationships. One of her subjects, Jill, sixteen, was somewhat unhappy with her thirty-three-year-old boyfriend, Carlos, because he was stern and volatile, making all the decisions and restricting her comings and goings. But she accepted this parentlike behavior as "overprotectiveness" appropriate to her age. Indeed, Jill believed that Carlos "had saved her from a life of abuse, drug abuse, and academic failure that were condoned by her mother and her grandmother."[14]

At the Kowalskis, it seemed, neither overweening concern nor its total absence was the problem, but simply a family coming asunder, hard put to support any more pressure. On television, Rob and Pauline were a strict but loving and united pair, and the press wrote the family's script as upright, solid, and unanimously heart-broken. "You did everything a family is supposed to do to keep your daughter—" Maury Povich fed Pauline Kowalski on the phone. "Correct," she interjected before he could finish his phrase, "away from this fellow."

But by many indications the Kowalskis were not the mutually supportive and intimate unit they presented on his show. In fact, according to records at the Providence County Superior Court, Rob and Pauline had been in conflict since 1994, had filed for divorce in July 1996, and were separated when Heather ran away. Although the bulk of the divorce records are sealed, filings regarding custody affirm Dylan's account that Heather's parents had feuded over their daughter's relationship with him. For instance, Pauline alleged that Rob "encouraged" Dylan and Heather by covering up their liaison and allowing them to talk on the phone and see each other in defiance of Pauline's "ban" on the relationship. The mother's next allegation, that "[s]ubsequently, Dylan Healy would get Heather out of school by pretending to be her parent calling for early release," implied that Rob had instigated—or at least inspired—that behavior, too. Pauline asked the court to suspend Rob's visitation with Heather, but it did not.

Heather was obviously at odds with her mother. It is unlikely that a thirteen-year-old would run away from home for three weeks "on a whim," as Pauline put it. At her press conference, Heather said she hadn't called home because she was afraid the phones would be tapped and she and Dylan would be found. "I didn't know if I really wanted to come home right then," she averred. Just before they took off, she wrote to Dylan of her misery at home: "You are the only thing left in my life to keep me happy."

The Kowalskis seemed to view their daughter in two ways: as a breakable china doll and as an unbending hellion. But it was as if these two images could not be seen at the same time. Rob presented himself as astonished that the girl who marched in the color guard would break rank so decisively with her family. Less imaginable, probably, was that his little girl could want so badly to be loved by a boy that she'd break the law for it. In the end, it was as if Heather felt forced to choose between good girl and bad, and like many girls since time immemorial, she elected bad. Dylan's attorney told me he wished the family had sought counseling instead of turning their frustration over to the police. Dylan's mother said, "If only her parents had called me. Maybe we could all have talked and . . ." Her voice trailed off. Instead, as if to clear away all the ragged contradictions of their family life, as if to legitimize their anger and fear, the Kowalskis turned to the law, which brooks no ambiguity at all.

But the Kowalskis' exasperation, and the way they handled it, was one thing. What the police and the courts did once they had the case was another. "It's perfectly understandable for parents to go crazy if their thirteen-year-old daughter is dating a twenty-one-year-old guy," said Sharon Lamb, a psychology professor at St. Michael's College in Vermont and the author of *The Trouble with Blame: Victims, Perpetrators, and Responsibility,* when she read a draft of this chapter. "But the legal system is supposed to sort things out rationally and justly."

Unfortunately, legislators and the courts have been behaving like freaked-out moms and dads discovering a thirteen-year-old in flagrante on the living room couch. Reviving laws that reduce consensual tradeoffs of love, lust, need, and power to alleyway assaults of vicious predator upon powerless victim, public officials in the 1990s increasingly attacked complicated social problems with the blunt instrument of criminal law and then applied hysterically heavy penalties.

In 1995, a California sociologist uncovered the datum that at least half the babies of unmarried teen mothers were fathered by men over twenty.[15] Suddenly everyone from the left-feminist columnist Katha Pollitt to the archconservative Family Research Council was crying rape. The American Bar Association convened a special committee to propose legal responses to the newfound problem. Both political parties vowed to attack this species of "child abuse" in their 1996 presidential campaign platforms, and the welfare "reform" law signed by President Clinton at the end of his first term urged that "states and local jurisdictions aggressively enforce statutory rape laws," required states' welfare plans to develop educational programs for law enforcers, counselors, and educators on "the problem of statutory rape," and directed the U.S. attorney general to study the link between statutory rape and teen pregnancy, with a focus on "predatory older men."[16] California governor Pete Wilson committed eight million dollars of a fifty-two-million-dollar teen-pregnancy-prevention campaign to invigorate statutory rape prosecutions with the goal of reducing the welfare rolls;[17] Texas, Florida, Georgia, Maryland, and a number of other states soon followed suit.[18] In 1996, Gem County, Idaho, prosecuting attorney Douglas R. Varier went one step further: he criminalized all teen sex that led to pregnancy. Exhuming a 1921 law against fornication, or sex between unmarried persons, he charged a group of pregnant teens and their boyfriends.

The California data on adult fathers and teen mothers were subsequently challenged by demographic experts, who said the publicized numbers were too high,[19] that the policy discussion vastly oversimplified, indeed misrepresented, the causes of childbirth among minor-aged women,[20] and the new initiatives had no demonstrable effect of deterring either sex or childbirth.[21] Asked by the American Bar Association, for instance, only one in five lawyers said they thought "holding males accountable [for relations with minors] through prosecution and child support enforcement is an appropriate response" to teen pregnancy.[22]

The laws forced people on the ground to make perverse choices among untenable options. In Orange County, California, after Governor Wilson's program went into effect, state social service agency workers surreptitiously arranged marriages between their pregnant clients, some as young as thirteen, and the adult fathers of their babies, in order to prevent prosecution that would break up intact relationships.[23] And among their intended beneficiaries, such laws met with near-universal scorn. "Let's say [the guy] goes to jail," a teen mother in San Jose patiently explained to a reporter. "She's not going to get any support. She's going to end up on welfare."[24] Queried about the antifornication crusade, Gem County high school kids called it preposterously intrusive, not to mention futile in preventing future pregnancies. The students, about half of whom had already had sex, proposed a less punitive strategy for ameliorating the pregnancy problem: in one survey 79 percent said they wanted better sex education.[25]

Do statutory rape prosecutions have any constructive effect on the "perpetrator," the "victim," or her family? Historically, "as their traditional forms of [familial, religious, and community] sexual regulation eroded, numerous parents—immigrant and native-born, black and white—sought court intervention to restrain their rebellious daughters," wrote historian Mary Odem, who studied cases that transpired in California in the 1880s and the 1920s.[26] But the court officials did not chase down the white slavers who parents believed had run off with their daughters; they did not issue back-stiffening judicial reprimands like "Listen to your mama and stay out of the dance halls." Instead, especially after the turn of the century, the stereotype of the sexual girl as victim was transformed into one of deviant or delinquent. The courts increasingly charged the girls with "precocious sexuality" (having sex or appearing to want to) and dispatched them to reform school, leaving families bereft of the daughters' much-needed earnings and household help.[27]

Whereas misbehaving boys found themselves in court for the same transgressions as adult men might commit—say, theft or assault—girls were punished more harshly than boys and for lesser, victimless infractions, especially for the crime of "precocious sexuality."[28] This "sexualization of female deviance" has persisted into our time, wrote criminologist Meda Chesney-Lind. By the 1960s, three-quarters of all arrested girls were charged with sexual misconduct,[29] tracked into the system as PINS, or "persons in need of supervision," or labeled incorrigible,[30] terms that called up images of sentinels at the bedroom window, guarding the irredeemable. At the end of the twentieth century, a girl like Heather was viewed as both victimized and incorrigible. She was both a nineteenth-century-like fallen woman in need of moral resurrection and a modern slut who should have known better. For such girls in an era of "tough love," punishment is protective reeducation.

Legal solutions neither offer emotional satisfaction (which shouldn't be the role of the law anyway) nor fix a bad situation. At the beginning of the twentieth century, "age-of-consent law and the juvenile court system merely perpetuated the stigma and supported the punishment of working-class females who engaged in unorthodox sexual behavior," wrote Odem.[31] At the end of the century, this is still true, with the additional fillip that the laws punish the unorthodox behavior of boys as well, if they are gay. But the law also perpetuates a stigma on behavior that is not particularly unorthodox—the "intergenerational" relationship. In fact, the coupling of a taller, richer, stronger, older man with the smaller, younger, less experienced woman is not only the romantic ideal, it is the norm. Research from the 1970s on has consistently found that whatever the law, a majority of girls lose their virginity to someone older than they.[32] At this writing, that means a tenth to a quarter of young women's chosen lovers are criminals.

Most important, as Lynn Phillips pointed out, such laws do nothing to address the needs for love and guidance, economic autonomy, respect, social status, or sexual agency that may lead some girls into such liaisons, nor do they redress the age and gender inequalities that prevent those girls from negotiating equally with their partners over safe sex, pregnancy, or money and that render them vulnerable to domestic violence and abandonment.

For Dylan, Heather, or their families, it is hard to discern what, if anything, enforcement of the law accomplished.

And Justice for None

In the brilliant autumn of 1997, Dylan Healy was sentenced, first at the federal courthouse and the next day in state court, at Providence's red-brick Licht Judicial Complex. The convict sat in flimsy leg shackles and prison orange, looking more stunned than repentant, while the clerk recited the convictions and penalties like a medieval Catholic litany, announcing each act of "felonious sexual assault with a minor," along with each separate period of penance. Dylan received twelve to twenty-four years on sixteen state charges, including twelve counts of felonious sexual assault, plus two federal counts of crossing state lines to have sex with a minor—the Mann Act, passed in 1915, at the height of the white-slavery panic. After the reading of each count and its penalty, the judge asked the defendant to affirm that he understood.

He did understand—literally, at any rate. But the statement Dylan's lawyer read for him spoke more of the tragedy of emotional ill health and immaturity than of criminal malice, more of misbegotten love than criminal misconduct. "I accept full responsibility," the statement began, insisting it was not meant "to excuse or minimize" Dylan's crimes. But as he told of a childhood and youth plagued by unbearable shyness and loneliness, redeemed by a girl who "made me feel happier than I had ever felt [and] who brought joy into my life," it did not appear that he understood or accepted the moral lesson his punishment was meant to teach. Indeed (a strategic misstep, taken against advice of counsel), Dylan seemed to be confessing that he'd do it all again. As the obstacles to their being together mounted, Dylan said, so did his obsession: "I loved her beyond reason and fled with the one I loved."

Dylan was incarcerated at Ray Brook Federal Correctional Institution, a medium-security prison in the Adirondack Mountains of upstate New York, to serve the first five and a third years of his sentence. His "roommate," who had shot a man, was doing less time and had a lower security-risk classification than Dylan.[33] When I visited him, it was clear that Dylan still loved Heather beyond reason. The usually reticent young man talked for four hours straight, mostly about her. Although his medication had quieted some of his obsessiveness, he had not abandoned his high-romantic notion of love, which is, after all, obsessive love. His mother told me his reading was limited mostly to self-help literature. But when I queried him about books he liked, he told me his all-time favorite was Emily Brontë's *Wuthering Heights,* which he'd read twice. "She starts getting delirious, she's so in love with him," he described the heroine, Cathy Earnshaw, who is almost demonically possessed by her love for the gypsy Heathcliff. "She says she'll wait for him forever, even though he's not that good of a guy—he's kind of evil." He grinned a little at this, perhaps comparing his own not-too-shabby reputation with the fictional character's towering badness. "Even if she does die, death won't stop her love; she'll be waiting for him." Dylan seemed to drift during our conversation from anchor-dragging depression (he told me he had been on suicide watch) to unmoored dreaminess. He explained his plan: to find another lawyer, get the prohibition lifted on his communication with Heather, and have his sentence reduced. When he got out she would be of age, and they could get married.

While Dylan sat behind bars, Heather returned to high school. It does not appear that this was easy for her, at least at first. Asked by the court what "may be different at school, in the neighborhood, or with your friends because of what has happened to you," Heather seemed to interpret what happened to her as what the press and her parents did, not what happened with Dylan. Nothing was different between him and her, she wrote. As for others, "some people treat me nice, & some just call me a slut. But mostly everyone just stares as I walk down the street."

Right after the arrest, Pauline Kowalski seemed wishful that her daughter's sojourn on the other side of the law was an aberration, that Heather had truly been lured away from regular life by a wicked adult, and now that the malefactor was behind bars, her girl would be home safe. She was willing to give Heather limited license. She'd allow her back on the Net, but for "homework projects" only: no chat-rooming. She hoped she and her daughter would talk more. "I want her to get back to being a normal thirteen-year-old girl," said Pauline.

But the demonization of Dylan Healy seemed not to have normalized much of anything for the Kowalski family. "Things have changed for the rest of my family though," Heather wrote in the statement. "They believe that Dylan tried to take me away and use me for sex. So now they are much more watchful at what I do, and my mom thinks she should make *every* decision for me." Every parent must balance permission with supervision—and perhaps Heather did need more supervision than she'd been getting. But Pauline's watchfulness seemed only to turn her daughter more vehemently against her. Rob contended in divorce filings that Heather wanted to live with him; Dylan said the same. But when the Kowalskis' divorce was finalized in February 1998, the court ruled that Heather's physical and legal custody would be shared and she would spend alternating weeks with each parent.[34]

When I last talked to Dylan's mother, Laura Barton, her declarations of optimism barely disguised her mourning and anxiety. "We love and support Dylan," she always said as she filled me in on his studies, his mood, and his diet. We never discussed his safety in prison, where "child molesters" do not fare well. Laura spoke with Dylan every few days but could rarely manage the eight-hour trip to visit him. And while she was trying to provide stability for her son far away in the Adirondacks, things had gotten shakier in her modest brick townhouse in Providence. Laura's marriage to Tom Barton, a soft-spoken, bearded road crewman, had been undone by the stress of Dylan's arrest and imprisonment. Longstanding fissures between them had widened, and the couple had separated shortly before their tenth wedding anniversary.

Creating Victims

"This court hopes with the love and support of her parents and her family that the victim will come to understand that what the defendant did was wrong, and that when she grows up, she comes to accept that this is something that was done to her and not because of her," intoned the Rhode Island judge who sentenced Dylan, fixing the girl with a stern half smile. Apparently the judge felt called upon to correct Heather's feeling, expressed in her court records, that she was not a victim, that Dylan had not harmed her physically or emotionally. Seated in the first row of the spectators' gallery between her temporarily united parents, wearing plain-teen jeans and sweatshirt and Dylan's necklaces, her hair cellophaned faintly red, Heather bit her lower lip and swallowed back tears as the sentencing was read. Now, as if being scolded, she looked at her hands, folded in her lap.

Many psychologists believe that adults' reactions even to certifiable sexual abuse can exacerbate the situation for the child, both in the short and in the long term. "There is often as much harm done to the child by the system's handling of the case as the trauma associated with the abuse," the National Center on Child Abuse and Neglect reported in 1978.[35] But the system's handling did not appreciably improve in the next two decades, especially as criminal proceedings increased against adults in adult-minor liaisons. When the youngster has had what she considers a relationship of love and consensual sex, it does no good to tell her she has been manipulated and victimized. "To send out the message that you've been ruined for life and this person was vile and they were pretending to care—that often does a lot of damage," commented Fred Berlin, a psychiatrist at Johns Hopkins University and a well-respected expert on treating sex offenders.[36]

How can harm be prevented rather than inflicted on youngsters? How can we even know what is harmful, so that we may be guided in guiding them toward happy and safe sexual relations?

The first answer is simple, said University of Georgia social work professor Allie Kilpatrick: Ask them. Have them describe their sexual experiences, without prelabeling them as abuse. In 1992, Kilpatrick published the results of a study based on a thirty-three-page questionnaire about childhood sexual experiences, administered to 501 women from a variety of class, racial, and educational backgrounds. Instead of employing the morally and emotionally freighted phrase *sexual abuse,* she asked specific questions: How old were you, how often, with whom did you have sex? Did you initiate or did the other person? What acts did you engage in ("kiss and hug," "you show genitals," "oral sex by you," etc.)? Was it pleasurable, voluntary, coerced? How did you feel later?[37]

Kilpatrick found that 55 percent of her respondents had had some kind of sex as children (between birth and age fourteen) and 83 percent as adolescents (age fifteen to seventeen), the vast majority of it with boys and men who were not related to them. Of these, 17 percent felt the sex was abusive, and 28 percent said it was harmful.[38] But "the majority of young people who experience some kind of sexual behavior find it pleasurable. They initiated it and didn't feel much guilt or any harmful consequences," she told me. What about age? "My research showed that difference in age made no difference" in the women's memories of feelings during their childhood sexual experiences or in their lasting effects.

Teens often seek out sex with older people, and they do so for understandable reasons: an older person makes them feel sexy and grown up, protected and special; often the sex is better than it would be with a peer who has as little skill as they do. For some teens, a romance with an older person can feel more like salvation than victimization. Wrote Ryan, a teenager who had run away from home to live in a Minnesota commune with his adult lover, "John was the first person in my life who would let me be who I wanted to be. . . . Without John I would have been dead because I would have killed myself."[39] Indeed, it is not uncommon for the child "victim" to consider his or her "abuser" a best friend, a fact that has led to some dicey diagnostic and criminal locutions. William Prendergast, a former prison psychologist and current frequent-flyer "expert" on child abuse, for instance, talks about "consensual rape" and young people's "pseudo-positive" sexual experiences with adults.[40]

Of course, there are gender differences in the experiences of early sex. The law did not invent these. Boys are used to thinking of themselves as desirers and initiators of sex and resilient players who can dust themselves off from a hard knock at love. So among boys, "self-reported negative effects" of sex in childhood are "uncommon," according to psychologists Bruce Rind and Philip Tromovitch's metanalysis of national samples of people who have had such experiences.[41] Girls and women, on the other hand, are far more often the victims of incest and rape than boys are, and gender compounds whatever age-related power imbalances an intergenerational liaison may contain. Phillips found that girls spoke of entering such partnerships willingly and often rationally and of satisfaction with the adult status they borrowed there. Yet they also often "let their guard down with older guys," agreeing not to use a condom, to drop out of school, or cut off ties with friends and families who could have helped them after the relationship was over. Her older informants offered another vantage point from which to view such relationships, often speaking disparagingly of their past older lovers and regretfully of their choices. Phillips pointed out that such bad behavior and twenty-twenty hindsight aren't exclusive to older-younger relationships. A younger lover might have been just as unfaithful and just as likely to leave a young woman with a baby and no help.[42]

The subjects of Sharon Thompson's *Going All the Way* represented such love affairs in far more positive ways. Just over 10 percent of the four hundred teenage girls she interviewed through the 1980s "told about actively choosing sexual experiences with men or women five or more years older than they." These girls "had no doubt that they could differentiate between abuse, coercion, and consent." They represented themselves as the aggressors, persisters, and abandoners in these relationships, adept at flipping between adult sophistication and childlike flightiness to suit their moods or romantic goals.[43]

Which story is true—freely chosen love or sweet-talked dupery? Both, said Thompson wisely when I asked her.[44] Phillips seemed to agree. "Rather than presuming that adult-teen relationships are *really* a form of victimization or that they *really* represent unproblematic, consensual partnerships—rather than maintaining either that willingness means consent or that an age difference means an inherent inability to consent—we need to step back and probe the nuances of adult-teen relationships from the perspectives of young women who participate in them," Phillips wrote. If we are going to educate young women to avoid potentially exploitative relationships, "those strategies must speak to [their] lived realities and the cultural and personal values that they, their families, and their communities hold regarding this issue."[45] Phillips admitted to ambivalence about age-of-consent laws.

"Scrambled Scripts"

"The 'life script'—our expectations of what we will do, and do next, and next after that in life—has been greatly scrambled in U.S. and Western Europe," Teachers College education professor Nancy Lesko commented in a 2000 interview. What Americans typically believed in the 1950s—that they would go to school, then get a job, then get married, then have sex, then have children—is no longer what youngsters necessarily have in mind. "None of that is certain any longer," said Lesko. "As a result, the sense of what youth or adulthood is comes into question and needs to be redefined."

Such redefinition is a subtle and never-ending task; it requires serious popular consideration and will never be settled for all time. In 1800, the age of consent was ten throughout America. In 1880, after the white-slavery panic, when a ten-year-old might be working fourteen hours a day in a factory, it was sixteen.[46] In the 1990s, the age of consent ranged, literally, all over the map: in Hawaii in 1998 it was fourteen; in Virginia, fifteen; Minnesota and Rhode Island, sixteen; Texas, seventeen; Wisconsin, eighteen. In New Hampshire, it was illegal for anyone to have sex with somebody under sixteen, even if both people were under sixteen.[47]

But sex is only one marker of social majority over which the law seeks dominion. The ages at which a person can drink, smoke cigarettes, drop out of school, get an abortion without parental notification, see a violent or sexy movie, or be incarcerated in an adult prison also are in dispute,[48] along with the question of whether parents should be held liable if their children break a law. Irrationally, as the age of sexual initiation slowly drops, the age of consent is rising.[49] And while "adult" sex becomes a crime for minors, it is only in the area of violent criminal activity that "children" are considered fully mature: in Chicago, in the late 1990s, an eleven-year-old boy was tried for murder as an adult, and at this writing prosecutions of minors as adults are becoming almost common.

There is no distinct moment at which a person is ready to take on adult responsibilities, nor is it self-evident that only those who have reached the age of majority are mature enough to be granted adult privileges. People do not grow up at sixteen, eighteen, or twenty-one, if they ever do. A three-decade study of thirty thousand adolescents and adults concluded that, cognitively and emotionally, both groups operated at an average developmental age of sixteen.[50]

Legally designating a class of people categorically unable to consent to sexual relations is not the best way to protect children, particularly when "children" include everyone from birth to eighteen. Criminal law, which must draw unambiguous lines, is not the proper place to adjudicate family conflicts over youngsters' sexuality. If such laws are to exist, however, they must do what Phillips suggests about sexual and romantic education: balance the subjective experience and the rights of young people against the responsibility and prerogative of adults to look after their best interests, to "know better." A good model of reasonable legislation is Holland's.

The Dutch parliament in 1990 made sexual intercourse for people between twelve and sixteen legal but let them employ a statutory consent age of sixteen if they felt they were being coerced or exploited. Parents can overrule the wishes of a child under sixteen, but only if they make a convincing case to the Council for the Protection of Children that they are really acting in the child's best interest. "Through this legislation, therefore, Dutch children of 12 to 16 years accrued conditional rights of consent to sexual behaviors, and parental authority was conditionally reduced," wrote David T. Evans in *Sexual Citizenship*. "Simultaneously it was recognized that all under 16 remained open to, and thus had the right to protection from, exploitation and abuse. . . . Overall, the legal message here is that children over the age of 12 are sexual and potentially self-determining, and they remain weaker than adults, and should be protected accordingly, but not under the autonomous authority of parents."[51]

The Dutch law, in its flexibility, reflects that late-modern script-scrambling, the hodge-podge of age and experience at the dawn of the twenty-first century. "If we admitted that we're not going to [live our lives] in the old order anymore . . . we could stop thinking of youth as deficient, as 'becoming,'" said Nancy Lesko. "We could begin to see them as capable, as knowledgeable. . . . It could be the starting point of attending to their sexuality differently."

5. No-Sex Education

From "Chastity" to "Abstinence"

There is mainstream sex ed and there is right-wing sex ed. But there is no left-wing sex education in America. Everyone calls themselves "abstinence educators." Everyone.
—Leslie Kantor, education director, Sex Information and Education Council of America (1997)

In 1981, the freshman Alabama Republican Senator, a Baptist with the apocalyptic given name of Jeremiah, came up with a way to wrestle down teen pregnancy at the same time as vanquishing what he believed were twin moral scourges: teen sex and abortion. In place of several successful national programs that provided birth-control services and counseling to young women, Jeremiah Denton's Adolescent Family Life Act (AFLA) proposed to stop teen sex by deploying nothing more than propaganda. AFLA would fund school and community programs "to promote self-discipline and other prudent approaches" to adolescent sex. Opponents quickly dubbed his innovation chastity education.

At first, the press and the public reactions were bemused. "Amazing," commented Zonker in Garry Trudeau's "Doonesbury," as he and Mike Doonesbury sat on their front porch on the comics pages, contemplating what the chastity bill might mean. ID checks outside Brooke Shields movies? Government-sponsored sound trucks cruising around on Saturday nights blaring *Cut that out*!? "Wow," said Zonker, stupefied by the thought.

But when Orrin Hatch, the powerful Utah Republican chair of the Labor and Human Resources Committee, signed on as AFLA's cosponsor, the bill suddenly gained gravitas. "This benighted piece of legislation is called the 'chastity law,' but it is no joke," said a *New York Times* editorial condemning the bill at the time.[1]

No joke indeed. AFLA was the first federal law specifically written to fund sex education, and it is still on the books. It has not yet accomplished its ambitious goals of eradicating teen sex, teen pregnancy, and abortion in one swipe. But for a triumphal New Right recently installed in Washington, under its imperial president, Ronald Reagan, the new law was a major victory. For young people's sexual autonomy and safety, though, it was a great blow—the first of a pummeling that has not yet ceased.

Over the next two decades, large, well-funded national conservative organizations with a loyal infantry of volunteers marched through school district after school district, firing at teachers and programs that informed students about their bodies and their sexual feelings, about contraception and abortion. These attacks met with only spotty resistance. Sex ed was a political backwater to begin with; hardly anyone paid attention to it. Unlike its opponents, sex ed's champions had a couple of national organizations but no national movement, no coherent cultural-political agenda. As the sociologist Janice Irvine points out, neither feminists nor the political Left rallied to the cause; gays and lesbians joined the fray only in the 1990s, when attacks began to focus more directly and hostilely on them. The most progressive and politically savvy sex educators were working outside the public schools, so they had limited say in public policy and little direct effect on the majority of kids. At the grass roots, the visible forces against sex ed were usually minuscule, often one or two ferocious parents and their pastor. But local defenses were feebler, and the already puny garrisons of comprehensive sexuality education began to fall.

Twenty years later, the Right has all but won the sex-education wars. In 1997, the U.S. Congress committed a quarter billion dollars over five years' time to finance more education in chastity, whose name had been replaced by the less churchy, more twelve-steppish *abstinence*.[2] As part of the omnibus "welfare reform bill," the government's Maternal and Child Health Bureau extended grants to the states for programs whose "exclusive purpose [is] teaching the social, psychological, and health gains to be realized by abstaining from sexual activity." In a country where only one in ten school-children receives more than forty hours of sex ed in any year,[3] the regulations prohibit funded organizations from instructing kids about contraception or condoms except in terms of their failures. In a country where 90 percent of adults have sex before marriage and as many as 10 percent are gay or lesbian, the law underwrites one message and one message only: that "a mutually faithful monoga-mous relationship in the context of marriage is the expected stan-dard of human sexual activity." Nonmarital sex, educators are re-quired to tell children, "is likely to have harmful psychological and physical effects."[4]

At first, there was a flurry of opposition to the welfare regula-tions. But every state eventually took the money. In many states, the dollars went largely to curriculum developers outside schools. But over the decade, right-wing propaganda and political action had been pushing public-school sex ed steadily toward chastity. Now that push was compounded by the financial pull from Washington, and the process lurched forward. By 1999, fully a third of public school districts were using abstinence-only curricula in their class-rooms.[5] Of a nationwide sample of sex-ed instructors surveyed by the Alan Guttmacher Institute, 41 percent cited abstinence as the most important message they wanted to convey to their students, compared with 25 percent in 1988. In the same dozen years the number of sex-ed teachers who talked exclusively about abstinence in their classes rose elevenfold, to nearly 25 percent from only 2 percent. The study's findings suggested "steep declines . . . in teacher support for coverage of many topics including birth con-trol, abortion, information on obtaining contraceptive and STD services, and sexual orientation," commented one report. "More-over, the proportion of teachers actually addressing these topics also declined."[6]

Today, the embrace of abstinence appears nearly unanimous. The only thing left to debate is whether abstinence is the *only* thing to teach. The Planned Parenthood Federation, for decades the Right's designated agent of Satan on earth, almost immediately rolled into bed with the abstinence mongers; only a few courageous chapters, such as Greater Northern New Jersey and New York City, buck the tide. Although it has been America's flagship advocate and a valiant defender of comprehensive sexuality education since 1964, the Sex Information and Education Council of the United States also publicly pledged allegiance to abstinence. "SIECUS supports abstinence. I repeat: SIECUS supports abstinence," began a typical mid-1990s speech by then-president Debra Haffner. "But SIECUS does not support teaching young people only about abstinence." Even Advocates for Youth, perhaps the single most progressive independent sexuality educator and sex-ed proponent in the country (in 1997 it told states to reject the welfare money "four-square"), now touts abstinence along with the more liberal messages in its publications. Today comprehensive sexuality education calls itself abstinence-plus education, to distinguish itself from abstinence-only.

Parents, when asked, overwhelmingly rise in favor of sexuality education covering a wide variety of topics, including contraception and even abortion and sexual orientation.[7] But, no doubt motivated by fear of AIDS, they like abstinence too. Of a national sample of parents surveyed in 2000 by the Kaiser Family Foundation, 98 percent put HIV/AIDS prevention on the list of desired topics to be taught in school, with abstinence following close behind, at 97 percent.

The idea that sex is a normative—and, heaven forfend, positive—part of adolescent life is unutterable in America's public forum. "There is mainstream sex ed and there is right-wing sex ed," said Leslie Kantor in 1997, when she was traveling the nation in her work for SIECUS. "But there is no left-wing sex education in America." She included her own organization in that characterization. Just fifteen years after Joyce Purnick's newspaper denounced the idea of chastity as antediluvian, the *New York Times* columnist felt compelled to insert a caveat into her critique of the new abstinence-only regulations. "Obviously," she began, "nobody from the Christian right to the liberal left objects to . . . encouraging sexual abstinence."[8]

There are two problems with this consensus. First, around the globe, most people begin to engage in sexual intercourse or its equivalent homosexual intimacies during their teen years. And second, there is no evidence that lessons in abstinence, either alone or accompanied by a fuller complement of sexuality and health information, actually hold teens off from sexual intercourse for more than a matter of months.

On the one hand, it seems obvious that American adults would preach to children not to have sex. The majority of them always have. But the logic that it is necessary and good to offer abstinence as one of several sexual "options"—the rationale given by the abstinence-plus (formerly comprehensive) educators—is more apparent than real. When asked a few years ago why her new curriculum's title now prominently featured the word *abstinence,* a progressive sex educator (who has herself worked to build a dike against the deluge of abstinence ed) said, "Because it is one way teens can choose to deal with sex." Her interlocutor, a saber-tongued sex therapist, replied, "Right. So's suicide." Abstinence education is not practical. It is ideological.

No Sex, Please. We're Sex Educators

Of course, Orrin Hatch and Jeremiah Denton did not invent sex education as an instrument of sex prevention. Throughout history, wrote Patricia Campbell in a historical survey of sex-education texts, "whether the tone is pompous or jazzy, the intent is always to teach [young people] the currently approved sexual behavior for their age group."[9] And the currently approved sexual behavior for any child's age group in almost any era has been no sexual behavior at all.

"[Sex instruction] should emphasize the perils of illicit coitus, moral and physical, without which . . . the instruction would be likely to have little deterrent effect," wrote one of the "progressive" fathers of the sex instruction in 1906, laying out the goals of his discipline.[10] By 1922, when the federal government undertook to publish its own sex-ed guide, *High Schools and Sex Education,* it practically eliminated sexuality from the courses altogether. Its accompanying medical examination forms, for instance, presumably employed to elicit some intelligence about the students' sex lives, steered clear of the subject and probed instead for such crucial information as "Do you masticate thoroughly?"[11] Evelyn Duvall's 1950s megaseller, *Facts of Life and Love for Teenagers,* rehearsed the stifling protocols of approved teen social behavior for decades to come, in minute detail: "When they reach the box office, Mary steps back and looks at the display cards while John buys the tickets." But life and love for teenagers meant "dating," which emphatically did not mean sex. At the end of the evening, Mary "is careful not to linger at the door."[12]

The founder of modern progressive sex education, Dr. Mary S. Calderone, pulled back from saying "no" but persisted in saying "wait." Addressing Vassar College's all-female class of 1964, Calderone, president of Planned Parenthood, world-renowned birth-control advocate, and soon-to-be charter president of SIECUS, neither moralized nor trafficked in fear. Yet she promised a youthful freedom and adult satisfaction that could be gained only by eschewing premarital sex. Hold off now, she told the students, and you will have "time . . . to grow up into the woman you were meant to be." The rigors of self-restraint would be repaid in more emotionally and sexually rewarding marriages, she said.[13]

Although her counsel seems moderate now, Calderone and her fellow sex-education advocates suffered bloodthirsty attacks from the Right, who smeared them with McCarthyist and anti-Semitic innuendo and implicated them in undermining the American way of life itself. "The struggle continues between those who believe in parental responsibility and those who seek to seize control of the thinking of America's youth," declared the deep-voiced narrator of an anti-sex-education filmstrip produced by the John Birch Society. "The future of your children and your nation is at stake."[14]

Calderone's disciples, who would become the founding generation of modern progressive and mainstream sex educators, were the first to hint that sex, if not always approved, was nonetheless normative teen behavior. A few were unabashed child-sexual liberationists. "Sex is a natural appetite. If you're old enough to want to have sex, you're old enough to have it," proclaimed Heidi Handman and Peter Brennan, in their 1974 *Sex Handbook: Information and Help for Minors*.[15] Psychologist Sol Gordon produced a stack of books that were not as radical as Handman and Brennan's but also respected young people's ability to make their own decisions. In *You* (1975), Gordon answered the perennial question "Are you ready [for sex]?" with more queries: "Are you mature? Are you in love? Are you using birth control?"[16]

Reading these books, one is struck by the total absence of the word *abstinence,* which did not enter the popular lexicon until the early 1980s (a Lexis-Nexis search of all U.S. magazines and newspapers brought up two citations in 1980, both of which were stories about the pope). Mainstream sex ed in the 1970s was still flogging the no-sex message, but books like Gordon's also represented an important strain of liberalism regarding child sexuality.

Chastity

Indeed, the 1970s were a banner decade for youthful sexual autonomy, not only in the streets and rock clubs, but also in schools, clinics, and the highest courts of the land. Following *Roe v. Wade*

(1973), liberals and feminists won a steady series of court cases guaranteeing poor and teenage women's rights to birth control information and services, and Washington and the states responded by establishing major programs to provide them.[17] This proliferation of clinics reporting to the government had an unexpected result, noted by the public-health historian Constance Nathanson: suddenly, there were mountains of data on teen sex, contraception, and pregnancy and its termination—information previously available only about the poor. The liberal family-planning establishment thought it could deploy the new data to gain support for its cause. So did the Right.

Then in 1976, some statistics dripping with propaganda potential arrived. The pro-family-planning Alan Guttmacher Institute released *Eleven Million Teenagers,* a report announcing a national "epidemic" of teen pregnancy. "Unwanted pregnancy is happening to our young women, not only among the poor and minority groups, but in all socioeconomic groups," the institute's president told Congress. "If I had a daughter, I would say [it was happening] to 'our' daughters."[18]

This was not accurate.[19] First of all, unwanted pregnancy, for the most part, was not happening to the daughters of demographers, doctors, and Washington bureaucrats. Now as then, more than 80 percent of America's teen mothers come from poor households.[20] And even among these young women, there was no epidemic. Eleven million referred to the number of people under eighteen who had had intercourse at least once. Teen pregnancies actually numbered fewer than a million a year, and of those teen mothers, six in ten were legal adults, eighteen or nineteen years old.[21] Yes, unmarried teens were having more sex in the 1970s than they'd had in the decades before.[22] But teen motherhood had hit its twentieth-century zenith in the mid-1950s, when one in ten girls between fifteen and nineteen years of age gave birth. Since then, the rate has steadily dropped.[23]

Still, the idea of the teen-pregnancy epidemic focused public anxiety about teenage girls' newly unfettered sex lives. Politically, it served both liberals and conservatives—the former arguing for reproductive health services and education for sexually active youth, the latter trying to rein in the services, the education, and most definitely the sex.

The 1980 national elections gave conservatives their chance.

Voters returned Republican control to the Senate, a Democratic stronghold for the previous twenty-eight years, and installed Ronald Reagan in the Oval Office. The new president appointed to every office related to sex education, contraception, or abortion someone who opposed all of the above.[24] "These people provided for the anti-abortion movement a forum in government that it had never had," said Susan Cohen, now a senior policy analyst at the Guttmacher Institute. For the reproductive-rights movement, added Bill Hamilton, then lobbying for the Planned Parenthood Federation, the 1980 elections were "a cataclysmic setback." For comprehensive sex education, it was the beginning of the end.

A few months into the 97th Congress, Orrin Hatch honored the president's request to demolish Title X of the Public Health Services Act of 1970, which provided contraceptive services to poor and young women. What Hatch planned to do was reduce the program's appropriation by a quarter and repackage the whole thing into block grants to the states. Bundled in with rodent control and water fluoridation and without a mandate that the legislatures commit any money to reproductive services, Title X might well cease to serve its reproductive-services mandate.[25]

Meanwhile, down the hall, the anti-abortion zealot Jeremiah Denton was chairing the subcommittee on human services of Hatch's Labor and Human Resources Committee and contemplating his role in history. With the help of some friends, including Catholic birth-control advocate Eunice Shriver, sister of Ted Kennedy, he arrived at S. 1090, the Adolescent Family Life Act. Soon, Hatch was on board, too.

AFLA was a trident: One prong promoted adoption as the "positive" alternative to unwed motherhood or abortion, although at that time 96 percent of pregnant adolescents were rejecting adoption as a cruel and unnecessary option.[26] Another prong prohibited government funds to any agency whose workers even uttered the word *abortion* to a teenager, much less performed the operation. "Chastity education" was the central, most controversial prong.

But public controversy and press ridicule, from the political cartoons of small city papers to the editorial pages of the *New York Times* and the *Washington Post,* seemed barely to ruffle Capitol Hill's confident new majority. With the National Right to Life and the American Life League barnstorming in the background and the family planners distracted in the rush to save Title X, S. 1090 zipped through the Senate. When it came up during the final budget reconciliation, California Democrat Henry Waxman, chair of the Commerce Committee's subcommittee on public health and Title X's most active defender, was forced to make a trade with Hatch and Denton. Waxman could keep Title X, but only with AFLA tied to it like a string of clattering cans.

"AFLA was the anti-abortion answer to Title X Family Planning," Judy DeSarno, president and CEO of the National Family Planning and Reproductive Health Association, summed it up seventeen years later. At the time, she added, most of the family-planning community was relieved. Had Title X been lost, millions of poor women would have gotten no reproductive health services at all, she said. "It was unfortunate," added Cohen of the Guttmacher Institute, "but the important thing is that the real preventive program has been able to survive over the last decade-plus, and AFLA has not really hurt that program."

Others disagreed strongly with the assessment that AFLA was doing little harm. Among the detractors were the lawyers at the American Civil Liberties Union's Reproductive Freedom Project, who believed that while the legislation might not hurt Title X, it would hurt sex education—and the First Amendment. In 1983, in *Kendrick v. Bowen,* they argued that the sex-education portion of the law was a Trojan horse smuggling the values of the Christian Right, particularly its unbending opposition to abortion, to public-school children at public expense. AFLA, they said, was a violation of the constitutional separation of church and state.[27]

The Supreme Court finally decided, ten years later, that AFLA was constitutional as written—"facially"—but that in practice the government was indeed promoting certain religions and discriminating against others. The bench appointed the ACLU to monitor the law's administration, which it unofficially had been doing throughout the litigation.

But, many now believe, it was too late. Some of the biggest federal grant recipients, including Sex Respect and Teen-Aid, had already turned their taxpayer-funded church-developed anti-sex-education curricula into big for-profit businesses. Respect Inc., which received more than $1.6 million in federal and state grants during the 1980s,[28] claimed in the early 1990s that its curricula were in use in one-quarter of American school districts.[29] Teen-Aid, which received AFLA grants amounting to $784,683 between 1987 and

1991,[30] became one of the major publishers of abstinence-only programs, which teach little more than "just say no."

This bankrolling—and the substitution of federal funds for contraception with dollars for chastity—was anything but surreptitious. AFLA "was written expressly for the purpose of diverting [federal] money that would otherwise go to Planned Parenthood into groups with traditional values," a *Conservative Digest* writer reported. "That noble purpose has certainly been fulfilled here. If it hadn't been for the seed money provided by the government, 'Sex Respect' might still be just an idea sitting in a graduate student's thesis."[31] Said former SIECUS spokesman Daniel Daley in 1997, "In those first years of AFLA, this money went directly from the government to Christian fundamentalist groups, who built the infrastructure of the organizations that are the most vehement opponents of comprehensive sexuality education today." Also born during that time was the discourse of teen sex that shapes policy to this day.

"The problem of premarital adolescent sexual relations"

In his July 1981 committee report on S. 1090, Denton quoted the statistics promulgated by the Guttmacher Institute[32] (he was probably unaware the organization was named for one of history's great champions of abortion rights). The senator declared that the government should address the "needs of pregnant adolescents" and proposed a prescription that the entire family-planning profession could applaud: *more prevention.*

But prevention of what? Poverty? Teen pregnancy? Unwed motherhood? Abortion? Denton claimed he could eradicate all of the above by preventing what he saw as the cause of them all: *teen sex.* In what would become the central maneuver in the conservative rhetoric of teen sexuality over the next decades, Denton collapsed four separate events—sex, pregnancy, birth, and abortion—into one "widespread problem." He attributed "serious medical, social, and economic consequences" to all four and then wrapped them into one whopper: *"the problem of premarital adolescent sexual relations."*[33]

This "problem" had been exacerbated by a decade of social policy, which he and Hatch summed up in a letter to the *New York Times* as "$1.5 billion of taxpayers' money [spent] on 'family planning.'"[34] Contraception and abortion, they reasoned, had led to teen sex, which led to pregnancy. The logical sleight of hand was impressive: contraception and abortion caused teen pregnancy.

But the real trouble, as the sponsors saw it, was not just adolescent sex. It was sex behind Mom and Dad's back. "The deep pocket of government has funded this intervention between parents and their children in schools and clinics for 10 years," wrote Hatch and Denton. "[I]t is little wonder that problems of adolescent sexual activity grow worse."[35] In other words, clinics that offered confidential services to adolescents, as the Supreme Court had ordered in 1977, were ripping the family apart by promoting children's liberation at the expense of a newly articulated subset of family values, "parental rights."[36] (Later, in conservative parlance, "parents" would become "families," implying a harmonious and cooperative unit without gender or generational conflict.)

For a decade, whether out of grudging realism or genuine support for the rights of young women, policymakers had gone along with the liberal family-planning establishment in regarding minor-age clients as independent actors in their own sexual lives. But by the 1980s, with AFLA inscribed as statute and political pressure rising from the Right, a time-tested theme was revived: parents should control all aspects of their kids' sexuality. "I am not opposed to family planning when we are planning families," Denton told the press. "However, unemancipated minors do not plan families."[37]

Family planning had long been a euphemism for contraception, which was a trope for modern, conscious, technologically enhanced sexual activity. To family planners, prevention had meant the prevention of unplanned pregnancy. Now prevention was the prevention of sex, and it would be accomplished not by the Pill but by diatribe and ideology. AFLA installed sex education under the aegis of "family life." And in the ideal family, parents kept their children safe by denying their sexuality and their autonomy, and children could feel safe by accepting the limits of childhood.

"Abstinence" Triumphant

Sexuality was "family life." And only families—that is, heterosexual married mommies and daddies—could have sex. In 1996, the man who brought extramarital fellatio and erotic cigar play to prime-time television signed into law a provision that would fiscally excommunicate sex educators who did not hew to this credo: Section 501(b): Abstinence Education, of the Social Security Act of 1997.

To receive money from Washington, states would have to match each federal dollar with two from their own coffers that might otherwise go to more catholic programs. Not only was the federal government encouraging abstinence-only; it was discouraging everything else.

The abstinence-only funding regulations were the platinum standard of conservative ideology about sexuality and the family. And like the AFLA-funded curricula that inspired them, their absoluteness made them easy for most Americans to dislike.[38] So at first, a number of health and education departments balked at using their limited dollars to preach abstinence in schools where half the kids were already having sex, and some already had babies or HIV. Some youth, sex-ed, and reproductive-rights advocates (most vocally Advocates for Youth) extolled their state bureaucracies to turn down the money. But many states already had similar, if not equally restrictive, laws. Of the twenty-three requiring sex education, fewer than half prescribed lessons on contraception, and all mandated instructing on abstinence.[39]

In the end, every state applied for the federal abstinence-only money in the first year, and all but two took it.[40] Five states passed laws requiring that sexuality education programs teach abstinence-only as the standard for school-age children.[41] In 2000, under the sponsorship of Oklahoma archconservative Republican representative Ernest Istook, the language of AFLA was brought into conformity with that of the welfare law, and an additional twenty million dollars were appropriated to fund AFLA's now seamlessly doctrinaire grant making. Organizations such as Advocates for Youth, SIECUS, and the National Coalition Against Censorship began campaigning that year to block the reappropriation of abstinence-only funding in 2001. But with George W. Bush in the White House and few Congress members willing to squander political capital opposing it, the program's healthy survival is almost assured.

In one way, the wide support for abstinence makes sense. Americans are still convinced that teen pregnancy is pandemic, and in a time of sex-borne death, containing the exchange of adolescent body fluids is an attractive notion to parents,[42] educators, and even to kids themselves.

In another way, however, it is senseless, and for the simplest of reasons: Comprehensive, nonabstinence sex education works. And abstinence education does not. In many European countries, where teens have as much sex as in America, sex ed starts in the earliest grades. It is informed by a no-nonsense, even enthusiastic, attitude toward the sexual; it is explicit; and it doesn't teach abstinence. Rates of unwanted teen pregnancy, abortion, and AIDS in every Western European country are a fraction of our own; the average age of first intercourse is about the same as in the United States.[43]

Abstinence programs, on the other hand, do not change students' attitudes for long, and they change behavior hardly a whit. By 1997, six studies had been published in the scientific literature showing that these classes did not accomplish their goal: to get kids to delay intercourse.[44] In one case, male students enrolled in a chastity-only course actually had more sex than those in the control group.[45] Following the implementation of the welfare rules, a study of 659 African American Philadelphia sixth- and seventh-graders, published in the *Journal of the American Medical Association,* returned the same verdict. A year after the classes, the kids who had undergone an abstinence-only program were engaging in intercourse in the same numbers (about a fifth) as kids who had received lessons stressing condom use, with the dangerous difference that the first group hadn't been taught anything about safe sex.[46] "It is difficult to understand the logic behind the decision to earmark funds specifically for abstinence programs," commented *JAMA*'s editors.[47] A consensus statement on AIDS prevention by the National Institutes of Health delivered an even more damning indictment: abstinence-only education was potentially lethal. The "approach places policy in direct conflict with science and ignores overwhelming evidence that other programs would be effective," concluded the group, whose members included many of the country's top AIDS experts. "[A]bstinence-only programs cannot be justified in the face of effective programs and given the fact that we face an international emergency in the AIDS epidemic."[48]

If it is difficult to understand the logic behind abstinence-only policy, it may be instructive to know that its proponents were proudly unswayed by logic. Although the law's impetus came in part from the continuing concern over nonmarital births, the House staffers who worked on the legislation admitted, in the commentary circulated in Congress, that "there is little evidence . . . that any particular policy or program will reduce the frequency of nonmarital births."[49] Now, this is not true: any number of policies, from contraceptive education to college scholarships for women, can reduce the frequency of nonmarital teen births. But the welfare law was not really intended to reduce teen births anyway. It was intended to make a statement: "to put Congress on the side of the social tradition . . . that sex should be confined to married couples." Like missionaries forcing the indigenous people to throw off their own gods and adopt the new dogma whole, the authors expected—indeed, seemed almost to relish—popular resistance to their ideas. "That both the practices and standards in many communities across the country clash with the standard required by the law," they wrote, "is precisely the point."[50]

Comprehensive educators, on the other hand, claim to be guided by reliable data, not ideology, or at least not conservative, antisexual ideology. So what was driving them to adopt abstinence?

Advocates were tired. They were worn down and in some cases financially broken by a decade of furious battering from the organized Christian Right, including hundreds of direct personal threats of divine retribution or its equivalent by human hands. (In one campaign, the conservative Concerned Women for America generated thirty thousand missives to Congress accusing SIECUS of supporting pedophilia and baby killing. "You will burn in the lake of fire," was only one of thousands sent directly to SIECUS president Haffner.) Classroom teachers were under increasing surveillance, which made them more cautious. Some got rid of the anonymous question box into which students used to place embarrassing queries, knowing they'd get straight responses; now, this was too dangerously unpredictable. Some told me their principals advised sending students who asked embarrassing questions that indicated they were sexually active off to the guidance counselor for a tête-à-tête (implying that sex is not only private but also a psychological and social problem). More and more dropped discussion of the controversial subjects, such as abortion, or stopped informing students about where they could get birth control.[51] In 1998 SIECUS published a handbook called *Filling the Gaps: Hard to Teach Topics in Sexuality Education.* The topics included safer sex, condoms, sexual orientation, diversity, pregnancy options, sexual behavior, sex and society, and (incongruously, but presumably because it could not be left off any list) abstinence. The "gaps," in short, were everything but sexual plumbing and disease.

But even those who continued to teach the "gaps" pitched abstinence too, whether they believed it was worthwhile or not. "The fact is, we all have to pay homage to abstinence before we can say anything else. Professionally, it is almost suicidal not to," Leslie Kantor, education vice-president of Planned Parenthood of New York City, told me ruefully. "The vast majority of adolescents in America and across the globe enter into sexual relations during their teen years. This is just a fact, and to talk about anything else is simply wasting time. [Nevertheless,] if you are not seen as a supporter of abstinence . . . you are not likely, if you are a teacher, to keep your job, and if you're from the outside, you won't get in to do any sexuality education at all."

The titles of the comprehensive curricula were white flags spelling out this surrender. "Living Smart: Understanding Sexuality," put out by ETR Associates, the nation's largest mainstream sex-education publisher, became "Sex Can Wait: An Abstinence-Based Sexuality Curriculum for Middle School." Planned Parenthood's 1986 "Positive Images: A New Approach to Contraceptive Education" was born again as "The New Positive Images: Teaching Abstinence, Contraception, and Sexual Health," even though the content is about as scant on abstinence lessons as its predecessor. A pamphlet on birth control education published in 2000 by the National Campaign to Prevent Teen Pregnancy was called *The Next Best Thing*. The title implied that contraception was the next best thing to abstinence, which the campaign had adopted from the start as the optimal defense against unwanted pregnancy. But to a skeptical observer it might signal the campaign's decision to champion the next-best method of sex education, because the best had become politically untenable.

Discouragement and realpolitik—these motivated the gradual retreat of the comprehensive sex educators. But there might have been something else operating, if not on the organizational level, then on the personal. By the 1990s, the Sexual Revolutionaries were parents, and, especially with AIDS in the picture, they were getting scared for their kids. "It's precisely because many of us experimented with sex at an early age that we know how problematic it can be," wrote New Mexico physician Victor Strasburger in the best-selling advice book *Getting Your Kids to Say "No" in the '90s When You Said "Yes" in the '60s*. "It's only now, when we are parents ourselves, that we are willing to acknowledge that perhaps we might have made a mistake in beginning to have sexual intercourse at too young an age."[52] He did not elaborate on the "problems" or the effects of that "mistake." Fourteen years after his book *You*, Sol

Gordon and his wife, Judith, wrote *Raising a Child Conservatively in a Sexually Permissive World,* which stolidly repudiated their former relativist stance on sexual readiness. "We think that young people should not engage in sexual intercourse until they are at least eighteen and off to college, working or living on their own," they advised.[53] (In the title of a later edition—as new marketing strategy or change of heart?—the authors changed the word *conservatively* to *responsibly.*)

Unlike the Gordons' earlier books, *Raising a Child* spoke not to teens themselves but to parents, now the designated guardians of their children's sexual lives. And like Hatch and Denton and the writers of the welfare regulations, these authors were speaking directly to parental fears. Those fears must surely have accounted for the lack of resistance among parents who supported comprehensive sex ed when those few (and it was almost invariably a very few) detractors started showing up at school board meetings. When educators Peter Scales and Martha Roper assayed the sex-ed battlefield in 1996, they discovered that "out of the glare of publicity, most 'opponents' and 'supporters' of sexuality education share many of the same basic values and hopes for children."[54]

They also shared the same anxieties. And progressive sex educators, most of whom were parents as well as professionals, had anxieties too. A joke circulating among them in the mid-1990s told the story:

> Q: What's a conservative?
> A: A liberal with a teenage daughter.

Abstinence-Only: Fear and Freedom

Here, according to the popular conservative-Christian-authored *Sex Respect,* are a few of the hazards of nonmarital sex:

> Pregnancy, AIDS, guilt, herpes, disappointing parents, chlamydia, inability to concentrate on school, syphilis, embarrassment, abortion, shotgun wedding, gonorrhea, selfishness, pelvic inflammatory disease, heartbreak, infertility, loneliness, cervical cancer, poverty, loss of self-esteem, loss of reputation, being used, suicide, substance abuse, melancholy, loss of faith, possessiveness, diminished ability to communicate, isolation, fewer friendships formed, rebellion against other familial standards, alienation, loss of self-mastery, distrust of [other] sex, viewing others as sex objects, difficulty with

long-term commitments, various other sexually transmitted diseases, aggressions toward women, ectopic pregnancy, sexual violence, loss of sense of responsibility toward others, loss of honesty,
jealousy, depression, death."[55]

"Sadness, not happiness, causes teen sex," declares a pamphlet
published by the same company, and "teen sex causes sadness."
The "Safe Sex" program marketed by the politically influential
pro-abstinence, antichoice Medical Institute for Sexual Health, or
MISH, packs seventy-five full-color slides of diseased genitals.[56]
And in the film *No Second Chance* a student asks the school nurse,
"What if I want to have sex before I get married?" She answers:
"Well, I guess you'll just have to be prepared to die."[57] It is not
for nothing that the comprehensive educators call these "fear-
based" programs.

But the writers of the abstinence-only curricula had a credibility
problem. Every kid knows that Mom and Dad, if they were like
more than 90 percent of baby boomer adults, did it before they tied
the knot, that they took the Pill, had abortions, and came through it
alive, well, and seemingly unharmed (unless premarital sex causes
baldness and a deafness to decent music). To overcome the con-
sumer's skepticism, not only did abstinence educators need to instill
in kids a reason to run from the lures of sex; they also had to point
them *toward* something worth having. So, believing that teen sex is
a form of self-destruction, the abstinence-only people (who are also
antichoice activists) ask kids to "choose life," not necessarily their
current lives but better lives further down the road. "Our goal
should be to instill hope for their futures: future marriages, spouses,
and families," read the MISH guidelines (sounding not so different
from Mary Calderone addressing the Vassar women).[58]

Thus, in alternately bleak and hearty language, the Christian
curricula coach their students to wrestle against desire. It is a match
worthy of Saint Augustine himself. "At one time in adolescence I
was burning to find satisfaction in hellish pleasures," confessed the
tortured supplicant. "If only someone could have imposed restraint
on my disorder."[59] Abstinence is not easy, yet the goal is attainable,
the abstinence-only educators cheer. And if you don't succeed at
first, you get another chance: you can pledge "secondary virginity."
If only Augustine had taken "Sex Respect." With that option, he
might have finessed his famous dilemma: the yearning to be chaste,
but not yet.

Of course, like the young Augustine, the modern teenager isn't usually thinking that far ahead. When neither stick nor carrot does the trick (disease and death seem improbable, and future happiness vague and remote) there has to be a sweeter, more immediate promise held before the students' noses. Chastity's advocates came up with a gold ring that glitters for both kids and parents: "freedom."

"Adolescent sexual abstinence offers the freedom to develop respect for oneself and others, use energy to accomplish life goals, be creative in expressing feelings, develop necessary communication skills, develop self-appreciation, achieve financial stability before having a family, and establish greater trust in marriage," says MISH.[60] In *Sex Respect,* one version is subtitled "The Option of True Sexual Freedom." And Teen-Aid claims: "Saving sex brings freedom."

The only "freedom" reserved for skepticism in these texts is "reproductive freedom," put between quotes by Teen-Aid's authors, who also note the feminist provenance of the idea and list it among the "myths of premarital sex" that students are encouraged to challenge. (*"Consider:* Who waits anxiously each month for her period? Whose lifestyle is drastically changed?") "Men" are directed to ponder, "Where is the freedom in worrying about getting a girl pregnant?"[61] As is common in abstinence ed, the gender-unequal burdens of sex are acknowledged, but claims to gender equality are dismissed, even denigrated—here, with the implication that feminists are fighting for pie in the sky and that "men" do best honoring their paternalistic obligation to "girls" by respecting their purity.

The idea of freedom, soaring like an aria over the ostinato of sexual peril, was a stroke of marketing brilliance, resonating with a major theme of American history and advertising. Freedom can mean anything from universal suffrage to a choice of twenty-seven flavors of Snapple, and bondage anything from chattel slavery to the discomfort of bulky sanitary pads. But as Aunt Lydia told the women whose lives were consecrated to breeding babies for the ruling classes in Margaret Atwood's dystopic-futurist novel *The Handmaid's Tale,* "There is more than one kind of freedom. Freedom to and freedom from." Referring to the democratic, gender-egalitarian period before the totalitarian theocracy that cannily resembles the one radical Christians might like to create in the United States, Lydia says, "In the days of anarchy, it was freedom to. Now you are being given freedom from. Don't underrate it."[62] The narrator, even as she cowers behind the fear that the aunts' protection has begun to instill in her, longs for the confusing but exhilarating "freedom to."

Like their fictional counterparts, the cleverest marketers of abstinence seem to intuit that teens vacillate between the attractions of the two kinds of freedom. With the popular culture pulling for "freedom to" engage in sex, and their teachers holding out "freedom from" all the sexual and emotional fuss and muss implied in growing up, students are by turns impressed by and dismissive of the dangers hyperbolized in abstinence education. Like advertising, which must continually jack up its seduction just to stay visible as other advertising proliferates, abstinence education had to make sex scarier and scarier and, at the same time, chastity sweeter. By neglecting the other information about pleasure that good sex ed could offer, fear and freedom had a fighting chance against teenage desire.

Family Life

If abstinence offers kids the freedom from growing up, it tenders to parents an equally impossible corollary, freedom from watching their kids grow up. That promise is fully consonant with what conservative parents want for themselves and their children, and sometimes it is fulfilled, at least temporarily. A woman I met at a convention of the conservative Christian organization Concerned Women for America told me that her fifteen-year-old daughter's "crisis pregnancy" turned out to be "a blessing." In renouncing her sexual relationship and pledging herself to "secondary virginity," the girl reconnected with her family. During her confinement, before she gave the baby up for adoption, she spent time with her mother shopping, talking, and praying; she played with her sisters, went to church midweek with her father. Literally unsteady on her feet, alienated from the pleasures that had pulled her toward her boyfriend and away from family and church, she was now thrown back to childlike dependence and gratitude, precisely at the age when she might otherwise have spurned her parents' best-meant solicitations in order to fly on her own.

For more moderate or liberal parents, the wish for such a "freedom" is more conflicted. The majority of American adults champion sexuality education at school: the very first Gallup Poll, in 1943, found 68 percent of parents favoring it,[63] and even the heaviest right-wing fire in the 1980s and 1990s didn't manage to blast away the base of that support, which consistently bested 80 percent.[64] But parents also embrace abstinence. Most concede that their kids will probably have sex in their teens, in other words, but surveying the dangers their children face, also wish they wouldn't.

Abstinence-plus speaks to these mothers and fathers. The *plus* addresses the rational concession that sex will happen. But the *abstinence* connects powerfully to that deep parental wish: to protect and "keep" their children by guarding their childhood. In this sense, abstinence is about reversing, or at least holding back, the coming of age, which for parents is a story of loss, as their children establish passionate connections with people and values outside the family.

Even for parents who revel in their children's emerging sexuality, it can mean loss. A strong feminist advocate of sexual freedom described watching her son, then about seventeen, standing side by side with his girlfriend at her living room window. "They were not hugging or kissing, but every part of their bodies was touching," she recalled. "The light from the window was all around them, but there was no light between them. Immediately, I knew they had made love." Twenty years later, the memory still brought a wistful softness to her face. "I went to the kitchen and burst into tears, because I knew I was no longer the most important woman in my son's life."

In some advertising copy in 1997, SIECUS president Debra Haffner criticized abstinence-only education as a kind of child neglect. "When we treat sexuality as adults-only," she said, "we abandon teenagers to learn about their sexuality on their own, by trial and error."[65] Her point was correct and crucial: accurate, positively communicated, and effectively transmitted information about sexuality makes the going happier, easier, and far less dangerous for young people. Abstinence-only education falsely promises parents it can eliminate the awfulness of watching children try and fail (because by the time they get to sex, they will be adults and able to handle it). But comprehensive education may also encourage a similarly unrealistic, but profoundly held, parental hope: that teen sexuality can be rational, protected, and heartbreak-free.

"The nature of teen romance is that it is tortured, and then it ends," the writer and former sex educator Sharon Thompson commented, laughing sympathetically. Thompson sees not only the avoidance of romantic pitfalls but also the knocks themselves as potentially "educative." She advocates "romance education," but she also knows that adults can't save their kids from *le chagrin d'amour*. Contrary to the implication in Haffner's plea that adults not "abandon" teens to sexual trial and error, the fact is that sexual relationships are by definition what teenagers do on their own, and the only way for teens to learn about them is to try—which usually means failing, too. "Maturity," including sexual maturity, cannot be attained without practice, and in sex as in skiing, practice is risky.

Haffner's statement fits with the contemporary belief that parents can be involved in every aspect of their children's lives, from soccer to sex. It is not surprising that this should be the direction in which sex education is turning. In the 1980s, sexuality ed was renamed family life education, even by Planned Parenthood, sending the message that sex belongs in the context of the heterosexual reproductive family. Along with sexual responsibility, students in many family-life courses learn the skills of householder and parent, the definitions of adulthood in centuries past. One course included a lesson on filling out a tax return. In almost all programs, parental consent forms are distributed at the start of the course. A tactic initially used to defuse community opposition, these forms also stack up as de facto acquiescence by sex educators to a parental "right" of control over their children's sexuality.

The comprehensives, who have long encouraged parents to talk frankly with children from early on, also have recognized that many won't or can't. Now, however, that balanced understanding is subtly drifting—with the gale force of political pressure from the Right behind it—toward more reliance on parents. With it have come many programs to educate them on how to be "the primary sex educators of their children," as the phrase always goes.

"Parent education" is a fine idea. But because the political goal is more about some liberal version of family values than it is about creating the highest-quality education, some of the courses get their priorities mixed up. One such curriculum is "Can We Talk?" a four-session video and discussion program for parents created by the visually inventive Dominic Capello under the sponsorship of the National Education Association and the Health Information Network. After a training session for educators, I expressed my concern to Capello that there seemed to be little guidance to parents about what they should say and that they therefore might well say inaccurate and bigoted things to their children—that masturbation causes blindness, for instance, or that Pop will beat you black and blue if you come home pregnant. "There's plenty of information in there," he countered, pointing to the twenty pages (with lots of white space and pictures) on puberty, reproduction, pregnancy, AIDS, and anatomy in the three-ring binder parent participants receive. (I suggested that in the next edition he add the clitoris to the list of relevant female body parts.) "But this is a first step," said Capello, an openly gay man who started his career as an art director for a radical queer magazine. "We're trying to help parents learn to communicate their values"—whatever those values may be.

Allies of comprehensive sexuality education have not ceased agitating for higher professionalism among sexuality educators (who are now, likely as not, the gym teacher or other reluctant draftee), through more rigorous training and accreditation. They have continued to lobby for compulsory school-based comprehensive sex ed taught by trained instructors. Yet the increasing propaganda and programmatic creep toward the kitchen table, at the very moment schoolteachers are being gagged in the classroom, amounts to a capitulation to the Right's agenda. Parent education, even well-trained parent education, affirms the new orthodoxy that parents possess the sex-educational will and competence whose very absence mobilized the founders of sex instruction nearly a century ago.

These recent moves toward parent education bespeak a contradiction inside sex ed. On the one hand, they are consistent with the historical conservatism of the discipline, which has always consigned sex to marriage and aimed to strengthen parental authority. On the other, they represent a retreat from the critique of the family implicit in school-based sexuality education, which endorses the sexual-intellectual autonomy of children and suggests that the family, with its hierarchical structure, its neuroses, ignorance, and taboos, is *not* the best sex educator after all.

Successes and Failures

After rising steadily from 1970, the rate of teen intercourse in America dropped a smidgen in the 1990s,[66] while the teen pregnancy and birth rates slid, by 17 percent and 19 percent, respectively (these were still the highest in the developed world, about comparable with Bulgaria).[67] Unsurprisingly, many link these two facts to a spreading conservatism among kids, including the embrace of virginity. The renewed popularity of virginity has been attributed to abstinence education.

Examined more closely, however, the causal relationship between abstinence education and a reduction in teen pregnancy is, at best, small. A major analysis by the Alan Guttmacher Institute attributes about a fourth of the decline to delayed intercourse but three-quarters to improved contraceptive use among sexually experienced teenagers.[68] In Europe, where kids have as much sex as they do in America, teen pregnancy rates are about a fourth as high as ours.[69]

In the Netherlands, where celibacy is not taught, contraception is free through the national health service, and condoms are widely available in vending machines, "teenage pregnancy seems virtually eliminated as a health and social problem," according to Dr. Simone Buitendijk of the Dutch Institute for Applied Scientific Research. Fewer than 1 percent of Dutch fifteen- to seventeen-year-olds become pregnant each year.[70] "The pragmatic European approach to teenage sexual activity, expressed in the form of widespread provision of confidential and accessible contraceptive services to adolescents, is . . . a central factor in explaining the more rapid declines in teenage childbearing in northern and western European countries, in contrast to slower decreases in the United States," commented the authors of another, cross-national Guttmacher study.[71]

There may even be an inverse relationship between abstinence education and declining rates of pregnancy. For one thing, because many abstinence programs teach kids that refraining from intercourse is the only surefire way to prevent pregnancy and vastly exaggerate the failures of contraception and condoms, students get the impression that birth control and STD prevention methods don't work. So they shrug off using them or don't know how to use them. Contraception education, on the other hand, works: teens who learn about birth control and condoms are 70 to 80 percent more likely to protect themselves if they have intercourse than kids who are not given such lessons.[72]

More fundamentally, though, it is a truth universally acknowledged among social scientists that attitude is one thing and behavior quite another. In one major recent government survey, only about a quarter of kids who hadn't yet had intercourse expected to do so while they were still in their teens. In reality, twice as many do.[73] Good intentions, moreover, are the paving-stones on the road to what public-health professionals call bad outcomes. In this case, the outcome proves another sad truth: "good girls get caught." A good girl, by definition, is not a girl with condoms and lube in her backpack. As Planned Parenthood's curriculum "Positive Images" points out, "'Abstinence' often fails, i.e., people who *intended* to be abstinent have sexual intercourse and don't use either a contraceptive or a condom."[74]

In a recent analysis of the massive National Longitudinal Study of Adolescent Health, Columbia University sociologist Peter Bearman looked at the success of "chastity pledges." The pledges, usually taken publicly as part of a Christian fundamentalist virginity movement, have indeed given several million teens the personal gumption and peer support to postpone intercourse—on average, eighteen months longer than nonpledgers. But in the end, such pledges are counterproductive to developing habits of lifetime sexual responsibility. When they broke the promise, as almost all did, these fallen angels were less effective contraceptors than their peers who had become active earlier.[75] The study of Philadelphia middle schoolers reported in *JAMA* educed the same results. When the abstinence-only students engaged in intercourse a year later, a third of them did so without protection. Fewer than one-tenth of the group who had been taught about condoms took that risk.[76]

Another little-publicized fillip in the statistics is this: when analysts at the Centers for Disease Control looked more closely at the diminishing teen-sex rates, they found that boys were having less intercourse (15 percent less from 1991 to 1997), but girls' rates hadn't slowed.[77] The practice that had declined among girls was *unprotected* intercourse.[78] Condom use, not chastity, more plausibly explains the encouraging news about declining teen pregnancy.[79]

In the end, sex education classes may be no more responsible for any sexual "outcomes" than the larger culture in which the classes are embedded. Advocates for Youth, which leads annual summer tours of the European sex-ed field for American educators, has observed that the Continent's relatively low rates of teen pregnancy, abortion, and sexually transmitted diseases are rooted most of all in Europeans' attitudes about sex. "Adults see intimate sexual relationships as normal and natural for older adolescents, a positive component of emotionally healthy maturation," a brief report of the early tours' lessons said. "At the same time, young people believe it is 'stupid and irresponsible' to have sex without protection and use the maxim, 'safe sex or no sex.' The morality of sexual behavior is weighed through an individual ethic that includes the values of responsibility, love, respect, tolerance, and equity."[80]

Of course, inculcating values is a large part of what sex education
is and has always been about. The Right is less shy than the Left
about saying this. Sadly, of the lofty list above, tolerance and equity
are not exactly majority values among American teens. But, Bearman found, neither are love and respect expressed through chastity.
Indeed, an interesting thing about chastity pledges is that virginity
must remain a minority value, and the pledgers a countercultural
clique, in order to succeed. As soon as more than about 30 percent
of a school's students climb on, the pledged virgins start falling off
the wagon.[81]

At any rate, most mainstream professional organizations have
deduced that declining rates of teen pregnancy can be attributed to a
combination of abstinence messages and contraceptive and safe-sex
information; in 1999 the American Medical Association and other
prominent organizations endorsed abstinence-plus education. And
to be sure, for many of these social-sexual changes the comprehensive, or abstinence-plus curricula, can take credit. Still, there is evidence that the most impressive gains of such programs lie in the
"pluses": students' tolerance toward sexual difference, increased
contraceptive and condom use, and improved sexual negotiation
skills.[82]

So how do the abstinence-plusers score in the main event, achieving abstinence from intercourse? Kids who get a taste of the full
menu of sex-ed topics postpone intercourse longer than those who
receive no such classes. But on a measure of virginity-guarding
months, the ab-plusers have done almost as pitifully as the abonlys. According to the evaluation of one "plus" plan, the length of
time students held off intercourse averaged seven months.[83] A kid
who resists on New Year's Eve, in other words, succumbs on the
Fourth of July.

"Criminal" Activities

As the decades plod on, some public-school comprehensive sex
educators work harder, taking risks to teach what needs to be
taught. Others toe the line and feel discouraged. Some quit their
jobs to move to alternative institutions—churches, community, gay
and lesbian, or AIDS-education groups, progressive chapters of

moderate national organizations like Planned Parenthood, or rare innovative outfits like New Jersey's Network for Family Life Education, which puts out the excellent teen-run publication and Web site Sxetc.com.

But nationally influential progressive sex educators are a dwindling crew. It's hard to say exactly how many there are—a few dozen or several hundred. But their voices have been largely lost in the mainstream discourse, with grave effect. Some "outsider" educators, seeing their ideas pushed further and further to the margins, have broached the possibility of shifting sex ed out of the public schools altogether in favor of invigorating public-service media and community-based educational strategies—an idea that others, including me, criticize as misguided.

Some formerly committed teachers have lined up at the abstinence-only trough, ethics be damned. A Minneapolis sex-ed consultant told me boldly one morning in 1998 that "we've been doing sex ed wrong for the past fifteen years." How so? "We say sex is bad for kids, and it isn't." The interview was rushed, because that afternoon she was slated to do a teacher-training workshop— on the city's new abstinence-only curricula. Huh? "It helps me get more business in town," the educator explained. If a woman with these beliefs was now concealing them in order to preach the gospel of chastity to young teachers, I despaired of the next generation of sex educators, not to mention their students.

The Minneapolis teacher was an extreme example of a slow but sure surrender by a significant portion of the sex-ed mainstream to the demands of a brazen right-wing minority. But not that extreme. In the fall of 2000, the super-mainstream National Campaign to Prevent Teen Pregnancy, in Washington, D.C., placed free public-service advertisements in youth-directed publications such as *Teen People* and *Vibe*. Each ad featured a photo of a teenager (ethnic and stylistic diversity dutifully respected) with a large word emblazoned across it: NOBODY, USELESS, CHEAP, DIRTY, REJECT, PRICK. Smaller, far less legible type softened these smears: "Now that I'm home with a baby, NOBODY calls me anymore"; "All it took was one PRICK to get my girlfriend pregnant. At least that's what her friends say." (The prick apparently was not the boy in the picture.)

Some people in the field, including Advocates for Youth president James Wagoner, were outraged by the resurrection of these ugly stereotypes of sexually active or pregnant teens and charged the campaign with blaming teens, whom "society" has denied "access to information and confidential sexual health services—and a true stake in the future." But in one of its mailings, the National Campaign held up as a shield the encomia of teens who (spontaneously?) wrote in to praise the advertisements. "They don't glamorize sex," one correspondent said. "They simply show the reality."

Yes, this campaign did show the reality at the turn of the twenty-first century: shame and blame still surround teen sexuality, and its prosecutors are not only Bible-thumpers but "responsible" sex educators and teens too. The Right also indicted the ads, by the way, for neglecting to pitch abstinence. But Focus on the Family could have blown them up and plastered them across the stage at their 2001 national convention. A pretty, pouty Latina with CHEAP slashed across her bare belly in big bright letters, a brown-skinned boy in a backward cap with the scarlet letters USELESS labeling him—these, better than anything their public-relations firms could have produced, proclaimed the conservative activists' good news: Victory!

The Right won, but the mainstream let it. Comprehensive sex educators had the upper hand in the 1970s, and starting in the 1980s, they allowed their enemies to seize more and more territory, until the Right controlled the law, the language, and the cultural consensus. Sad as the comprehensive sex educators' story is, they must share some of the blame for what the abstinence-only movement has wrought in the lives of the young. Commenting on its failure to defend explicit sexuality education during an avalanche of new HIV infection among teenagers, Sharon Thompson said, "We will look back at this time and indict the sex-education community as criminal. It's like being in a nuclear power plant that has a leak, and not telling anybody."

6. Compulsory Motherhood

The End of Abortion

Johnny and Janey sitting in a tree,
K-I-S-S-I-N-G.
First comes love,
Then comes marriage,
Then comes Janey with a baby carriage.
                    —children's rhyme

Abstinence education is the good cop of conservative "family re-planning," by which human relations are restored to what the Right views as a "traditional" structure (Dad on top, Mom next, kids below that) and sex to its "traditional" function, procreation. But if a teen cannot be persuaded to tarry in celibate, parent-controlled child-hood and insists on being both young and sexual, the Right has a bad cop. Its job is to barricade the option of abortion. This imposes a sentence of immediate and irrevocable adulthood on any "child" who crosses the sexual line and makes a mistake. Compulsory moth-erhood can be effected in two ways, legally and culturally.

On the legal front, the anti-abortion movement has had a mixed record, with many of its initiatives found unconstitutional. Never-theless, its record over nearly thirty years shows a dogged climb to-ward success. Almost from the moment the Supreme Court legal-ized abortion in *Roe v. Wade* in 1973, lobbyists and activists have kept up a steady presence in every legislative chamber, including Congress. Only four years after the ruling, President Jimmy Carter

117

signed the Hyde Amendment prohibiting federal Medicaid funding for abortion, which hit the youngest and poorest women—who also happened to be women of color—especially hard.[1] Hyde's first fatality was Rosie Jimenez, a twenty-seven-year-old single Texan mother receiving welfare and Medicaid while working in an electronics factory and going to college part time. She died after an illegal abortion, with a seven-hundred-dollar scholarship check in her pocket, having chosen her education over paying for a legal procedure.[2]

By 2001, thirty-two states required parental involvement, either notification or consent, in a minor's getting an abortion[3] (in one of the last holdouts, Vermont, a Republican takeover of the House of Representatives released a bill from the committee where it had been locked up by Democrats for a decade). That year, the Supreme Court ruled unconstitutional Nebraska's law prohibiting so-called partial-birth abortion by a slim five-to-four majority, but anti-abortionists went immediately back to work in the states to craft legislation that would pass constitutional muster. The next Supreme Court appointment, which is likely to occur during the antichoice George W. Bush administration, could bring the fragile edifice of abortion rights down.

When they aren't walking the statehouse halls, anti-abortion activists are on the pavements, outside the clinics, shouting and praying.[4] Their protests are not always lawful. From 1993 to 1997, the Justice Department recorded more than fifty bombings and arson attacks at abortion clinics,[5] and from 1993 to 1999, seven people, including clinic workers and doctors, were killed by anti-abortion terrorism.[6]

Still, considering the amount of clamor it raised, the antichoice movement has achieved a monumental, and paradoxical, triumph in the decades after *Roe*: *it has wrought a near-total public silence on the subject of abortion in the discourse of teen sex.*

Moral Rights

In spite of the significant increases in expense, danger, and worry that their laws have exacted on young women seeking abortions, antichoicers have not achieved their main goal: to stop teen sex and abortions. Studies in the 1990s showed that the majority of girls throughout the world have sex in their teens,[7] and, while abortion rates are dropping, primarily because of increased use of condoms to prevent HIV transmission, American teens still get abortions at almost the rate they did just after *Roe*;[8] women under twenty are involved in about 30 percent of all surgically terminated pregnancies.[9] Moreover, women continue to procure abortions at strikingly similar rates worldwide, whether or not the procedure is legal[10]— just like American women before *Roe*, who put their lives in the hands of barbers and gangsters to terminate unwanted pregnancies. (In the 1950s, illegal abortions killed an estimated five thousand to ten thousand women a year.)[11] In most developed countries, the surgical termination of a pregnancy is a legal, normal part of women's reproductive lives.

Even opponents of abortion have abortions. According to the Alan Guttmacher Institute, "Catholic women have an abortion rate 29% higher than Protestant women, and one in five women having abortions are born-again or Evangelical Christians."[12] Yet the American Right's unceasing condemnation, expressed in sentimental language, illustrated with mutilated viscera, and enforced with fatal bullets, has transformed the emotional and moral conception of abortion no less than the practicalities of getting one. By the beginning of the twenty-first century, one can hardly speak of abortion without a note of deep misgiving or regret, if one speaks of it at all. "Abortion on demand and without apology," a feminist demand before *Roe*, is as rare in 1999 as it was in 1959. What this means for unmarried teens is that unwanted pregnancy has regained its age-old resonance of sin and doom, and motherhood again has come to feel like the near-inevitable price of sexual pleasure.

Although the right to terminate a pregnancy is still protected by the Constitution and polls show that support for choice has not significantly waned overall,[13] the support is more qualified.[14] Most important, according to an annual study conducted by the University of California at Los Angeles, among incoming college freshmen (the very women most likely to need abortions) support for choice has declined every year except one since 1990.[15]

A quarter century after *Roe*, the grassroots pro-choice movement is all but moribund. A splashy Feminist Expo for Women's Empowerment sponsored by the Feminist Majority Foundation in the mid-1990s could find no room for a speech or panel about women's right to choose. In an influential article in the *New Republic* in 1995, "power feminist" Naomi Wolf scolded middle-class women for those putatively blithe "suburban country-club rite-of-passage abortions; the 'I don't know what came over me, it was such good Chardonnay' abortions" and extolled feminists to reconsider abortion within the "paradigm of sin and redemption."[16] At a clinic in Texas, where the Christian "crisis pregnancy center" opened next door and Right-to-Lifers held prayer vigils almost daily, journalist Debbie Nathan observed besieged front-line workers succumbing to a kind of Stockholm syndrome, adopting their captors' doubts as to whether abortion was such a great idea after all.

The Australian pro-abortion activist Marge Ripper called this new tone the "awfulisation of abortion." Under its influence, abortion's proponents become its apologists, espousing the arguments of their antagonists, slightly softened: abortion is an evil, though a "necessary evil." It is a deeply private "family" affair and never preferable to contraception. As the journalist Janet Hadley commented, this last argument implies, incorrectly, that contraception is always reliable and "safe," as opposed to abortion, which is not. This makes contraception the "responsible" option and abortion therefore "irresponsible."[17] (In fact, according to a study by the Alan Guttmacher Institute published in 1996, six in ten abortion patients had been using contraception, but it failed.)[18] As early as 1980, American pro-choice feminists started to cast themselves as "pro-family," some even implying that if the state provided good child and health care, everyone would want babies, and abortion would become obsolete.

By the 1990s, the pro-choice lawyers were still in court, the doctors were taking the bullets. But few advocates of choice seemed willing to defend the ethical position *for* abortion itself—as complex as any serious ethical position—that women's right to terminate a pregnancy is a *moral good*. Few argued that women's right to control fertility, the biological handicap of the female sex, amounts to full existential equality with men; and that the use of one's body against one's will amounts to nothing less than slavery. The only moral argument for choice was made on children's behalf: that wanted children fare better in the world, which is already overpopulated with hungry, neglected, and abused kids.[19]

Liberal Hollywood sure isn't defending choice. Pregnancy panics have long been melodramatic staples, for their obvious tear-jerking potential, and so, for dramatic resolution purposes, are false alarms and miscarriages. But if a pregnancy lasts on screen, abortion is never an option and always a tragedy. Indeed, the A-word is rarely even uttered. On *Beverly Hills 90210,* a young woman and her boyfriend vow not to make "the biggest mistake of our lives" by doing "something we'll regret" forever (terminate her pregnancy). On the CBS lawyer drama *The Practice,* the ambitious, sensible thirtyish African American office manager confesses, unable even to utter the forbidden word: "I got pregnant when I was fifteen. . . . I couldn't take care of a baby. . . . Yeah, I did it. . . . But there's not a day goes by I don't think about it." Whole movie plots turn on babies who in the real world would never get a chance to gestate. Even the ultracynical, penniless, baby-hating, Machiavellian antiheroine of *The Opposite of Sex* and her gay boyfriend reject abortion.

Anti-Abortion Syndrome

These plots enact a psychological "syndrome" invented in the late 1970s by anti-abortion "scientists": "postabortion syndrome" or "postabortion psychosis," a condition of lasting guilt, regret, and physical damage allegedly caused by abortion.[20] Postabortion syndrome has been proven nonexistent. When nearly fifty-three hundred women, about half of whom had abortions, were administered annual questionnaires over eight years, their levels of emotional well-being were found to be unchanged by the procedure.[21] Claimed links between abortion and breast cancer have also been discovered to be unfounded.[22]

But the idea that abortion is inevitably awful has taken hold, particularly among teenage girls. For those too young to have experienced the panic and peril of an unwanted pregnancy before *Roe* (or, in many cases, after it), the high melodrama and black-and-white morality of the anti-abortion script holds particular appeal. A fourteen-year-old black Brooklyn teenager who miscarried told me, "I *never* would have an abortion, because I'd be thinking about that baby the rest of my life." A pregnant sixteen-year-old in El Paso, a wealthy white girl who was a star runner and honors student (and whose maid was going to take care of the child), was having a baby for the same reason. "My mom wanted me to [have an abortion]," she told me. "But oh, I couldn't live with that. Every year I'd be wondering, like, my baby would be this many years old and what would he be like?" Even a teen leader of the youth caucus of the left-wing, militantly pro-choice Refuse & Resist! at the podium of a pro-choice speak-out in 2000, wondered out loud whether her recent abortion "was the right thing or the wrong thing to do." She went on, accompanied by hip-hop hand movements, to acknowledge that her doubts were "probably planted in my mind by the antichoice fascists." She suspected she was being brainwashed to feel guilty, in other words. But she felt guilty all the same.

The little quantitative research on the subject suggests that these girls' feelings are widespread. In the early 1990s, Rebecca Stone and Cynthia Waszak ran focus groups on abortion with thirteen- to nineteen-year-olds. On the whole, the youngsters expressed "erroneous and anecdotal evidence about abortion more often than sound knowledge, portraying the procedure as medically dangerous, emotionally damaging, and widely illegal." The source of this information, said the researchers, was largely anti-abortion propaganda, which was abundant and often targeted expressly at suggestible teens. Pro-choice opinions, they believed, were less widely propagated and less likely to be pointed directly at teens.[23] In 1998, concerned about this imbalance, the Pro-Choice Education Project surveyed sixteen- to twenty-four-year-old women nationwide with an eye toward designing a pro-choice public-service advertising campaign. The project found that while almost two-thirds of their respondents selected "pro-choice" when given the options of "pro-choice" and "pro-life," the proportion of support dropped to half when the women were asked if they supported abortion. "They're for women's rights," commented spokesperson Marion Sullivan, "but not necessarily for abortion."

Young men are also affected by anti-abortion propaganda, which may reinforce the masculine pride of paternity and their belief in paternal privilege, whether or not they want to be active fathers. A significant minority of Canadian and American young men—about a third—told researchers that they believed a father should have a legal prerogative to prevent a partner from having an abortion.[24]

Schoolbook Blackout

If kids are learning about abortion in school sex ed at all, they learn that it is a bad thing. The 1995 survey of state laws on sexuality education conducted by the National Abortion Rights Action League (NARAL) found that only nine states specifically named abortion in their sex-ed statutes. Of these, only Vermont required giving students neutral information on the procedure; the others either forbade teachers from talking about abortion as a reproductive health method or allowed discussing its negative consequences only.[25] In the quarter of American school districts that "Sex Respect" purportedly reaches, kids learn that abortion means "killing the baby" and that its risks include "guilt, depression, anxiety," as well as "heavy blood loss, infection, and puncturing of the uterus."[26] In fact, after *Roe,* abortion's risks plummeted, with 0.3 deaths per 100,000 abortions. In 1990, pregnancy termination carried one-eleventh the risk of childbirth, one-half the risk of a tonsillectomy, and one-thousandth that of a shot of penicillin.[27]

At this writing, you can barely find the word *abortion* in the pages of the "comprehensive" sex-ed curricula, either. Girls Incorporated's *Taking Care of Business,* for "young teen women ages 15–18," recommends using birth control and discusses the relative effectiveness of various methods but does not discuss the medical solution if the condom breaks or the diaphragm fails.[28] ETR's "abstinence-based" curriculum, "Sex Can Wait," tells instructors to discuss the stresses of handling marriage, school, work, and parenting and to suggest the "often overlooked" option of adoption. But abortion zips by in one ominous (and in my view, inaccurate) sentence: "Abortion, adoption, and single parenting are equally complex options."[29] The thorough *New Positive Images,* written by two dedicated advocates of adolescents' reproductive rights, names every contraceptive method, including "emergency contraception" (also called the morning-after pill), but skims over the word *abortion.*[30] (Its authors at Planned Parenthood are working on a new text on teaching about abortion, though it is hard to imagine that many public schools will adopt it.)[31]

Programs for boys, finally understood as the missing link in sexual responsibility, often instruct teens in birth control methods, but especially those aimed at inner-city youth zoom right past abortion to put the emphasis on marriage and fatherhood. With cozy names like Dads Make a Difference, these programs transmit the warning, *If you're going to have sex, get ready to support a baby.* While this might be the right message to young couples who choose to have a child, it assumes they will make that choice, especially if they are poor, black, or Latino. Statistics bear out this assumption: Whereas almost three-quarters of higher-income teenagers who get pregnant have abortions so they can they can go to college, establish a career, and marry before having children, teenagers from poorer families with narrower prospects have less incentive to delay starting a family. So only 39 percent of poor and 54 percent of low-income adolescents terminate unplanned pregnancies.[32] Still, the propaganda aimed at young men jumps too quickly to the conclusion that, because poor teens are likely to *have* the children they conceive, they therefore *want* to conceive them and therefore must be dissuaded of that desire. Hector Sanchez-Flores, who runs Spirit of Manhood, a program with young Chicano men in San Francisco, refuted this notion soundly. At a Planned Parenthood conference in 1998, he reported that fully three-quarters of the guys in his program did not want their partners to get pregnant, and four out of five wanted to share the responsibility for contraception.[33]

If it is curious that comprehensive sex educators, almost universally pro-choice, have seemed willing to throw abortion overboard, perhaps there's an unspoken reason. Besides the bigger holes bored by the Right, there is another, less visible leak in their boat. As we saw in chapter 5, by the 1990s the comprehensives were engaged in a contest to be best at preventing teen sex, not preventing unwanted pregnancies or unwanted children. In such an atmosphere, a call for abortion is almost an admission of defeat.

Access Denied

If abortion is disappearing as a reproductive "freedom," with all the emotion that word entails, it is also a fleeting right, especially for teenagers. By the late 1990s, there were no abortion providers in nearly a third of the nation's metropolitan areas and in 85 percent of American counties, according to NARAL.[34] Almost a third of obstetrics and gynecology residencies failed to teach abortion procedures in 1992 compared with just 8 percent that did not in 1976.[35] And while young women's right and ability to get an abortion declined steadily, their parents' prerogative to stop them increased. As of 1999, parental notification or consent laws were in effect in forty states.[36] Two-thirds of girls talk voluntarily to their mothers or fathers before choosing to end a pregnancy, and even more than that percentage of parents are supportive.[37] But girls who do not inform their mothers or fathers usually have good reason: many have already experienced violence at home and, when they tell, are met with more.[38] Parental notification statutes do not increase family communication, as they are meant to do.[39] Rather, they greatly increase the risks to the pregnant young women by delaying their abortions.[40] In all, the American Medical Association reported in 1993 that "minors may be driven to desperate mea-

sures" by such laws. "The desire to maintain secrecy has been one
of the leading reasons for illegal abortions since 1973."[41] Yet propaganda claiming that parental consent and notification laws protect
minors has been effective. A majority of parents and young women
endorse these laws.[42]

In the late 1990s lawmakers fenced pregnant young women into
an even smaller familial corral, forbidding any unrelated person,
whether a close friend of the family, a trusted minister, or even a relative who was not legally the young woman's guardian, to help her
terminate a pregnancy. A Pennsylvania woman was convicted in
1996 of "interfering with the custody of a minor" when she drove
the thirteen-year-old girlfriend of her nineteen-year-old son to New
York State, where there are no parental consent rules, to get an
abortion. (The young man was convicted of statutory rape in the consensual relationship.)[43] In the summer of 1998, legislation was introduced in Congress making it a federal crime to take a minor across
state lines, from a parental-consent state to one without that regulation, to get an abortion. Sponsors heard testimony from public-
health professionals who called the bill "harmful and potentially
dangerous" and from Karen and Bill Bell, an Indiana couple whose
daughter, Becky, had died from complications of a back-alley abortion because she was abashed to tell them of her situation.[44] Promoters touted the bill as a child-protective measure anyway,[45] but
the name of the proposed law, the Child Custody Protection Act, unwittingly revealed its real intent. The bill, which passed the House in
1998 and 1999, would protect not the child but custody itself.[46]
When abortion is involved, the bill's authors implied, the life of a
pregnant girl is less valuable than an abstraction called the family.

A Premodern Tale

Throughout most of the developed secular world in the twenty-first
century, abortion is considered a normal part of women's reproductive lives. But in the United States, a link between sex and babies,
uninterrupted by contraception and abortion, is now assumed by
policymakers at every level. What has resulted are coercive, ineffective "solutions" to nonmarital pregnancy, single motherhood, and
the welfare dependency that is presumed to go with it, including
resurrected "jailbait" laws and the old-fashioned shotgun wedding.
The political center has shifted so far rightward and the symbolic
time frame so far backward that even mainstream organizations are

adopting anachronism and calling it innovation. At its three-day Roundtable on Adolescent Pregnancy and Prevention in 1998, the venerable social-service behemoth the Child Welfare League took up pregnancy termination in none of the scores of workshops and panels. Instead, the league devoted a special series of sessions to running that staple location of 1950s melodramas, "homes for unwed mothers."

Without abortion, the narrative of teenage desire is strangely, and artificially, unmoored from modern social reality. Instead of sound policy, the anti-abortion movement has rewritten a premodern parable, in which fate tumbles to worse fate, sin is chastised, and sex is the ruination of mother, child, and society. Gone is premeditation in sex; gone too the role of technology, of safe contraception or "planned parenthood." Gone far away is the relief, even joy, of ending an unwanted pregnancy and women's newfound power to decide what they want to do with their bodies and their lives and when they want to do it.

But modern social reality has not gone away, and girls are caught in the middle. In that bizarre match over the morality of single motherhood between a fictional television character and a real-life politician, single mom Murphy Brown KO'd her censurer, Dan Quayle. Asked by pollsters in 1994 whether they would become mothers if their childbearing years were waning and they hadn't yet married, more than half of teens said they would.[47]

Yet on the other, shadowy side of the culture, the taint of "unwed motherhood" grows to a deep, bloody stain. Desperate girls, including middle-class high schoolers with every opportunity before them, hide their pregnancies, give birth in hotel rooms, then swaddle their babies in Hefty bags and deposit them, alive or not, in closets and Dumpsters.[48] For these young women, "getting caught," both as sexual beings and as dumb-luck mothers, is fraught with shame and denial. Abortion has moved beyond the pale, a terrible secret worse than any imaginable fate. For these teenagers, there are no reproductive "options" at all.

7. The Expurgation of Pleasure

It is dangerous to suggest to children, as certain books do, that there is any pleasurable sensation resulting from manual manipulation of the organs, for the force of suggestion or curiosity has led some children to experiment with themselves until they formed the habit.

—Maurice Bigelow, *Sex-Education* (1916)

In 1989, reviewing the definitions of healthy teenage sexuality that she had collected from hundreds of professionals over the years, the veteran progressive sex educator Peggy Brick noticed "a profound gap in adult thinking about adolescent sexuality. Several concepts central to human sexuality [were] missing," she said, "notably pleasure, sexual satisfaction and gratification, and orgasm. Even adults who discount the usefulness of 'just say no' are unlikely to advocate *good* sex for teens."[1] In 1994, SIECUS reported that fewer than one in ten courses mentioned anything about sexual behavior, and only 12 percent of sex-ed curricula "suppl[ied] any positive information about sexuality" at all.[2]

Around the same time as Brick was lamenting the arid state of sex educators' thinking, sociologist Michelle Fine was observing it in practice in city high schools. Struck, too, by what wasn't there, Fine wrote an article in the *Harvard Educational Review* called "Sexuality, Schooling, and Adolescent Females: The Missing Discourse of Female Desire." The piece showed how the official line of sex ed was that girls want love but they'd rather not have sex, and that they consent to sex only as a ruse to attain love. Because this quest was presumed to put girls at risk of exploitation by callow boys and caddish men, classroom conversation concerned itself exclusively with female victimization, sexual violence, and personal morality. On the rare occasion female desire did come up, it was only a "whisper" emerging from the girls as "an interruption of the ongoing [official] conversation."[3] Symptomatic of the problem it was critiquing, for years Fine's article remained the only citation on the subject of desire in the sex-educational literature.

Nothing much has changed in a decade. While desire swirls around teens in every aspect of the popular culture and social life, in the public school curricula it is still a "hidden" discourse. But this hiding, paradoxically, makes desire very much the subject of sex education. Any half-awake student knows what to infer from all those lessons about chlamydia and early fatherhood: desire and pleasure are dangerous, and teens must learn how to keep them resolutely at bay.

A near-universal classroom exercise consists of students "brainstorming" the reasons kids might have sex ("Uh . . . to get a better grade in biology?"). Almost every curriculum includes a printed list of such reasons, similar to that of "Will Power/Won't Power," the Girls Incorporated's abstinence-plus program for girls twelve to fourteen. Whereas the abstinence-only curricula recognize only reprobate reasons for sex, "Will Power" offers motivations both authorized and condemned: "to communicate warm, loving feelings in a relationship; to keep from being lonely; to get affection; to show independence by rebelling against parents, teachers or other authority figures; to hold on to a relationship; to show that they are 'grown up'; to become a parent; to satisfy curiosity."[4] Not on this list or almost any other: *to have pleasure.*

While these texts teach that sex is compelled by emotional need and social pressure, the body they represent is that of puberty and reproduction—one of sprouting hair, overactive oil ducts, egg-shedding uteruses, and wiggling zygotes. In them, physical desire is an animal response to increased hormone production and the species' imperative to preserve itself; at the same time, it is represented as an intellectual and emotional response to powerful propaganda: MTV made me do it. The closest the texts come to recognizing the body of longing and sensation is to deem "sexual feelings" and "curiosity" natural or normal (a small minority tell students that some people are attracted to people of the same sex, usually leaving it to the students to decide whether such a taste is natural or normal). But the ways such feelings might be experienced physically are rarely described; they remain elusive, almost metaphysical. The deletions create a bizarrely disjoint sense of sexuality's relationship to the body. A student might know what ejaculation is and be able to catalogue the sexually transmitted bugs that can lurk in semen but never have discussed orgasm in class. She may come away expert in the workings of the vas deferens, yet ignorant of the clitoris.

Curiously, while most curricula overlook desire or pleasure as a reason to have sex, and while the physical signs of desire are rarely addressed, all classes supply students with a repertoire of "refusal skills" and "delaying tactics" to combat the urge, along with plenty of time to rehearse them in structured role playing. (These tactics don't inspire much confidence in this skeptical observer. ETR's "Reducing the Risk," for example, suggests chewing a cough drop to prevent deep kissing and, to cool down a heated moment, leaping up to exclaim, "Wow, look at the time!")[5] Desire, when acknowledged, is as often as not someone else's or that of the crowd, which seeks not pleasure but, rather, conformity. "Peer pressure" is uniformly high on the list of reasons to have sex.

As for gender, the abstinence-only curricula continue to exhibit what Michelle Fine described a decade ago: the peer doing the pressuring is male; the refuser-delayer is female. Some mainstream publishers set out to fix this bias in the 1990s. "Reducing the Risk," for instance, employs a novel approach: it names one of its fictional couples Lee and Lee, who evince no obvious gender traits and take turns aggressing and thwarting aggression. In Lee and Lee, the ideology of chastity has trumped women's liberation. Now, boys are expected to desire as little as girls.

"The Sex Act"

If the focus of abstinence-based education is the risks of pregnancy and disease, it makes sense that the sexual behavior students learn about is the one that carries the most risk: intercourse, which, unless specified otherwise, means penile-vaginal intercourse. Many of the abstinence-onlys assiduously exclude specifying otherwise. I attended meetings in the late 1990s of a New York City Board of Education committee packed with conservatives by Republican mayor Rudolph Giuliani and charged with revising a sex-ed curriculum authored by the previous, Democratic administration. A large part of one session was devoted to striking the words *vaginal, anal,* and *oral* wherever they appeared modifying *intercourse* in the text. Said one board member, who identified himself as a father, "We don't have to give children any more ideas than they already have."

For educators with a conservative agenda, teaching that sex means heterosexual intercourse is part of the point. For straight unmarried boys and girls, according to them, anything more than holding hands is treacherous and sinful; homosexuality is beyond consideration. (Even for married folk, sex beyond intercourse can be dicey. In their megaseller *The Act of Marriage,* fundamentalist Christian marriage counselors Tim and Beverly LaHaye caution that a vibrator "creates an erotic sensation that no human on earth can equal," putting a woman who gets used to one at risk of finding her "major motivation to marry . . . destroyed." They also warn that the jury is still out on the potential dangers of oral sex.)[6]

For the comprehensives, as we saw in the previous chapter, the censorship of classroom conversation is not deliberate in this way. It represents for some instructors a resigned surrender to pressure from the opposition (the banishment of Surgeon General Joycelyn Elders, for suggesting that masturbation might be discussed in the classroom, stands as a sort of cautionary parable). For others, the shrinking repertoire of topics they are willing to discuss signals a gradual, not-so-conscious absorption of the values behind that conservative pressure. In either case, though, the abstinence-plusers haven't given in all the way. They don't foment fear of all sex or try to persuade kids that sex is a privilege of married couples, like the joint income-tax return and the preprandial martini. In abstinence-plus programs, *abstinence* means refraining from risky behavior, which is to say from intercourse.

That said, abstinence-plusers don't spend much time, if any, discussing the more sophisticated aspects of lovemaking (say, a hand job), because, ironically, a straightforward conversation about a hand job can get a teacher into more trouble than talking about the Good Housekeeping–approved must-to-avoid, even though the former has far less potential of getting its practitioners into serious trouble. The easily inferred message: hand jobs are as illicit as intercourse. Throughout the 1980s and 1990s the comprehensive curricula featured recitals of what sex therapists call outercourse, but most such lists were vague, dull, and short. One suggested to students only that they "explore a wide range of ways to express love and sexual feelings," excluding going all the way. Romantic practices were often specified, such as sending billets-doux. But more clearly erotic pursuits, even hands-off practices like talking dirty on the phone or masturbating in front of a partner, were not.

Erotic creativity in educational writers is decidedly not rewarded in the abstinence era. The author of the first version of a 1997 Planned Parenthood pamphlet entitled *Birth Control Choices for Teens* was brave enough to inventory, under "Outercourse," reading erotica, fantasizing, role play, masks, and sex toys (with the warning to keep them clean and cover them with condoms). But, even though the brochure would not necessarily be used in the public schools, these suggestions were too hot for the organization to handle, and the pamphlet was revised to omit them, leaving only the more staid options of masturbation, erotic massage, and body rubbing. Then, according to a source at Planned Parenthood, the warehoused originals were burned.

Even progressive educators can unwittingly find themselves endorsing intercourse as *the* sex act. Teacher Joan Rappaport, who led a wide-ranging series of discussions called "Adolescent Issues" at a Manhattan private school, was mystified when she heard the course evaluations of her middle schoolers. When asked what they'd learned, said Rappaport, "one girl said, 'Basically, like, *Don't have sex*.'" The other kids concurred. Rappaport spent a weekend contemplating how a program that treated sexuality in a balanced, tolerant, and, she thought, enthusiastic way could have metamorphosed into "just say no."

Finally, she figured it out. "You know," she said, "we talk a lot about AIDS and STDs, we talk about emotions and sexual identities, about different kinds of families, about, well, most everything. We say masturbation is normal and they shouldn't be ashamed or worried about it. And yes, we do discourage intercourse. But we never, ever talk about masturbation as *pleasure* or any other ways of having sexual pleasure."

Now, American sex ed was never conceived as erotic training. Quite the contrary: Most in the field today and in the past have presumed that kids get more than enough of that. These people view the classroom experience as an antidote to the "oversexualizing" commercial media and a coercive peer culture; their own role is as an advocate of informed forethought against the merchants of impulsiveness and of the soberer pleasures of childhood, such as sports and friendship, against the premature pull of genital sex. It is the rare pedagogue who breaks out. The week after that revealing review, Rappaport gave her sixth-grade girls an assignment: "Go home and find your clitorises." The teacher, who was then the mother of two teenage boys, chuckled recalling her students' shocked faces and also understood the hazards of what she'd done: "If I were in a public school, they'd have fired me."

In the end, while the abstinence-plus teachers do not impose the Right's embargo on talking about sex outside heterosexual monogamous marriage, their focus on intercourse as *the* verboten act, coupled with the bowdlerization of nonpenetrative sexual experiences, has an ironic and ultimately harmful effect. Much as they try to *de*emphasize intercourse, it comes to take up the whole picture. The infinitive *to have sex* is restored by default to the exact meaning it has long held for American kids (and presidents)—that is, what the penis does inside the vagina.[7] "To kids, 'to have sex' means 'to have intercourse,'" Rappaport reflected, echoing what many other teachers told me. "So when we say 'Don't have intercourse' and leave out the rest, it's as if the rest doesn't exist. What they get is, 'Don't have sex.'"

When curriculum writers started to comprehend this confusion, they inserted exercises in which students would discuss just what abstinence means. But the main message, planted deep in the vernacular, endures. A Minneapolis sex educator paraphrased his students' definition of abstinence this way: "We did the things with our hands and our mouths and the trapeze and the pony—but we didn't have sex."

In representing intercourse as the ultimate—and, by implication, uniquely "normal"—sexual experience, educators do more than increase the odds their students will have mediocre sex until they stumble upon some other source of erotic enlightenment. Consciously or not, they also communicate the assumptions that sex is primarily heterosexual and reproductive and, above all, that it is always perilous.

Such uninformed sex, moreover, *is* perilous. "When adults deny the full range of human sexual expression and regard only intercourse as 'sex,' students are denied an important educational opportunity," wrote the sex educator Mary Krueger in 1993. "Many young people believe there is no acceptable form of sexual behavior other than intercourse. Operating under that assumption, students may put themselves at risk from unwanted pregnancy or sexually transmitted disease by engaging in intercourse when less risky sexual behavior would have been equally fulfilling."[8] In *Fatal Advice,* the author and AIDS activist Cindy Patton agreed strenuously. The dissemination of information crucial to containing the AIDS epidemic among young people was "made virtually impossible by the restrictions that prevented the discussion of condoms or instruction in non-intercourse forms of sex," she wrote.[9] By 2001, the omissions in abstinence-only education seem to have left a fair number of teens with the impression that anal intercourse carries no risk. The practice, at any rate, appears to be more common than in previous generations, especially in communities that attach a high value to vaginal virginity and among young urban gay men, an alarming number of whom report practicing the riskiest act, unprotected anal intercourse.[10] Such "prevention" of sex prevents real prevention: of disease. As a result, young people are dying.

Bad Sex

The Minneapolis student playing with the pony and the trapeze suggested what the findings of scant behavioral research show. Sexual experience, in kind, frequency, and age of engagement, differs according to a youngster's race and class, as well as her gender and whether she lives in the city or the country. But it can be generally said that fear of AIDS is increasing the incidence of nonpenetrative sexual practices among teens and preteens. By the preteen years, most children have started pursuing eroticized romances. In 1997, a quarter of fourteen-year-old boys said they had touched a girl's vulva, and 85 percent of teenagers had kissed somebody romantically. Almost a third of high schoolers in one California study had masturbated someone else, and a quarter to a half engaged in heterosexual fellatio or cunnilingus. Although they admit to a dearth of statistical data, some social scientists believe that journalists are overestimating the amount of oral sex among teens, especially young teens.[11]

In addition to what kids are doing, though, equally interesting is what the things they are doing mean to them. Whereas their parents' generation tended to regard oral sex as more intimate than intercourse, many kids see it the other way around. One fourteen-year-old boy told a reporter that intercourse implied a "real commitment," but oral sex didn't necessarily mean a relationship at all.[12]

With all that touching and sucking, are youngsters having sexual pleasure, even if their teachers neglect to mention it? That's hard to know. For, while evaluators of sex education programs can measure the impact of contraceptive instruction on birth-control practices or exposure to HIV-transmission information on condom use, they rarely ask the kinds of questions that would help them assess the effect of schoolhouse prudery (or *Buffy the Vampire Slayer,* for that matter) on how sex *feels* to young people sensually or emotionally.

Research on the quality of youths' sexual experience is virtually nonexistent. Getting funding to ask adults about their sexual attitudes or behavior is hard enough; asking minors the same questions is nigh on illegal. Congress has repeatedly blocked surveys of young people that mention oral sex.[13] Imagine what it would be to apply to the National Institutes of Health to find out about sixteen-year-olds' fantasies, their desires, their arousal or orgasm? That, in the eyes of many influential Congress members, would border on sexual abuse.

Still, there's no reason to believe kids are different from adults in this regard. Under the best of circumstances, pleasure takes practice. And sexual ignorance, coupled with sexual guilt perpetrated by parents, clergy, teachers, and public-service announcements, contributes to crummy sex, and to all the emotional "harms" with which the abstinence-only educators impugn adolescent sexual activity. Said sexologist Leonore Tiefer, "It is impossible to separate issues of coercion and consent, regret, neurosis, harm, or abuse from a culture in which there is no sex education."

Some people I've talked with conjecture that current teen sex might be worse than that in previous generations. The stock explanation is confusion: the media say, "Just do it"; school says, "Just say no." My own feeling is, it's more complicated. For one thing, popular culture is nothing if not eclectic in its sexual messages. On one channel the boys in *Queer as Folk* are buggering each other at the back of the disco; on another, the characters can't escape the surveillance of angels. Ally McBeal spends half her day in orgasmic fantasies about her clients and the other half being seduced by her law partners, yet she becomes apoplectic when her roommate sleeps with a man on the first date. The only consistent media message—about hamburgers, headache relief, or a high return on investments—is get it now. Americans of all generations expect immediate gratification of desire, for everything.

This demand to have it all right now may be a leftover from a Sixties culture of unapologetic hedonism. But that culture offered the tools and some instruction in the art and craft of immediate and long-lasting pleasure: drugs, leisure time, and a widespread popular education in sexual technique, from erotic massage to the clitoral orgasm. In one sense, these cultural and erotic changes have taken permanent hold; just peruse the self-help shelves if you don't think so (not to mention the pornography shelves in any small-town video rental store). But the reveling in excess that characterized that era has turned to penitence. The Right indicts the counterculture as the handbasket in which we are all being carried to hell, and everyone else nods in sheepish assent. A result: Young people probably feel the sexual urgency their parents felt at their age.[14] But since they get little true pleasure instruction from any source, they are less likely to find gratification.

Although many "sexually active" youngsters actually have intercourse only intermittently, anecdotal evidence suggests that when intercourse is possible, it happens fast, and oral sex is an equally hasty affair. "We used to do all this slow kissy, touchy stuff," a seventeen-year-old who had recently lost her virginity told me. "But now it's like, the minute we start, he's looking for that condom." (At least he's looking for that condom. While 75 percent of teens use a condom their first time, only 60 percent say they use them regularly.) Long Island, New York, middle school guidance counselor Deb Rakowsky asked one ninth-grade girl what sex was to her. "It's, like, the boy puts it in you and moves around for about three minutes," she replied. How does it feel to her? The girl shrugged. "If that's her idea of sex," Rakowsky told me, "I think it's pretty sad."

Regret

Of at least one phenomenon we have plenty of evidence: kids are having sex they don't want, and the ones who say they don't want it tend to be girls. In the late 1980s, the prominent sex educator Marian Howard announced that the greatest wish expressed by the eighth-grade girls entering her Atlanta sexuality-ed program was to learn how to say no without hurting a boy's feelings. In the two decades that have followed, study after study has been released demonstrating that girls are having sex they don't want, that girls who feel good about themselves don't have sex, and that girls who have had sex don't feel good about themselves. In the mid-1990s, it was reported that one in four teenage girls said she'd been abused or forced to have sex on a date.[15]

Girls are indisputably the more frequent victims of sexual exploitation and violence. But the gender assumptions articulated by Fine play not only into young people's feelings about themselves and sex but also subtly into the ways these research data are obtained and interpreted. One way gender biases are smuggled into research is under cover of a study's definitions, or lack thereof. In one of the above studies, conducted by the prestigious Commonwealth Fund, the questionnaire the girls answered did not define "abuse" at all. The other, from the highly respected Alan Guttmacher Institute, described abuse as "when someone in your family or someone else touches you in a sexual way in a place you did not want to be touched, or does something to you sexually which they shouldn't have done."[16] These studies, in other words, left about an acre of space for unarticulated cultural assumptions to creep in, both the subjects' assumptions and their interpreters'.

If girls are not supposed to feel desire and are charged with guarding the sexual gates, were Marian Howard's students able to conjure any self-respecting, self-protective self-image besides saying no? What, to the Guttmacher respondents, was "something . . . they shouldn't have done"? Nancy D. Kellogg, at the pediatrics department at the University of Texas, San Antonio, has pointed out that teenagers may use the term *abuse* for wanted but illegal sex, such as that between an adolescent girl and an adult man.[17] Or might these girls desire to be touched by a boy but worry that if it comes to intercourse he won't put on a condom? If he forces her anyway, it is rape. But fearing the consequences of arousal is not the same as not wanting to be touched.

In 2000, a poll of five hundred twelve- to seventeen-year-olds conducted by the National Campaign to Prevent Teen Pregnancy found that nearly two-thirds of those who had "had sex" wished they had waited (the report used the unclear terms *had sex* and *sexually active*). Of the girls, 72 percent had regrets, compared with 55 percent of the boys. More than three-quarters of the respondents thought teens should not be "sexually active" until after high school.[18] A spokesperson for the campaign said the poll was evidence that "many teens are taking a more cautious attitude toward having sex."[19] If a cautious attitude were all, and if caution were to translate to safer sex, that would be great. But these data reveal more than caution; they reveal shame. Teens get the message that the sex they are having is wrong, and whenever they have it, at whatever age, it's too early.

The findings inspire many troubling questions. Are these expressed feelings akin to "postabortion syndrome," a second-thought sadness brought on not necessarily by the experience itself but by the barrage of scolding messages from teachers, parents, and media? And why do girls feel them more than boys do? Again, might this be related to the still-thriving double standard? How much of that sexual regret is really about romantic disappointment? Might real pleasure, in a sex-positive atmosphere, balance or even outweigh regret over the loss of love? Even if the sex isn't satisfying, Thompson has found, a young person may look back on the experience with happiness, pride, or secret rebellious glee. But my instinct is, bad sex is more likely to leave bad feelings.

If nothing else, the blank spaces in these data remind us that most pencil-and-paper tests reveal only the slimmest minimum about sexuality. As for informing us about desire or pleasure, that shrug of Deb Rakowsky's student may be as eloquent as all the statistics we have.

The banishment of desire and pleasure is not exclusive to the sex education classroom, of course. As we've seen in the first half of *Harmful to Minors,* the notion that youthful sexuality is a problem pervades our thinking in all arenas. If images of desire appear in the media, critics call them brainwashing. In the family and between people of different ages, sizes, or social positions, sex is always thought of as coercion and abuse. At best, youthful sex is a regrettable mistake; at worst it is a pathology, a tragedy, or a crime. In the secular language of public health, engaging in sex is a "risk behavior," like binge drinking or anorexia. In religion, it is temptation and a sin.

All the while, from the political right to the left, adults call child sexuality normal. What's abnormal, or unhealthful, is acting on it. In "responsible" circles, it is nearly verboten to suggest that youthful sex can be benign—and heretical to call it a good thing. When Naomi Wolf, in her otherwise rather pursed-lipped book on teen sex, *Promiscuities,* endorsed erotic education and offered a few cross-cultural examples of same, reviewers ridiculed her. As you may remember from the introduction to *Harmful to Minors,* an erstwhile editor of this book—the liberal, highly educated mother of a grade-school boy—thought it wise to hold off using the word *pleasure* as far into the text as possible or eschew it altogether.

In the end, there is something giddily utopian in thinking about sexual pleasure when danger and fear loom. But idealism is just the start. How can we be both realistic and idealistic about sex? With toddlers, children, or adolescents, how can we be protective but not intrusive, instructive but not preachy, serious but not grim, playful but not frivolous? Part II will suggest some ways of rethinking our approaches to kids' sexuality and offer some examples of sensible practice by educators, parents, and friends of youth, practice that is based on a simple belief: erotic pleasure is a gift and can be a positive joy to people at every age.

II
Sense and Sexuality

8. The Facts

. . . and Truthful Fictions

I do not know it—it is without name—it is a word unsaid,
It is not in any dictionary, utterance, symbol.

Something it swings on more than the earth I swing on,
To it the creation is the friend whose embracing awakes me.
                    —Walt Whitman, "Song of Myself"

For Freud, childhood sexuality was a relentless quest for intelligence. The desire for information didn't supplant the desire for physical pleasure; it complemented it. From the very start sexuality seeks language to explain itself, the child psychologist Adam Phillips said, explicating Freud, and the experiences of the body inspire more words, more "theories" and "stories."[1]

In a censorial era, Freud endorsed providing children with that language—with information about their body parts and processes, about how babies are made and born. His heirs, the Progressive Era "sex instructors," set out to rescue kids from the ignorance and negligence imposed by Victorianism, mostly in the form of parental reticence, and things more or less opened up as the twentieth century wore on.

Now, as the twenty-first century dawns, as AIDS still threatens and kids need information most, the tide has turned toward telling them less. A strategy of censorship has arrived disguised as counsel to parents to speak more, to embrace their role as children's primary sexual teachers. Here is a "family value" the mainstream sex-ed establishment can get behind, something no one, least of all their conservative antagonists, can disagree with. But a seemingly harmless, parent-friendly idea is likely to have a less than child-friendly effect. I can't help suspecting that the adversaries of school-based sexuality education have been gleefully aware of what would happen if the task of sexual enlightenment were relegated entirely to families: almost nobody would do it.

Polls bear out that suspicion. Parents talk the talk: most agree that sex ed is their job. But when it comes to talking the *sex* talk, few can bring themselves to do it. Among the 1,001 parents surveyed in 1998 by the National Communication Association, sex was the subject they felt "least comfortable talking about" with their children. Kids reveal similar discomfort and often evaluate their parents' efforts less generously than their moms and dads might hope. "The pattern that stands out first is the difference in parental and teen perceptions" of at-home sex talks, wrote the sociologist Janet Kahn in 1994. When she interviewed both generations of the same families, the kids consistently remembered talking about fewer topics than their parents did.[2] The 1998 National Longitudinal Study of Adolescent Health found that more than half of teens believed their parents understood them pretty well. The bad news was that almost half thought Mom and Dad got it only somewhat or hardly at all. The same survey discovered that nearly 85 percent of mothers disapproved of their teens having sexual intercourse and had communicated this value to their sons and daughters.[3] Under the circumstances, not every mom makes the perfectly askable confidante for a sexually active young person.

Even sexually "progressive" parents aren't problem-free. In the late 1960s, when my mother started suggesting I get a diaphragm, I did not quite need a diaphragm. But rather than explain to her that while I was sleeping with my boyfriend, I was still a "technical virgin," I instructed her in full-decibel fury to mind her own bleeping business. Laudable protective parental instincts notwithstanding, an intimate consensual sexual relationship, including one between minors, is private business.

Children absorb from their families attitudes toward love, the body, authority, and equality; they are trained in tolerance and kindness or their opposite at home. A few live in families comfortable enough to discuss the nitty-gritty details of sex. But the vast majority learn these from the wider world. In Uganda, the *Denver Post* reported, an ambitious national AIDS-education campaign asked rural villagers to overcome their modesty and "talk straight" to their kids. Skeptical about this expectation, the reporter pointed out that "mothers across the globe . . . find it difficult to talk to their children about sex." But the Africans, she reported, already had a custom that circumvented parental embarrassment. A Zimbabwean mother explained: "The aunties talk to the children."[4]

While teens tell people carrying clipboards that they wish their parents would discuss sexuality more, I believe that given the choice, they'd rather talk to the aunties. Chalk it up to the incest taboo: children don't want to know about their parents' sex lives and, from the moment they might conceivably have a sex life, they usually don't want Mom and Dad to know about theirs. This is why "sex instruction" was invented a hundred years ago. Sex-ed teachers are the aunties, professionalized.

Will the real sex educators please stand up? Mom and Dad aren't talking, and as we saw in chapter 5, the federally funded aunties aren't talking, except to read from their two-sentence script, "Just say no. Get married." Where is a youngster to turn? The bookstores and libraries hold pitifully few sex and relationship advice books that are comprehensive, sex-positive, and fun to read, even though the market is crying out for more. (On amazon.com, which retails hundreds of thousands of titles, such volumes as Mavis Gallant's funny, unfettered *It's a Girl Thing* consistently achieved sales rankings in the top few thousand, even years after its first publication. Wrote one young reviewer: "The best book I ever read!")[5] Some teen girls' magazines offer straightforward contraceptive and sexual-health information, but their messages of autonomy and body-acceptance are marred by self-esteem-busting photos of skinny models, features about dieting, and a general editorial bent toward boy-craziness. Editors are also constrained by threats of ad boycotts from religious conservative organizations; such a boycott was the coup de grâce that put *Savvy* under. For boys—who, publishing wisdom holds, do not read about relationships or themselves—there's almost nothing on the newsstands.

The Facts

Luckily, just as the sources of information about sex dried up in the earthbound institutions of the public school and publishing house, they started proliferating in cyberspace, where kids are wont to read anyway. The cheap and wide-open World Wide Web began to offer a bounty of witty, hip, pleasure-positive, credible, comforting, user-friendly sites on sexuality for kids and by kids, as well as those not specifically targeted to youngsters but useful to anyone engaging in sex or contemplating it. (In fact, at this writing the two best recent sex-ed books are compilations of the contents of Web sites: *The "Go Ask Alice" Book of Answers,* from the Columbia University Web site of the same name, and *Deal with It!* from gURL.com.)

Yes, any twelve-year-old with a jot of computer literacy can quickly click to a postage-size photo of a man in scuba gear forcing a female amputee to have anal intercourse with a sea cucumber (well, the sea cucumber is blacked out unless you type in your credit-card number). "Boy, I go on the Web and I'm seeing stuff that makes me feel *Amish*!" exclaimed a member of a group of not exactly prudish propagandists called the Safer Sex Sluts. But in his job as a freelance sex educator, this man, Rob Yaeger, encourages kids to search out all the sexual information they can find. And he knows they can find it, up-to-date and uncensored, on the Web.

Because Web sites are here today and gone tomorrow, the designation of any sort of a sex-educational cyber-canon is impossible. Instead, I'll name names of sites extant at this writing as exemplars of what a good resource should be.

Detailed, Playful, Egalitarian

Go Ask Alice, Columbia University's sex and health information site staffed by a half dozen writers in occasional consultation with the university hospital's doctors, answers hundreds of questions a day from nervous first kissers and unsure bisexuals, HIV-positive teens and those wishing to avoid becoming so, virgins and pre-orgasmic lovers in more than fifty countries.[6]

> I am 16 years old and I have never been kissed and I have so many questions about it, but I am very nervous about it because I think I am really going to mess up," writes Freaked Out About First Kiss. "What is the common age for a girl to be kissed? When you kiss someone, do you both move your tongue at the same time? And where do you move your tongue? God this is driving me crazy. And since I have never kissed anyone, I am afraid to go out with a guy because what if he freaks out when I tell him that I have never been

kissed, and, if he tells a whole bunch of people, I would feel so stupid.

Calm, reassuring, and authoritative, Alice replies: "No need to get your knickers in a twist over your very first kiss—the more relaxed you are, the more enjoyable this event will likely be for you *and* your lucky partner. Nor does Alice see why you need to tell any potential partner about your kissing, or non-kissing, history."

Typically thorough and gently humorous, Alice proceeds through more precise suggestions for kissing practice. She resolutely resists defining normal behavior, even though "Am I normal?" lurks beneath many of the questions she, and every other "expert" receives (particularly the perennials about masturbation, penis size, and homosexuality). "Each kiss will be a little different, depending on many things, such as who you are kissing, how you feel about the person, and what is going on at the time," she says. "Kissing is not a science."

Alice's values are those of democracy, equality, communication, and mutual consent: "Your tongue will most likely be met by the other person's, and the both of you can go from there—figuring out what pleases each other and what is, and is not, comfortable." Although she does not dispense over-the-counter behavioral or medical prescriptions, questions about intercourse or oral or anal sex are accompanied by safe-sex tips. Information on contraception and abortion, STD testing, homosexuality, HIV prevention and treatment, and sexual violence are ubiquitous on the site, along with links to other resources.

Sex-Positive, "Graphic"

Like Alice, and like the best classroom teachers and texts, the superior sex-ed sites combine realism about the likelihood of youthful sexual activity with enthusiasm, but not boosterism, for sex—a sort of sexual pro-choice position. This balance is struck nicely on the home page of Chicago's adult-and-youth Coalition for Positive Sexuality and in its slogan, "Just say yes."[7]

> Just Say Yes means having a positive attitude about sexuality—gay, straight or bi. It means saying "yes" to sex you do want, and "no" to sex you don't. It means there's nothing wrong with you if you decide to have sex, and nothing wrong with you if you decide not to. You have the right to make your own choices, and to have people

respect them. Sex is enjoyable when everyone involved is into it, and when everyone has the information they need to take care of themselves and each other.

Even while they espouse such wide-open values, many of the sex sites post warnings that their discussions might occasionally be "graphic" (this may be to mollify fretting moms and dads or zealous politicians or federal agents). What this means is that the information is detailed enough to be useful to someone who actually intends to use it. So, unlike abstinence-plus educators, who might teach condom application using the ever-firm banana, or the abstinence-only educators, whose goal is to make the condom sound so icky and unreliable that students will reject the whole ordeal of penetration, the designers of safe-sex pages proceed as if the condom is going to be rolled onto a penis, which is then going to be inserted into a bodily orifice of another person. These sites universally discuss a crucial, and too often neglected, component of condom use: lubricant, which renders the latex prophylactic more pleasurable in sensation and less likely to tear. On Just Say Yes's site, an animated limp penis stands up to receive its rubber hat, applied by someone else's hands, then goes limp and starts all over again, endlessly. "Get it on," the text advises, noting the other vital detail that the penis has to be erect before the condom goes on it. The organ, by the way, is healthy-looking but not intimidatingly large.

Youthful, Compassionate

Equally important in the interactive universe of the Web are the kid-to-kid chats and personal stories featured on many sites. On gayplace.com, a site maintained by the SAFETeen Project for GLBTQ (that's gay, lesbian, bi, transgendered, and "questioning") youth,[8] "Jason—A Story of Love, Determination, Hope, and Death," tells the autobiographical (and possibly embroidered) tale of a fourteen-year-old, "innocent, young, [Mormon] boy . . . struggling to understand myself and my sexuality," who falls in love with Jason, a twelve-year-old in his Boy Scout troop. After some months their "relationship bloomed into a powerful bond of love. We became one in spirit, soul, and often enough, body." Kicked out of his house, Jason runs away, becomes a porn actor, and eventually kills himself. A melodrama, perhaps, but judging from the number of similar stories online, a direct arrow to the hearts of isolated gay and lesbian kids.

Of the estimated five thousand young people who commit suicide annually, 30 percent are gay, lesbian, or desperately "questioning."

Chat on Coalition for Positive Sexuality's "Let's Talk" bulletin board wheels freely, from sadomasochism ("Okay, so here's the question. im [sic] interested in becoming a submissive and then maybe a slave. do any of you know any websites about that? mainly informative, not porn") to a plea for help from a religious boy, "overwhelmed by my hormones," who wails, "Is there any kind of pill I can take or something else I can take to totally stop this sex drive or at least curb it?" He received only one practical response: "All I can say is avoid spicy food."

gURL.com, a Webzine for teenage girls, was founded by two women not so far into adulthood that they'd forgotten either the pain and humiliation ("Those Yucky Emotions") or the sweetness of teen-girl life, including the discovery of sexuality. Along with straight-on info about such physical subjects as the clitoris and vaginal discharge, the zine's interactive Sexuality Series challenges the mainstream media's tyranny over young people's sexual tastes and expectations. "[I]n the world of thinking about sex, anything can be sexy," wrote the Webmistresses in one installment. "This is sometimes difficult to remember while being bombarded with images and what-not from the world which try to tell you 'WHAT SEX(Y) IS.'" Visitors' contributions to a page on kissing included, for instance, "Kissing people's eyelids is really nice, too."

A publication that comes both on paper and in pixels is Sex, Etc. (www.sxetc.org), an award-winning newsletter produced for teens by teens under the aegis of the Network for Family Life Education at Rutgers, State University of New Jersey.[9] Treating issues from open adoption to parental consent for abortion, from depression to whether masturbation can "hurt you in any way" (answer, in short: no), the well-written, good-looking pub strikes a balance between uncertainty and knowingness, feeling and fact. Its racially, sexually, and economically diverse editorial board ensures a wide range of language and opinion.

Anonymous

Although adults have posted Danger signs all along the byways of cyberspace, the online world is actually one of the safest sexual zones. If a young person is inclined to try her typing fingers at cybersex, she can experiment with sexual poses and fantasies without worrying about pregnancy, STDs, or even, for the most part, emotional involvement. If the action gets too hot, she can politely absent herself or delete an overanxious suitor.

The same anonymity that gives cybersex its fluidity and safety also lubricates the dissemination of sexual information. The namelessness of its correspondents, usually flagged as the Web's inherent peril, shelters youngsters from the mortification of appearing klutzy or uncool, slutty or prudish. Questions that are virtually unaskable in person are easily asked virtually. One boy queries Alice about the etiquette of oral sex, specifically, whether to come in his girlfriend's mouth and how to talk about it. The correspondent closes his letter, "I realize this question may sound rather juvenile, but who else can I turn to?" Alice's answer: Discuss it beforehand. Then, when the big moment arrives, say, "Where would you like me to cum—in your mouth, or somewhere else? . . . I'll tell you when I'm about to go . . . or I'll bark . . . or something." Alice congratulates the writer for his maturity in being so considerate of his partner.

And then there are the postings whose responses might save a young person from more than embarrassment. "My boyfriend hits me." "I am turning tricks and want to know if I have to use condoms every time." "My parents hate me because I'm gay. I want to kill myself." On the Web, the lonely can get fast companionship; the clueless, compassionate, nonmoralistic support and crucial practical help. At best, a kid in need can find a community of kindred souls struggling with a marginalized sexual identity, with violence or date rape, hostile parents or depression—and then bookmark it for the next time.

Plentiful, Accessible

Many adults would argue that there's too much sexually explicit material on the Web, in the form of pornography. Doubtless, there's lots. Will it hurt kids who look at it? I asked the constitutional lawyer and writer Marjorie Heins, who has probably reviewed the literature on this subject more thoroughly than anyone else in the United States. Her response (replete with lawyerly and scholarly qualifiers): "As far as I'm aware, there's very little psychological research on the effects of viewing pornography on children at all. And to the extent one can even talk about scientific proof in social-science research, it's my opinion that it has not been proved that there are widespread or predictable adverse psychological effects on kids from exposure to pornography." My own reviews of the literature, scant as it is, come to the same conclusion. Pornography doesn't hurt the viewer, and, especially for a young person trying to figure out his or her sexual orientation, it can help in exploring fantasies and confirming that other people share the same tastes.

But porn offers only one kind of information: rudimentary images of physical parts and the permutations of their display and contact, blessedly free of judgmental commentary (if you don't count "Jessica's perfect boobs," etc.). In my opinion, the problem with sexual information on the Net is not that there is too much of it but that too little of it (at this writing, anyhow) is any good. That's what David Shpritz, a high school cyberwizard at the Park School in Brooklandville, Maryland, found when he went online in the late 1990s, prospecting for resources on sexuality for his classmates. Under the keywords *sexual health*, he turned up some information on AIDS and HIV that he thought might be intimidating to teenagers, a few good pages for gays and lesbians, and a preponderance of advertisements for sexual aids, mostly for impotence. "One disturbing observation," he wrote, was "that even out of the sites that seemed helpful for teens, there were very few that dealt at all with topics like communication or relationships." All he found on this score was "Teen Love Connection," run by two sixteen-year-olds, but it was more like "a dating game or 'singles bar'" than a source of information. When he queried, "How do I know if I am in love?" (incidentally, an extremely frequent FAQ from teens), he received no answer. Said Shpritz, with endearing humility, "I guess it's a good thing I didn't really need to know."[10]

Finally, what's on the Net is simply unavailable to too many kids. While the percentage of American households with Internet access is soaring, and Internet penetration is increasing rapidly, alongside that growth exists a persistent, even widening racial, ethnic, and economic "digital divide." More than half of American households owned computers and 41 percent were going online in August 2000. But fewer than a quarter of black and Hispanic households had Internet connections, a bigger gap between these families and white and Asian American families than existed two years earlier. Not surprisingly, income also accounted for disparities in Web access. Whereas more than three-quarters of households with incomes over fifty thousand dollars had Internet accounts in 2000, only 12.7

percent of those making less than fifteen thousand dollars and 21 percent between fifteen thousand and twenty-five thousand did.[11]

Government and privately funded efforts to provide Internet access to schools and libraries in poor neighborhoods may do little for sex education anyhow. For, under community and political pressure, many of those institutions have installed filtering software, and Congress has required it on every publicly owned computer accessed by minors.[12] Such filters, as we saw in chapter 1, block the very information that might forestall a pregnancy or HIV infection or help a kid extricate herself from an abusive relationship. To get the facts, kids need freedom.

Truthful Fictions

Another thing Freud observed was that when factual information is unavailable or improbable, the child's sexual impulse turns to the invention of explanatory "theories." Child sexuality, commented Adam Phillips, "partly took the form of a hunger for coherent narrative, the satisfying fiction."[13]

Such narratives are more than stand-ins for the truth. Because so much of sexuality resides in the interstices between the body and what can be said about it in a textbook, these inventions are also the truth. Children need two kinds of information: the "facts" and the truthful "fictions," the stories and fantasies that carry the meanings of love, romance, and desire.

The purpose of this book is not to exegize sexuality in commercial culture at the turn of the twenty-first century. Suffice it to say, images of the erotic are myriad and complex enough to allow critics to decry the dearth of sexual "realism" and, simultaneously, the surfeit of explicitness in prime-time TV and Hollywood, including such teen-steam dramas as *Dawson's Creek, Buffy the Vampire Slayer,* and *Felicity.* Television sex, it is true, is "unrealistic" in one way: nobody is fat or disabled or even pimply (even old people are beautiful), nobody pulls out a condom in the heat of passion—and the passion is almost always heated. On the other hand, the young people on these programs are engaging in "realistic" sex practically full-time, including awkward kisses, pauses to ask for permission (on *Felicity*), unwanted pregnancies, and, needless to say, betrayals, heartbreaks, and postsex postmortems at regular intervals.

Yet, notwithstanding the prodigious quantity of sexual jokes and stories, the quality of the product is drudgingly uniform—

"either a romantic greeting card . . . or a nasty, brutish act of aggression," as the critic Stephen Holden described Hollywood's limited fare.[14] Advertising is equally niggardly, leaving consumers wishing they lived inside perfect bodies engaged in perfect seductions, like those Calvin Klein swimmers who kiss and touch underwater and need never even come up for air.

Perhaps, like pornography, Hollywood and popular music should be expected to provide little more than the crude elements of fantasy, leaving the viewer or listener to fill in the feelings. My own first sex-educational text, deciphered (not always successfully) at great length with my sixth-grade best friend, was *Peyton Place.* A few years later, I pored over the more instructive, but in its way no less melodramatic, *Penthouse,* left in plain-enough sight by the enviably worldly family in whose modern, art-filled house I babysat. Of course, like every other person in the developed world in the twentieth century, I learned to kiss from the movies.

But if most of the commercial culture speaks the language of the erotic like a tourist thumbing through a phrase book, there is more for kids to read and see. In school, sex education can surely be integrated into the whole curriculum, not just into biology and "health." If sexual education is an education in speaking and feeling as well as doing, then sex ed should fall under what is now called language arts. I offer here a short, though hardly complete, reading list.

For their high-heartthrob quotient, I'd suggest not only the super-canonical poets like Shakespeare and Donne, but Whitman, the joy-brimming democrat of love, Emily Dickinson, who cloistered her longing between the dashes of enigmatic lyrics, and contemporary women poets such as Muriel Rukeyser, Adrienne Rich, and Sonia Sanchez, who sing the cadences of the body while chronicling the struggle to balance dignity with desire, equality with the compelling surrender of love and sex.

To satisfy the teenage greed for romantic narratives, the publishing industry pumps out thousands of "young-adult" novels. But these conform roughly to the same script (as synopsized by my local bookstore clerk and two-years' young-adult awards panelist): "Will he ask me to the prom? No, he won't. I'm going to die. Yes, he will. I'm saved! What should I wear?" But the classics are also plump with melodrama. Cathy and Heathcliff, in *Wuthering Heights,* are not exactly your perfect role models of the egalitarian love relationship, but for longing and passion—phew! Flaubert's description of Madame Bovary's trysts may be obscure to many teenage readers. But never mind. They can gorge themselves on the anticipation and frustration, jealousy and deceit, the despair and ecstasy of forbidden love (not to mention the clothes), as good as anything on *As the World Turns*.

The language of the erotic, like the erotic itself, can be subtle or rough. "When the writer doesn't hit the nail on the head with full-frontal language, it sends the reader back into herself to discover similar complexities," commented the poet and teacher Barry Wallenstein. He recommends, for its veiled sexuality, Elizabeth Bishop's poetry. Chuck Wachtel, a novelist and writing teacher, extolled full-frontal language, which he calls the "ordinary, domestic language of eroticism," such as the bawdy jokes and songs of his Italian Jewish working-class childhood, which ring through his own fiction. In the classroom, Wachtel says, he is constantly reminded of the evergreen capacity of erotic art "to acquaint ourselves with ourselves," no doubt the endless appeal of *Romeo and Juliet* in its many incarnations.

Concerns about exposing kids to sexual materials before they are "ready" were dispelled for me when I watched the firecracker of a poet and impresario Bob Holman teaching a Sappho fragment about erotic jealousy to a group of sixth- and seventh-graders at a middle school literary festival. The kids got it—got the extravagant disarray of emotion distilled into a few bracing lines—enough to craft their own imitative verses. And for youngsters who aren't up to the challenge of "adult" literature, the late 1990s produced a few rare works for young people that explore the nuances of love and sexuality with power, humor, and style. One outstanding author is the hippie surrealist Francesca Lia Block, whose eponymous heroine Weetzie Bat describes with the kind of florid verbosity that many young readers seem to appreciate: "A kiss about apple pie à la mode with the vanilla creaminess melting in the pie heat. A kiss about chocolate when you haven't eaten chocolate in a year. A kiss about palm trees speeding by, trailing pink clouds when you drive down the Strip sizzling with champagne. A kiss about spotlights fanning the sky and the swollen sea spilling like tears all over your legs."[15]

Visual art opens the door equally wide, if not wider, to the feelings and mysteries of sexuality. Pictures can be literally erotic, with bodies in sensual or religious ecstasy or pain. But they don't need to be figurative to move sense and sensuality. When Vanalyne Green, a child from a working-class home, saw and made her first paintings, it was a revelation. "Art gave me a language for things I couldn't feel other ways," including sexual things, said Green, now an award-winning video artist and professor at the School of the Art Institute of Chicago, whose work often explores sexuality. Ann Agee, a ceramic artist in her forties, described with perfect visual recall a dress of her mother's that hung in a garment bag in the attic. "It was a gorgeous turquoise and green, a watery pattern, silky," she told me. At the age of four or five, "I used to go up and unzip the bag and look at the dress and touch it and smell it. It was beautiful and special and secret. I didn't have the language for this yet, but I think that was when I first knew what sex was."

These are seminal developmental experiences. Yet as schools have turned utilitarian, organizing their curricula to produce the high-paid computer scientists of tomorrow, the arts and humanities are being shoved off the program. And when religious zealots search the public libraries like mine-sweepers for every *breast* and *screw,* every scene of masturbation or sex without retribution, and replace them with their dry sermons on abstinence, they do not deprive children of erotic information. Instead, they abandon the younger generation to a broad but shallow slice of sexual imagery—to the Hollywood hokum of puppy love and rape, the soulless seductions of the sitcom, and the one-size-fits-none spandex beauty of MTV. It makes sense to offer an alternative.

Does reading Jane Austen reduce teen pregnancy? Or increase orgasmic capacity? One reviewer of these pages worried that this chapter is too anecdotal, that I don't make a strong enough case for the sex-educational value of literature and art. Apparently studies show that listening to Mozart makes kids better at math, which presumably helps them become those future techno-millionaires (maybe I'm a statistical outlier, but I listened to Mozart as a kid and I'm terrible at math). So perhaps research exists; I confess, I didn't look for it. The point of this chapter is somewhat different: that the pleasures of artistic eros are self-evident, and it also seems self-evident that a rich imagination is the soul of good sex.

The Right, as it often does, understands this well. It is not overreacting to all those art exhibits it deems harmful to minors. The arts are dangerous. That is why painters and poets are in prison under every repressive regime in the world. There is no getting around the fact that the martyred Christ of a Renaissance painting, languid as a lover in postcoital exhaustion, can provide transgressive inspiration.[16] Or that *Romeo and Juliet* deserves the X-rating conservatives want to slap on it.[17] Teenagers who have passionate sex, disobey their parents, take drugs, and commit both murder and suicide—these are decidedly bad role models, engaging in high-risk behavior!

The poet's tongue is that of the lover. He does not pause, when celebrating the realm of the senses, to consider if the content is "age-appropriate." Quite the contrary. I give you Yeats:

> O love is the crooked thing,
> There is nobody wise enough
> To find out all that is in it.
> For he would be thinking of love
> Till the stars had run away
> And the shadows eaten the moon.
> Ah, penny, brown penny, brown penny,
> One cannot begin it too soon.[18]

9. What Is Wanting?

Gender, Equality, and Desire

There is a powerful norm of heterosexuality, and a powerful double standard. Girls focus largely on appearance and boyfriends, boys focus on machismo and sexual gains. To deviate is not accepted.
—**Laurie Mandel, Dowling College, on suburban middle schools (1999)**

Gender starts cutting down kids' experiential options early: a preschool teacher told me the boys in her class refuse to use the red crayon because "red is a girl's color." By middle or junior high school, the gender codes have been cast in steel, enforced both by the "hidden gender curricula" of school programs and by the "feeling rules" kept in check by both adults and other children.[1] Kids, especially during the jangled early- and midadolescent years, are urgently concerned with what sociologist Gary Fine calls "impression management," the personal effort to control and monitor what other people think of you. For the vast majority of young people, social survival is a matter of conformity. And one of the safest survival strategies is to toe the line of gender, assiduously acting the part assigned to the body you're in and steering clear of people who don't.

In school, perhaps more than at home (which is why parents are sometimes appalled when they catch their kids unawares among their friends), both masculinity and femininity are narrow balancing beams, easy to tumble off. Girls must appear amenable to sex but not too amenable. If a girl is standoffish or proud, she is a "bitch."

But if she talks too dirty or behaves too lasciviously, she's a "slut" or a "ho." A boy who does the latter is admired as a "player."

If he does the latter toward girls, that is. Because if a boy is shy or insufficiently enthusiastic about, say, discussing the size of a classmate's breasts, he can find himself ostracized as a "faggot." Masculinity is policed chiefly by boys against other boys, and homophobia is its billy club. "Anything that is feminine, boys learn to reject—sensitivity, empathy, vulnerability," said Deborah Rakowsky, a guidance counselor in a suburban middle school. But this is not just a phenomenon of lockstep suburban conformity. Carol Kapuscik, the mother of a seventeen-year-old male skateboarding fanatic named Max, described how her son participated in casual gay-bashing, even though he had grown up in the sexually iconoclastic Lower East Side of New York, with many gay and lesbian family friends and neighbors (the waitresses at the corner restaurant are drag queens). "Everything they denigrate is 'faggot,'" said Carol. "That's a 'faggot' movie, 'faggot' pants, a 'faggot' video game. I've even heard them refer to certain foods as 'faggot.'" She did not think her son uses the term against other boys but said, "Even though they throw the word around like it was nothing, when a kid is called a faggot, it really has the power to sting."

No wonder few gay or lesbian kids have the wherewithal to be "out" in junior high or high school. As a straight boy who graduated from high school in rural Vermont told me, "Everybody called everybody 'faggot' or 'queer.' But there were no gay people at school." I imagine his second observation was wrong.

The Australian sociologist Bob Connell has pointed out that masculine and feminine styles differ from school to school and among social classes, races, or ethnic groups. Michael Reichert, a Pennsylvania sociologist whose work on boys has taken him both to Philadelphia housing projects and to an elite suburban boys' prep school, noted, for instance, that a working-class boy might assert his dominance by beating up another kid, whereas an upper-class boy would do the deed verbally, with sarcasm (verbal "dissing," of course, is a high art of hip-hop as well).[2]

Teens even stick to gender roles when they dissemble about sex. "Three times more junior high school boys than girls say they have had sex, at an earlier age and with more partners. What does this mean?" asked sociologist Mike Males. "Are a few girls really getting around? Are boys having sex with aliens? Each other?"[3] (In his incredulity that the last could happen, Males isn't unlike the kids he's talking about.) Another study found that when kids lied, boys tended to state falsely that they had had sex, whereas girls said they were virgins.[4]

What may be most consistent about gender norms is the degree of their totalitarianism. A child, said Connell, does have the option to "collude, resist, or conform" when faced with the prevailing gender codes. If he resists, he may reap the benefits of pride, integrity, and a certain liberation. But he will also pay a price. As sociologist Laurie Mandel put it, "To deviate is not accepted."

None of this is good for kids—or for sex. For while young people are doing their damnedest to avoid rocking the boat of gender, there's evidence that gender is sinking the ship, with girls and boys clinging to the gunwales as it goes down. Interestingly, it's not just gendered behavior (what cultural theories call the *performance* of gender) but even gendered *thought* that narrows the sexual experience, to individuals' detriment. Research shows that strong belief in the ideologies of masculinity and femininity makes for bad and unsafe sexual relations. Joseph Pleck, a research psychologist at the University of Illinois at Champaign-Urbana and one of the founders of the pro-feminist men's movement, discovered that young men who subscribe to traditional ideologies of masculinity (for example, who agree strongly that men should be sure of themselves or that men are always ready for sex) are less likely to use condoms. Evidence of dating violence between teenagers is spotty but troubling. Although a certain number of young couples report relationships of frequent mutual violence, girls are much more likely to be the victims than the instigators or perpetrators; they report, along with extreme physical injury, emotional hurt and persistent fear following the incidents.[5] Extreme masculine identity, including the sort that is socially rewarded, has also been linked with violence. In 1986, the FBI found that college football and basketball players, the masculine elite, were reported to the police for sexual assault 38 percent more often than the average male student. Members of prestigious fraternities were also disproportionately involved in sexual violence against women.[6]

Nor does femininity stand girls in good stead for taking care of themselves sexually. According to Deborah Tolman, a senior research fellow at the Wellesley College Center for Research on Women, "Feminine ideology is associated with diminished sexual health." The more concerned a girl is with looking pretty and behaving tractably, the more likely she is to bend to peer pressure from older guys, to have sex while high on drugs, and to take sexual risks such as unprotected intercourse. The "rejection of conventional feminine ideology," on the other hand, "is associated with more agency," said Tolman. The less "girly" a girl is, the more she'll take hold of her own sexual destiny, having sex when, with whom, and in what ways she wants.

Gendered sexuality goes far deeper than social attitudes or behavior. It shapes our very fantasies, which are the wellspring of desire, not only what we believe we should want, but also what, in our hearts and groins, we do want: the silent, menacing male stranger; the reserved but sexually yielding, then voracious, girl next door. Without alternatives to these ingrained fantasies (and again, particularly in the hyperconformist adolescent years) these caricatured desires can impede the process of discovering and accepting the idiosyncrasies of what a person might really want in sex and of finding emotional fulfillment in relationships.

Desire and Excess

Desire is probably the least studied, least understood aspect of sexuality. Where does it come from, how is it sustained, how does it affect sexual response or satisfaction? These questions have largely escaped the inquiry of sexologists, whose main, dubious contribution to the subject in recent decades has been to delineate two modern disorders relating to desire's quantity: "insufficient sexual desire" and "sex addiction" (the former looks a lot like "frigidity," the latter like "nymphomania," though unlike their predecessors these modern versions are said to afflict men as well as women). "Too much" or "too little" according to whom, for what purpose, and compared with what? Sex researchers and clinicians rarely consider the social, historical, and political complexity of these questions.[7]

As historians have shown, the notion of pathology pressing in on the borders of normalcy informs the entire discourse of sexuality. And, just as nymphomania has lurked around the edges of our conceptions of female sexuality, the very definitions of child sexuality from infancy to adolescence also have implied the imminent danger of excess. From polymorphous perversity and that pesky infantile "curiosity" right through raging hormones, childhood sexuality seems always to threaten outbursts of irrational, uncontrolled sexual need. The ruling Freudian narrative concerns the necessity of the sublimation of the sexual instinct: in it, the animal-like infant becomes a civilized adult and enters the humanity-sustaining project of culture. Conventional sexuality education, born at the dawn of the Freudian era, offers rationales for moderation and methods of resistance to this "naturally" pathological, or at least disorderly, infantile desire. And if the current orthodoxy holds that optimal sexual "health" is to be achieved through abstinence, adolescent desire itself is a "risk factor," an early symptom of sexual maladies to come, including not only viruses and pregnancies but also the emotional trauma of sexual relationships, which are by definition "premature." As the federal abstinence-only education funding guidelines put it, nonmarital, nonheterosexual sex is "likely to have harmful psychological and physical effects."[8]

Sex radicals of the 1970s, après Wilhelm Reich, took the opposite tack, arguing that the repression of desire was bad for everyone, from children to entire societies. The goal of liberationist sexuality education, therefore, was to free the flow of sexual energy. But there are few such radicals around anymore, or at least few willing to voice their opinions out loud. Progressive sex educators, whose hearts may beat to the dangerous rhythms of sexual liberation but whose heads strategize for safety, offer a compromise between ideological poles: "The initial step in the sexual limit-setting sequence involves acceptance of one's own sexuality," wrote Deborah Roffman and William Fisher, two progressive sex educators. "Because sexual norms still stress that it is improper for teenagers to be sexually active, acknowledging sexual desire requires teenagers to admit that they are contemplating violation of an important social rule. . . . [But] adolescents who cannot acknowledge their own sexuality obviously will be unlikely to plan for prevention."[9] Know your desire, lest danger get the best of you.

Accepting one's sexuality is no mean task, though. A "desire education" may be in order. And that brings us back to gender. Because gender so profoundly affects both the nature of desire and the ability to acknowledge it, which then affect a person's confidence in acting on it happily and responsibly, such an education would need to be gender-specific. If the following precepts seem obvious, the necessity of stating them is evidence of the current state of sex education and popular opinion. Indeed, simply guiding young people to explore their desire may be, at the moment, a radical idea.

What Girls Can Learn

Desire resides in the body

"How do I know when I want to have sex?" Melissa, the thirteen-year-old daughter of a Washington, D.C., union officer asked her mother. "When you want it so much that you feel you can't not have it," the mother, Andrea Ely, answered. She went on to say that you could always have sex in the future, but once you'd had it, it would change the way you felt about the other person and you could not undo what you had done or unfeel what you felt. Consider your decision, she was saying. It will have emotional consequences. But she was also telling her daughter that the call of the body, if strong enough, was worth listening to—that desire is worth taking seriously.

For some girls, like some Deborah Tolman interviewed, the signals of desire are palpable and recognizable. These girls describe feelings of great urgency and "unmistakable intensity," Tolman wrote.[10] "The feelings are so strong inside you that they're just like ready to burst," one girl said. Said another: "My body says yes yes yes yes" (but her mind, no no no.) Teen girls' desire can have almost flulike symptoms, reported guidance counselor Rakowsky, laughing and shaking her head. "They tell me it makes their stomach hurt, it makes them sleepy, it gives them a headache."

But desire doesn't always speak clearly. Listening requires interpretation. And, sadly, many girls tell us that they don't know if they're feeling sexual desire or pleasure at all.

Writer and former sex educator Sharon Thompson believes it is imperative for girls to learn to identify and analyze desire, because it fuels much-needed female independence. "Here's a young girl and she's feeling excited. She might be excited just in general, about the idea of becoming involved with someone or some kind of person, about being in her body at that time of life." Whatever the feelings, she told me, "it's really important for girls to recognize and expect that feeling and understand there is a sexual component of that feeling. To sit back quietly in their bodies and their minds, and get a sense of all the factors and become at ease with it."

Masturbation, said Thompson, is the first step toward understanding, and owning, one's desire. "One of the things that masturbation teaches is that much of what you feel is in your own body. So many girls elide all the feelings they have in a relationship with one person. They don't recognize that a large part of those feelings are really there already, and they can have those feelings without that person. A girl can realize, 'Oh, I had something before this [relationship].' That [realization] is good and sustaining. It can carry someone through romantic disappointment," as well as help a girl extricate herself from an abusive or destructive, but sexually compelling, relationship.

I asked Thompson if girls should be taught, through books and films or conversations with adults or each other, how to name and classify the sensations of arousal. "It's essential," she said. "A large number of girls have those feelings and have no idea what they are. They only suspect they have to do with sex." When arousal occurs, "they go into a sort of trance state and absent themselves from themselves; they have no idea what happens next. They've been educated to believe they won't have those feelings, and it sends them into this hysteria. If only there was some foreknowledge about the feelings and a permission to have them, they could be recognized, and they could make decisions to protect themselves." Thompson tells educators to take advantage of the feminine culture of "girltalk," the intense, minutely detailed, and endless conversations among girls about love and romance—but rarely, specifically, about sex. "Girls will spend hours and hours discussing what everyone wore," she said, "but does anyone ever ask, 'And did your vagina get wet?' Now *that*," she said, laughing, "would be a useful conversation!"

Crucial to getting that useful conversation going between girls is the explicit message from adults that girls *do* desire and that their feelings can be just as pressing as boys'. The writer Mary Kay Blakely was the dean at a Catholic school in the 1970s where the headmaster each year gave a lecture on sex. "He'd have two glasses on the podium," she recounted. "He'd drop an aspirin into one, and it would just sit there. He'd say, 'This is how girls feel about sex.'" Into the other, the headmaster, a priest, would drop an Alka-Seltzer, to illustrate boys' sexuality. "After that, I'd have a stream of desperate girls in my office," said Blakely. "They'd tell me, 'I'm the Alka-Seltzer, not the aspirin! Is there something wrong with me?'" Blakely assured them that, no, there was nothing wrong with them. In fact, she implied, they were lucky to have those effervescent feelings, and encouraged them to come back and talk more when they were thinking about how to express them.

Fantasy is a way of exploring transgressive desire

As a child, the dancer and poet Flora Martin, daughter of permissive but not libertine parents, had heard little but positive, accurate things about sex. But of course she had no way of knowing what it was really like. So she imagined the parts she knew about, in the imagery of her own childish experience. "I thought intercourse must be great," said Flora, who was thirty-three when we talked. "To have part of another person inside of you, that seemed so . . . comforting. Like being hugged from the inside."

She also had an active, early fantasy life. "When I was about seven, I would lie in my bed and have fantasies about growing up and getting to live on my own. In my favorite one, I had a big apartment with one room. The room was empty except for two things: a huge bed with thousands of pillows and beautiful covers on it, and a refrigerator filled with ice cream and cake. My idea of being a grown up was that you could have sex and eat ice cream and cake all the time."

To me, this fantasy seemed so luscious, but also so *wholesome*, befitting the product of the sensual but eminently sane and upright family I knew. Then I learned from her younger sister that Flora's thoughts ran afoul of one of the Martin family's values. If the Martins held both food and sexuality in high regard, they were snobs about the former. In their house, overindulgence in food was looked upon with disapproval, and store-bought sweets were beneath contempt. For Flora, the cake and ice cream—not the sex!—supplied what the sex therapist Jack Morin calls one of the "cornerstones" of eroticized desire: the violation of prohibitions.[11] In a family atmosphere of sexual openness and liberty, which nonetheless transmitted a sense of boundaries, this daughter was reaching toward what sex can be at its best: a permissible transgression, a forbidden but guiltless pleasure.

A girl can be both a "sex object" and a sexual subject

"My main problem has to do with women being seen as sex objects," Linda Bailey, a nurse, told me and a group of mothers who had gotten together in a Berkeley, California, living room to talk about sex and child raising. "I still have a really hard time with the idea that Olivia might be flitting from one relationship to another sexually, because to me somehow that seems like she would be viewing herself as a sexual object, as opposed to being a whole person. . . . I don't know how she will reconcile being tough and feisty and independent with all the sexy stuff about being a girl." Bailey said that even at five, her daughter was learning at school that girls are (or should be) beautiful, first and foremost.

Can a girl care about beauty and also be tough and feisty? Can she be a "sex object" and also a "whole person"? Unlike many other feminists, Sharon Thompson doesn't worry too much about girls who primp and vamp. "They are trying on different ways to be an adult woman," she said of the problem of "objectification." "It's almost an extension of dress-up. It's not necessarily [developmentally] definitive or bad. When you try on acting sexual, at least it's an admission, a taking possession of a sexual self." Of course, she'd like to see a much wider range of what it is to be sexy in American culture, including lesbian styles, butch, femme, fat, thin, and in between, and so would I. "It's a misfortune that we don't like the styles of being sexual that are most prevalent in our culture," she said, meaning "we" feminists. "But when you put on one of those images, it doesn't mean you can now pretend you don't have a mind. You can still possess other parts of yourself."

Patricia Villas, forty-one, is the Peruvian American mother of a boy and two girls and a food service manager. She lives not far from Linda Bailey (but on the other side of the tracks) in Oakland. She says she's worried about her thirteen-year-old daughter, Moira, who is beginning to hate her body because she is plump. Villas is trying to help her daughter eat more healthily rather than diet or become obsessed with her size. Unlike Bailey, Villas is more concerned that her daughter will find her own body insufficiently sexy instead of overly so. In talking with Moira, she emphasizes the positive value of female sexual subjectivity over the dangers of masculine sexual objectification. Villas believes that knowing herself sexually will help Moira make the right decisions. "I wanted to have sex as a teenager. . . . I want Moira to understand how I learned about my body, what it feels like. I masturbated, I fantasized, and I had sex with boys. Sex is learning about yourself, in the same way as learning about all the other things you like. . . . I told her about the clit. I pointed it out: there it is. I tell her, 'You demand that [satisfaction]. You have needs. You have them fulfilled. And you have pride, you have dignity. You make the choices.'"

Desire alone does not guarantee sexual satisfaction

We are all trained to think that sexual pleasure goes without saying—
and that everyone knows sex is pleasurable. That's why so many
people feel there's something wrong with them when sex doesn't
"work."

But girls don't always have a pleasurable experience of sex. And
too many begin to suspect that it isn't what it's cracked up to be and
that there's not much you can do about it except lower your expectations. "It's not love, it's not even a relationship. It's not really always, like, fun. It's just something that you do," a fifteen-year-old
suburban girl said of "hooking up," which means anything from
light petting to anal or vaginal intercourse. Emotional detachment
such as she describes isn't the only cause of adolescent sexual ennui,
though. Pleasure isn't automatic, even when affection and desire
are plentiful. "It hurt, but it was beautiful," was a common description of first intercourse among girls Thompson interviewed in
researching her book *Going All the Way.*

Asked what messages young people need to hear about sex,
California sex and marriage therapist Marty Klein told me: "Sex
shouldn't hurt. If it hurts, you're doing it wrong." But how do you
get from "sex shouldn't hurt" to doing it "right"? The answer:
Young people need to learn that desire isn't enough, love isn't
enough. Sexual desire is cultivated, and technique is learned.

"This is the thing I am trying to do differently," said Sally Keirnan, one cool California afternoon in late August 1997, when we
talked with her friend and longtime business partner, Terry Rorty,
about raising their daughters, River Keirnan, fourteen, and Heather
Rorty, thirteen. "I grew up in Boulder, with liberal parents. My
mother talked to me about the mechanics of sex—the penis goes in
the vagina, you know—but she didn't talk about pleasure. She did
say, 'You'll like it when you get there.' But I couldn't imagine anything pleasant about it." Sally pushed her blond hair behind her
ears and continued: "The other thing my mother never told me
anything about was that there was movement, or ejaculation."

The two women, both in their forties, live in a wealthy Bay Area
suburb, where they run an import-export business. Recently, they
had taken their girls out to a special dinner, during which they im-
parted some of their experience, wisdom, pleasures, and doubts
about sex, love, and desire. Sally had one "main message": "It isn't

like there's just the act, and you know what to do. It's a matter of discovery. I told them about masturbation. That it's good to do, that I was ashamed and felt bad, but that I did it [anyway] throughout my teenage years." Much later she learned "that it is part of that discovery process. It took me fifteen years to learn to experiment, to figure out what worked for me."

Terry, sturdy and tall where Sally is petite, told River and Heather about the first time she had intercourse. "I had waited until my boyfriend's twenty-first birthday. The thing was, I was in love. But it was awful and painful anyway. I broke out into hives. We had no idea how to do it."

Still, Terry convinced Sally that detailing the techniques of how to do it would be too mortifying for the girls to hear from their mothers, especially in a restaurant. ("My daughter dies of embarrassment if your hair is parted the wrong way," noted Terry.) So while Sally refrained from her intended hip-thrust demonstration, she did mention "movement" during intercourse. The reaction: "They both chuckled, as if they knew that already," said Sally. In spite of the girls' feints of sophistication, said Terry, "we could tell they were sopping it up," and the girls had since come back to their mothers with questions.

At the restaurant, however, they employed every time-honored teenage tactic of deflecting embarrassment. "River's demeanor was like benevolently listening to two old aunts," said Terry. "Heather had a straw up her nose."

Even if the desire for a storybook romance is likely to be disappointed, the desire for sex that accompanies such fantasies is neither wrong nor harmful

"Most early" (meaning high school) "sexual experience in our culture is harmful to girls," declares clinical psychologist Mary Pipher in her best-selling *Reviving Ophelia: Saving the Selves of Adolescent Girls.*[12] In a kind of feminine Peter Pan story of the Little Lost Girls (and also an iteration of work by Harvard social psychologist Carol Gilligan, who saw a decline in female self-confidence starting at around the age of eleven) Pipher argues that girls have an authentic core, which is the flat-chested, soccer-playing preadolescent self. Once inside the adolescent body, inside American culture, however, all the piss and vinegar of that "true self" drain out, leaving girls vulnerable to depression and self-destruction, in need of rescue. The premise of *Ophelia* also underlies much popular advice about and for girls: that sex gets in the way of what they want and need in order to grow up happy and healthy.

There is no disputing that American girls must struggle with all their might to feel good about themselves once they start having women's bodies. But sexuality is both a blessing and a curse in that fight for self-love. In her book, Pipher paints it as a near-unremitting curse, describing the girls who engage in sex as "casualties."

"Lizzie," seventeen, strays from her steady high school boyfriend and loses her virginity to an older, more worldly male counselor at camp. When Boyfriend Number One finds out, he enlists his (and her former) friends in taunting and ostracizing Lizzie. Meanwhile, attention from her summertime lover fades. Lizzie is wrecked, but after a while, she recovers. She returns to her studies and finds solace in solitude and her loyal friendships. She starts dating again, this time "stop[ping] short of intercourse" because, according to Pipher, "she wasn't ready to handle the pain that followed losing a lover."[13]

But Lizzie did handle the pain, quite well. And it's hard to say, as Pipher reflexively does, that it was sex that hurt Lizzie. The lion's share of her grief was inflicted by her fickle, conformist, and sexist so-called friends. She may have been temporarily gun shy after her disappointment, but, as Pipher admits, she had also learned "to take care of herself and withstand disapproval" and "to take responsibility for sexual decisions."

What else might she have learned? Something useful about sex itself from the devilish camp counselor (who was, after all, a more practiced lover than she)? The beginnings of discerning what felt good to her, what made her comfortable enough to receive pleasure, or what might give pleasure to another person? If, according to her therapist, Pipher (and to the canon of advice literature), sex was the trauma and semichastity the recovery, then she had to repudiate anything positive about the sex she'd had with this young man in order for her to heal.

Thompson thinks this orthodoxy is backward, and I agree. Girls, she says, are far more likely to be ruined by love than by sex. A better lesson for Lizzy might have been to moderate her romantic expectations the next time. Then she might be able to glean self-esteem and enjoyment from the sex and emotional closeness of the relationship. Teen romances end, says Thompson; that is their nature. If sex educators and therapists could drop the bias that long-term commitment is the highest goal and the only context for sexual expression, they might be able to help youngsters (especially girls, who are more burdened by romantic illusion) relish such relationships, protect themselves while they last, and bounce back when they are over.

Love and lust are not the same thing, and love doesn't always make sex good

Because girls receive so many messages that what they really want is love (and thus interpret the urge for sex as love), adults who care about girls "should make knowing about and understanding girls' sexual desire central, rather than bury the possibility of girls' sexual desire and agency under relational wishes," writes Deborah Tolman.[14]

The problem is, of course, that sexual desire is not buried under relational wishes only in theory or only by adults. To many girls much of the time, love and lust feel mixed together, inextricable. That's how they feel to many grown women, too, which makes educating their daughters a tough job.

"I understood love as the thing I always was trying for," said Terry Rorty. "I did not understand sex [well enough for it to be] a super way to have love and express love." Twenty-five years after her first sexual experience, which was sexually unsatisfying in spite of deep love, Terry still finds it difficult and painful to sort out love and sex. In fact, she said, she and Sally had been planning the "girls' dinner" for two years, but they kept putting it off. "And really," said Terry, "the reason was that I was waiting to have something intelligent that would be worthy of a mother telling a daughter—and I felt stupid." Her eyes filled with tears. "I still feel stupid." Like many women, Terry struggles between the pull of romance and a solid sense of herself as a sexual agent. When I asked about desire, she admitted, "I don't know if I know when or what or who I desire, really, even now."

She continued: "I realized that after all these [sexual] stripes, I don't feel I have a comprehensive, empowering conversation to have with my daughter. And that was a source of grief. I think what I am upset about is that I am afraid that my daughter is already programmed to make all the mistakes I made, defining herself in terms of a man's love." She went on, with difficulty. "I am still compelled by romance. What do I know about the distinction between sex and love? I can't find a distinction. It's troublesome. It ends me up not very happy a lot of the time."

Sally watched Terry tenderly, then said, "I think that's your ultimate goal: that the combination of the two is the best." Terry glanced back doubtfully. Then, after a while, a look of tentative triumph crossed the planes of her wide Irish face. "We wanted to give the girls a little about what to expect, to tell them some things that were useful. Sally saying it takes some time to get sex right. And me saying love was worth it, but loving someone doesn't always make sex good."

What Boys Can Learn

Boys, it is assumed, are brimming with desire. And, from my vantage point at the back of the auditorium of a residential facility for delinquent boys, during an eighth- and ninth-grade sex-ed class, that certainly looked true. The instructor was a talented young Planned Parenthood educator named Matthew Buscemi, who specializes in working with boys. The curriculum for the day was fairly standard: information about the female reproductive system, the menstrual cycle, pregnancy, and at the end, a film on childbirth. But alongside the official discourse, an unofficial one, a discourse of desire, was asserting itself. From girls, Michelle Fine had heard "whispered interruptions." In this room, the boys' announcements of lust were delivered fortissimo (though they were also interruptions). But like Fine's girls, these boys also communicated something about what was missing. In their case, it was a language that allowed for nuanced emotion, including doubt about sexuality.[15]

Striving for maximal comfort, Buscemi joked, elicited participation from the shyer kids ("What do you start getting on your face when you reach puberty?" I heard him ask a class of sixth-graders and their fathers in another town, another evening. A tentative reply from a boy at the back: "Acme?"). He answered all questions without scolding or moralizing.

In a reform school, where every minute is regimented, such license, coupled with the subject at hand, stirred nervousness that kept threatening to erupt into wildness. The minute Buscemi took out his poster-board diagrams, the wiry kid wriggling in the metal chair beside me was supplementing the lesson with his own supposedly firsthand knowledge, just audible enough for his neighbors to hear. After a while, his zeal grew too great for this private performance, and when Buscemi mentioned the vagina, the boy shot up his hand and shouted, "That the pussy, right?"

"Right, the vagina is the pussy," answered Buscemi evenly, clearing up possible confusion and maintaining his free-floating control.

With this and a patter of similar questions, the boy was surely challenging Buscemi's authority (finally it earned him a threat of expulsion from the room by one of the regular teachers). He was also playing out the perennial conflict in the sex-ed classroom between the teacher's agenda to transmit necessary, nonerotic information and students' yearning for "carnal knowledge." He was dirtying up the sanitized clinical discourse with the recognizable cadences of the street.

But he was also expressing something positive about the masculine relationship to sex (one that, I might add, is often held against boys): its enthusiasm. With each remark, this boy scored a round of sniggers from his peers, along with their own comments, a mixture of appreciation and aggression ("Ooh, I'd like to get my dick in . . ."). But signs of another kind of ambivalence toward women and their bodies also emerged. During the section on pregnancy, a student inquired with touching concern about whether intercourse hurts a pregnant woman or her fetus. Then, during a short, explicit film on childbirth, virtually the whole possible spectrum of thirteen- and fourteen-year-old masculine responses to the female body came pouring out. First, the boys jeered as the couples gazed into each other's eyes and talked about love and babies. Then they whooped with amazement and relish as the camera focused on a woman's spread, naked crotch, which looked indistinguishable from a pornographic pussy. The whoops quickly turned to howls of disgust, or maybe terror, when that pussy transmogrified to an educational, reproductive vagina and the baby's bloody head emerged, followed by a gooey plop of afterbirth. The cozy family scenes that concluded the film brought mostly groans and chortling, as if the boys were either exhausted from the intensity of the foregoing or ashamed to reveal they were moved. I had noticed a few watching the birth raptly, entranced.

Boys learn that they should want sex, always be ready for it, and also be "good" at it. They learn early to pay attention to their sexual parts and to name at least the grossest manifestation of arousal (hang around any group of male seven-year-olds and you're sure to pick up the word *boner* or its local equivalent). But adults give them almost no clue about the potentialities of their own bodies, much less women's or other men's, and even fewer strategies for sorting out the mélange of curiosity, ardor, awkwardness, fear, and awe they feel. As I witnessed at the Long Island school, those feelings too often devolve into thin bravado and sexist cant.

Boys' desire education, then, would be different from girls'. Simply put, the emphasis might fall on the other side of the love-lust divide.

Boys are more than hormone-pumping bodies

While boys feel permission to experience their sexual bodies, they may hardly be closer to knowing the full range of that experience than girls are. From the get-go, they are expected always to want sex. "There is a pressure all around boys to commodify sex. Sex is an 'it,' a thing to get," said Tolman, when we spoke at the early stages of her long-term study of boys' feelings about sexuality and masculinity. She suggested that these demands require a kind of alienation not only from feelings but from the body as well. "Boys are considered all body. But if we really try to understand what their experience is, I would bet they are observing sexuality in a profoundly dissociative way. They are watching, not feeling. I don't think boys are having incredibly wonderful sexual pleasure, even though they are supposed to. They may have orgasms more than girls. And coming is pleasure. But performance is such a big part of it, too. That stinks for women and for men."

Helping boys to connect feelings with sexual performance may contribute to sexual equality, implies Harvard psychologist William Pollack in *Real Boys: Rescuing Our Sons from the Myths of Boyhood*. Rather than charge girls with resisting and boys with refraining from sex, we should recognize that boys are not "sexual machines" any more than girls are sexual doormats, says Pollack.[16]

A girl can be both a sexual object and a sexual subject.
So can a boy

Boys' apparent sexual voracity is not really sexual, Pollack implies. It is a cover for boys' fear of sexual humiliation: "Their behavior is a compromise between a desire for connection and the fears of rejection, additionally fueled by unconscious shameful fears of early abandonment."[17] Well, maybe. Maybe sometimes.

The achievement of equality does not require that we desexualize boys as we do girls. The masculine self-recognition of sexuality is something to be celebrated. Rather, the message to boys about their own as well as girls' sexuality should be that it is as variable as the people in whom it resides, and that any individual girl can be expected sometimes to want sex with a particular person, and sometimes not to. Placing girls on a pedestal of purity is not the same as respect. It only perpetuates the division of the female population into virgins and whores, a division upheld with dreary diligence by our nation's schoolchildren. The task for boys is to listen and discern a partner's clues. (These lessons apply equally to a male partner, if that is the boy's choice. The difference is, other boys don't arrive with a veil of mystery around them.) Boys can also expect girls to listen to them. In this way, neither gender is cast as the permanent aggressor or resister, expert or innocent.

We have evidence that this is already happening and that practice in listening bears fruit over time. A heartening study of sexual consent conducted by Charlene Muehlenhard and Susan Hickman at the University of Kansas psychology department showed that while college women and men often make their willingness to have sex known in different ways, they almost universally understand the cues from a partner of the other sex. And—good riddance to bad myths—"a direct refusal (saying 'no') was not perceived as representative of sexual consent by either women or men," Muehlenhard wrote me. "They seemed to agree that 'no' meant 'no.'"[18]

This is surely good news. The next task is for boys to hear yes and, even more complex, the expressions of desire between absolute no and absolute yes.

"Dirty talk" need not be derogatory

Because boys feel permission to "talk dirty" and girls do not, boys own sexual slang, at least in the coed public. Taught that girls' sexuality is both hotly desirable and repulsive and that their own sexuality must be dominant and cool, boys (and men) deploy "obscene" language simultaneously to express desire and to deny the intensity of that desire by communicating contempt for the girl (or woman) who inspires it. Similar ambivalence may play into the use of feminized obscenities, such as *bitch* or *pussy,* to insult boys deemed insufficiently masculine or cool. Suspecting that for young men dirty talk is mostly a way of strutting and a vocabulary of hostility, most teachers confronting the word *pussy* would criticize and prohibit its use.

Yet in the privacy of their bedrooms, these very same teachers, male or female, might utter the same word with passion, humor, and affection. Sexual language, formal or slang, attains meaning in context. "To me, the word *slut* is a compliment," said therapist Klein. "It simply means a woman who likes sex and isn't ashamed of it."

The point is not to strip boys' vocabularies of "obscenity" but to broaden the meanings they can assign to the erotic vernacular. This can be accomplished only if the context in which that language is used—sex and relationships—becomes more egalitarian, a far harder, longer-term project than expurgating "bad words" from the language. In the meantime, perhaps teachers should not jump to conclusions about the intent behind the use of any given word. By translating *pussy* to *vagina,* without further comment, Matt Buscemi may have succeeded in transmitting the message that sexual slang can be used neutrally.

Sex causes vulnerability. And vulnerability has its benefits in sex

Being tough and casual about sex may protect boys from deep hurt, but it also insulates them from deep satisfaction. The process of opening oneself begins with desire. Of course, boys long for love and for particular love objects, and when they're being honest most admit to fewer hits than misses in their pursuit. Of his first (and in his opinion long-overdue) sexual experience in the early 1960s, a male friend told me, "Oh, I had been thinking a lot about breasts for years—*years*. But it never occurred to me in my wildest imagination that I'd ever have *access* to them." This masculine anxiety that one will be completely excluded from the possibility of gratifying desire has hardly disappeared in the allegedly promiscuous 2000s.

Still, as long as boys are expected to cultivate and express an attitude of "What the hell, why not?" whenever sexual opportunity knocks, they may miss out on learning discernment about what they really want and, in the process, dull the sexual experiences they do have. Wanting more, or wanting something or someone specific, means having more to lose. But potentially, more may also be gained. The vulnerability entailed in true desire has its benefits.

"We like to retell the story of Thetis and Achilles," said Niki Fedele, a therapist who, along with colleague Cate Dooley, heads the Mother-Son Project at Wellesley College's Jean Baker Miller

Training Institute, in Massachusetts. In the myth, the mother Thetis dips her son Achilles into the River Styx to render him invincible as a warrior. But she grasps him by the heel, and it is Achilles' heel that Paris's arrow finally finds, fatally wounding the hero.

The classical interpretation of the myth is to blame Thetis for Achilles' downfall: mother-love makes a man weak, not strong; it is accountable, indeed, for his fatal flaw. But Fedele and Dooley apply a feminist spin. "She gave her son a gift," Fedele explained to a group of mothers in a Saturday workshop about raising sons. "She allowed him to be human. We say, let boys have vulnerability and become fully human."

Whereas Fedele and Dooley assign the nurturing of boys' tenderness to mothers, fathers can certainly do it too. Mauricio Vela, a Salvadoran American youth worker in San Francisco, worried about the pressure on his junior high school sons to be macho. As an antidote, he offered the example of a sweet and soft, though strong, man. "I kiss my boys and hug them all the time. I try to tell them I love them as much as I can." And he tells them in, quite literally, a tender language. "I speak Spanish to my sons because there is more *cariño* in it." *Cariño* means "loving care," literally, "dearness."

Emily Feinstein, a sculptor who drives her beat-up Toyota pickup truck around the boroughs of New York City to teach conflict resolution to middle schoolers, sees their toughness more as a ruse than a deep-seated personal reality. Its origins, especially in the poorer boys she works with, she says, are social and political. "I see these incredibly tender-hearted people who want to make a difference, who want to love each other, and who are systematically taught not to show that," said Feinstein. "They are constantly being put down by the school and the culture. They don't want to be vulnerable to what's coming at them . . . [and] if you don't want to feel criticized, belittled, and humiliated, you take on this posture that nothing matters to you." Adults, she says, often mistake a pose of not-caring for cynicism and universal disdain. She believes the opposite is true. "They feel too much, there's no room to show that, so the posture says, 'Nothing is going to get to me.' They have certain things they care about passionately, where [all the need for belonging and appreciation] has gotten lodged. Clothes, music, hair: these things are desperately important to them. It's where they get to show they want to be loved."

One of Feinstein's main exercises in the classroom is the open expression of caring for friends—what she calls "put-ups," the antonym of "put-downs." Homophobia stands foursquare in the path of boys' showing their affection to each other. But she persists, and the put-ups get closer to the intended mark. "At first, the boys will think and think and say something like, 'You play sports good.'" Eventually, though, they begin to use the exercise not only to assess another person positively but also to acknowledge a *relationship*. "More and more, they'll say things like 'You've helped me with math. You've been a good friend.'" Feinstein thinks the homophobic restraints on masculine affection might also thwart boys' playfulness and tenderness in heterosexual sex—and that learning to express closeness openly could do the opposite.

Tolman echoes this contention, more explicitly about sex. "Boys are given so few tools to be conscious of connection between sex and love—that they, too, are involved with that connection." Still, she is hopeful. "I've just got to believe that it's a human thing to be profoundly connected to another person. And that is part of what we get in sexuality."

Not-knowing isn't unmanly. It can unlock the clues to desire

"If the average male has difficulty asking directions while driving, you can imagine how hard it is to set aside his bravado and ego to ask about sex," commented Alwyn Cohall, director of the Harlem Health Promotion Center at the Columbia University School of Public Health, at a Planned Parenthood conference in the late 1990s.[19]

Months later, in a conversation in a minuscule office at the Columbia Presbyterian Hospital Young Men's Clinic, Cohall's colleague Bruce Armstrong agreed. "There's so little talking among us," said the physician, sighing. That's an understatement. A survey in the mid-1990s of sexually experienced teens found that only a third had talked with their partner about contraception and 40 percent had talked about safe sex, but of those, one in five waited until after the fact to have that discussion.[20] "We hardly ever get an opportunity to hear from each other in a tension-free atmosphere," said Armstrong. Apparently, in bed at the moment of sexual intercourse is not a tension-free atmosphere for lots of teens.

The clinic, which Armstrong directs, provides that atmosphere. "One of the things that's really fabulous about our clinic is that when guys want to talk to a woman about their bodies, our female staff is here for them to do that. They want to know what a woman's orgasm feels like, what does it feel like to have a baby." He paused to talk to one of the interns who help staff the clinic, a young Pakistani American woman, then returned to our conversations. "These are not especially 'sensitive' guys. They're your typical macho-looking, baggy-pants-wearing guys from Washington Heights and North Harlem," the mostly Dominican and African American low-income section of upper Manhattan that the hospital serves. He paused in appreciation of the young men he refers to as "our fellas." "But they ask such piercing questions."

These young men, it seems, have found few adults to talk frankly with them about sex, least of all their families. As I've noted, families who are willing and able are few. But they exist. For one such family, the bottom line is creating an atmosphere where it is okay not to know. That family is the extraordinary ménage that raises Jeremy Pergolese, who was eleven when I met his parents. In two separate, single-sex-couple households, Jeremy's mother, Carol, and her partner, Beth Stein, coparent Jeremy along with their friends (and now legal coguardians) Jed Marks and his partner, David Booth. Three of the four parents are engaged in sex-related professions: Carol and Jed are employed by the same reproductive-health clinic, and David is a psychotherapist and professor of human sexuality. Because of the unconventionality of their family and the fact that they are lesbians and gay men, these mothers and fathers have found it necessary, and more or less natural, to raise an emotionally expressive, sexually informed boy. The ground rule, said Jed: "Whatever he asks, we tell him the truth. And we also tell him stuff he doesn't ask."

What does he ask? "I heard that you can have sex with more than two people at the same time. How do you do that?" (Jed's answer: "Picture three men, six hands, three penises. Jeremy goes, 'Ohhh, I get it.'") Other, more oblique queries have revealed Jeremy's anxieties about his fathers' sexuality. "Dad, do you have AIDS?" he asked Jed in a pizzeria when he was seven. "It was the first time he'd every brought up our gayness on his own," said Jed, explaining his theory of why this was the first such question: Jeremy had learned to associate gay sex with condoms, which his dads keep out in the open, so that the boy can handle them and consider them a normal part of life. But at school the only thing Jeremy had learned about condoms was that they prevented AIDS. And he'd learned from his friends that gay men got AIDS. Although

Jed was surprised and saddened that he and David had missed getting the message across earlier and that Jeremy had had to wonder and worry, the father assured his son that both he and his partner were healthy.

In a midtown restaurant, Carol told me that Jeremy's family offered him ideas of how to live and love in a more conventional sense, too. "In our two homes, he sees two radically different models," she explained. "Beth and I are really domesticated. Over there [at Jed and David's], there's freedom and independence. Jeremy doesn't want me to break up with Beth. He thinks a couple is normal." She is thankful to "the guys" for being so explicit about sex, which she feels shyer about discussing. But, she added, "I'd rather he be ready for the emotional part. What if the girl falls in love? Or if you do? Do you just want to do it, or is it in the context of an ongoing relationship? The brutal fact is, he is not going to wait until he is ready. Most people start having sex when they aren't ready."

Simply being the son of parents rehearses a boy in the comedy and tragedy of loving, Carol thinks. "All the power, love, and fear—the elements that go into making things sexy later—these are there with parents." Saying this, her face softened, like a woman thinking of her lover or like a mother, of her son. "It's a weird setup, but we must be doing something right. Or maybe we're just lucky. Jeremy is a laughy, huggy, kissy, funny, interesting kid. He is not afraid to feel."

David gives Carol and Beth and Jed and himself more credit than this nod to accident. He had parents, too, he reminded me, and didn't end up as open to a range of feelings as Jeremy appears to be. A parent's accessibility to being asked any questions about sex is about much more than sex, David insisted. "If a child learns it is not okay to ask about sex, that translates into 'Don't ask about other not-okay stuff that may come up,'" he said. "It goes way beyond sex. It allows open communication about what is known and what is not known. The child learns that it is okay not to know, to lose face, to be puzzled, to have ambivalent feelings."

Growing up in homes where marginalized desire is "normal" while attending school where it isn't, Jeremy may already be more comfortable with ambivalence and conflict than most children are. ("Your father's gay," a kid jeered at him on the playground. "Yeah, I know," he replied. "So what?") Because he has witnessed a variety of sexual styles and expressions among his parents' friends, and because he may or may not follow sexually in his fathers' foot-steps, he is learning that desire is unpredictable, personal, protean, and broad in possibility.

Gender provides fixed points of reference and defenses against ambiguity and the unknown sexual future. It's not hard to understand why most kids cling to the strictly conformist styles of masculinity and femininity. Challenging the certainties of gender may discomfit young people in the short term, but it can enrich their lives for the duration. Comfort with the unknown may be the most important ally in the interrogation of desire and in its fulfillment throughout a lifetime.

10. Good Touch

A Sensual Education

> I confess
> I love that
> which caresses
> me.
> **—Sappho**

Touch is good for children and other living things, and deprivation of touch is not. Baby mice who snuggle with their mothers grow fatter; lambs who are not licked fail to stand up and may soon die.[1] And what Psych 101 student can forget biologist Harry Harlow's doleful infant rhesus monkey, clutching a clown-faced, towel-chested, light-bulb-hearted surrogate mother, and when forced to choose, preferring to cuddle rather than eat?[2]

Human infants who are not held "fail to thrive," and if they survive, they may become social misfits. In 1915, visiting children's hospitals and orphanages, the pediatrician Henry Chapin discovered that the infants under age two, though fed and bathed adequately, were perishing from marasmus, or "wasting away." It took several decades to identify the other minimum daily requirement: touch. Because this was a presumed distaff function, women were dispatched to the institutions to perform the task of "mothering" (holding the infants) and death rates plummeted.[3] Since then, lack of touch in childhood has been implicated in pathologies from ecsema to anorexia.[4]

Loving touch seems to promote not only individual health but social harmony as well. Tiffany Field, the director of the Touch Research Institute at Miami University's medical school, compared children on the playgrounds in Florida with those in Paris and found that adult touch from parents, teachers, and babysitters was correlated with peaceful and cooperative play among the children.[5] The neuropsychologist James W. Prescott made even grander claims. Analyzing information on four hundred preindustrial societies, he concluded that a peaceful society starts with touch. "Those societies which give their infants the greatest amount of physical affection were characterized by low theft, low infant physical pain . . . and negligible or absent killing, mutilation, or torturing of the enemy," whereas those with the lowest amounts of physical affection were characterized by high incidences of the above. Prescott claimed, rather sweepingly, that his findings "directly confirm that the deprivation of body pleasure during infancy is significantly linked to a high rate of crime and violence." This link is biological, he implied: low touch programs the body to a short fuse and a quick punch.[6]

Anthropologists concur that America is an exceedingly "low-touch," high-violence culture.[7] But America's diversity, mobility, and high immigration probably belie any biological relationship between the first characteristic and the second. A more likely interpretation of these facts and Prescott's other findings is social. A culture that lavishes gentle attention on its young also may encourage tolerance of the vulnerable and discourage physical power-mongering. People brought up to be aggressive and suspicious of intrusions against their own body's "boundaries," on the other hand, will be more self-protective and territorial and thus more belligerent, both socially and sexually.

Sociobiology, in particular the kind that compares humans with other beasts, is of even more limited utility when explaining children's sexual development. Harlow's monkeys might have been like us when it came to clinging to Mama, but they also masturbated in public and would have as soon copulated with a partner half their age as with a peer. Behave that way in America and you could get sent to your room without supper, or to jail.

In other words, human touch acquires *meaning* in a culture, and primary among those meanings is whether or not a given touch, response, or even body part is sexual. Before a Western child has been "civilized," the penis, clitoris, vagina, or anus may be sources of pleasant feelings, like the knees or back, or interesting orifices into which to poke things, like the mouth or ears—not secret or thrilling "sexual" parts. Even claimed evidence of the biological "natural-ness" of child sexuality is surreptitiously meaning-laden. Psychologists and sex educators are fond of pulling out ultrasound photos of erect fetal penises to demonstrate that children are sexual before birth. But what they call a prenatal "erection," thus lending it sexual connotation, may be nothing more than a nervous response to the warm amniotic waves inside the uterus. Alfred Kinsey named a certain combination of infantile bucking, straining, and relaxation "orgasm,"[8] but he could just as easily have observed a baby's face scrunching in consternation and its body tensing in exertion, then resolving into beatific calm while he discerned a distinct odor emanating from the diaper.

Recent fierce contests over sexuality can be read as disputes over the meanings of touch—more precisely, over whether certain touches between certain people are sexual and, if they are sexual, whether they are "inappropriate" and therefore "harmful." Will intergenerational bathing or nude swimming, or sleeping in a "family bed" when a child is small, harmfully stimulate a child sexually? The scant available data on these practices generally say no: in fact, such relaxed family touch and sight are usually found to be benign or even propitious to later sexual adjustment.[9] Yet, in these conservative times, many popular advice columnists counsel parents against them, just in case.

Even people who are skeptical about claims of "oversexualizing" touch cannot entirely ignore them. Parents and teachers know they could face real legal trouble, including the loss of a job, a reputation, or even the custody of a child if they engage in innocent but unorthodox practices, such as breast feeding past toddlerhood or photographing children nude. In Champaign, Illinois, a thirty-two-year-old mother's five-year-old son was removed to foster care in the summer of 2000, after the babysitter called the local child-protective agency and claimed the child wanted to stop nursing but the mother wouldn't let him.[10]

More pernicious, adults begin to suspect themselves of deviance when they enjoy the touch of a child's body. In the early 1990s, a Syracuse, New York, mother was picked up by the police and briefly jailed after she phoned a local hotline because she was panicked by the slight arousal she felt while nursing her daughter.[11]

"That is really weird territory, right?" Chris Carter, a thirty-eight-year-old Chicago Web designer, asked me rhetorically as he glanced over at a photo of his bright-faced eighteen-month-old daughter in a yellow frame beside his computer. "Where culture intrudes about what's proper and what's not, what's healthy and what's not." He shook his head in befuddlement. "I take baths with Lily, and I'll hold her and soap her; she'll look at my penis. Okay. But it has brought up all these anxieties about what is good for her. I don't know. It's good for her to see a healthy enacting of sexuality and ease with one's body, comfort, acceptance of one's differences. Then I am thinking, *Am I doing something harmful to my child?* Like, is she going to grow up and tell her shrink she was sexually abused? And another part of me is thinking, *Boy, am I fucked up, thinking like this!* I keep trying to tell myself, *Just relax!*" Just relax: He might as well consult Mel Brooks the "psychiatrist," who counseled a patient who compulsively tore paper into shreds, "Don't be crazy! Don't tear papers!"

Not only parents but teachers too have been terrorized about touching by the child-abuse hysteria of the 1980s and 1990s that began with false allegations of abuse by teachers at the McMartin Preschool in Bakersfield, California. Preschool teacher Richard Johnson was just starting his career in Hawaii when the papers began to fill with stories of bizarre sexual torture at other schools.

"What a stifling effect this moral panic held over a young male teacher who until this time worried mostly about establishing warm, trusting relationships with all the children in his care," Johnson wrote. "I started to worry and second-guess myself when I went about my once taken-for-granted routines of changing diapers, wiping runny noses, unbuttoning and buttoning a two-year-old's 'Button Down 501' jeans. . . . I wondered about holding and attempting to calm an out-of-control three-year-old in a 'football hold,' as I was skillfully instructed to do during my master's practica. Suddenly, the sense of touch, which has always been such an integral part of my relationship with children (my own or any other I care for) was being called into question."[12] Johnson became increasingly demoralized as he saw such paranoia harden into policy, and he finally left the classroom.

Although most of the earlier sex-abuse convictions of day-care providers have been overturned (and all have been discredited), that terrified and terrifying period left an enduring legacy: a body of policy at all educational levels to guard against even the appearance of sexual touch in school. If student teachers take any courses in child sexuality, they place more emphasis on abuse than on unremarkable child development.[13] As a result, young teachers are on the qui vive for pathology. "My students, who are in their twenties, are shocked when a five-year-old reaches for a teacher's breast. They think he's 'oversexualized,'" Jonathan Silin, a professor of preschool education at New York's Bank Street College, said. "They don't realize this is a perfectly common and normative behavior." These students then get jobs at schools whose rules write those prejudices and misconceptions into "no-touch" policies forbidding male teachers from changing diapers or being alone with children and prohibiting caregivers, both male and female, from holding children in their laps while reading or even hugging a child who has fallen off a tricycle.[14]

Children, for their part, are trained to look for sexual malevolence in every adult touch. Programs such as the popular "good touch/bad touch" curricula have been shown to have no positive effects and plenty of negative ones. They reinforce kids' prejudices against "bad" people (i.e., people of different races or those who wear ragged clothing) and raise general levels of anxiety, particularly in young children.[15] A kindergartner refused to utter a word to her new teacher for weeks. Why? She'd been taught not to speak to strangers.[16] Not surprisingly, the programs make children especially wary of sex, teaching them, in the words of psychologist Bonnie Trudell, that "sexuality is essentially secretive, negative, and even dangerous."[17] They may even make children wary of their own parents. "We're in the kitchen," said a Chicago mother of a preschooler, "and Celia says, 'Don't touch my body, Daddy. Don't touch my vagina.' And I said, 'Geez, where'd she get this from?'" She'd gotten it from school.

Richard Johnson is a member of a small but growing group of educators intent on turning this trend around. The group's writing, collected by Joseph Tobin, a professor of early-childhood education at the University of Hawaii, into an anthology called *Making a Place for Pleasure in Early Childhood Education,* constitutes a powerful, often emotional critique of "no-touch" teaching. Reading it, one is left with the strong feeling that too little touch may be just as harmful as or worse than too much—whatever "too much" means—and that the losers are both adults and children.

This chapter advocates a "sensual education" for children at home and at school. An education in the body's physical responses can and should be mostly autodidactic, but adults play a crucial role. That role consists of two parts. The first, active, part is to touch children lovingly, though never intrusively, throughout their childhoods, including adolescence, and to transmit in word and deed the messages that pleasure is a good thing but that touching others must be done with their consent. The second, perhaps more difficult job involves restraint—stepping back and "making a place" for children's autonomous sensual and sexual pleasure. In that space, children of all ages may engage in masturbation without shame and consensual child-with-child sexual touching without adult interference. As they get older and their sexuality becomes more purposeful, genitally focused, and orgasm-directed, they may explore "outercourse," the techniques of nonpenetrative sexual pleasuring with one another, and finally engage in protected penetrative sex. Information on the pleasurable parts and practices of the body should be freely available but not forced on any child.

While it's important to keep major developmental stages in mind (two six-year-olds playing doctor are not the same as two seventeen-year-olds exchanging oral caresses), I avoid the commonly used term *age-appropriate,* which I find both too specific and not specific enough. As I discussed in the chapters about "children who molest" and statutory rape law, the term can be used specifically to codify "permissible" behavior (in fact, the term *appropriate* often stands in for *licit*), which is then used to indict children: a seven-year-old touching the vagina of a five-year-old is assumed to be coercing her; an eighteen-year-old is, legally, "raping" his consensual sixteen-year-old lover. At the other end, *age-appropriate* is too vague to apply to any specific person: it blurs not only the differences between individual children in emotional maturity, intelligence, or physical development but also the great variety in American family, community, and cultural values.

Masturbation: The Fundamental Sexual Pleasure

Western culture despises masturbation. This goes without saying. Since 1700, when the antimasturbation tract *Onania or the Heinous Sin of Self-Pollution, and All Its Frightful Consequences, in Both*

Sexes Consider'd, &c became an instant best-seller in England, Europeans and Americans have been indicting "self-abuse" as a scourge upon individual souls and bodies and the annihilator of whole races and societies.

In adults, masturbation is derogated as the default practice of the immature, undesirable, and desperate. In children, it represents everything grown-ups envy and dislike about the young: their dreaminess, hedonism, fidgetiness, solipsism, secrets, and endless excretion of slimy body fluids. As sex, it is disreputable. Not quite homosexual but even less heterosexual, masturbation is extramarital, nonfamilial, nonprocreative, meaningless, and eminently casual. And it is antisocial. "The emphasis in the solitary vice should perhaps be less on 'vice,' understood as the fulfillment of illegitimate desire, than on the 'solitary,' the channeling of healthy desire back into itself," wrote the historian of sex Thomas Laqueur.[18]

Over the last fifty years, a few revisionists have held their noses and found something good to say about the solitary vice. The child psychoanalyst Alice Balint in 1953 assured parents that masturbation was "not a deliberate naughtiness, but a help provided by nature against yearning, misery, fright, loneliness, or the excitement induced in a child by overdone fondness."[19] Some brave progressive educators in the 1960s put a more positive spin on the practice. "Parental attitudes that affirm the joys of sexual self-stimulation can help a child to develop a favorable sense of his own body," counseled Planned Parenthood's Mary Calderone. Benjamin Spock started out as relaxed about children touching their genitals as he was about other bodily functions. But in the 1976 edition of *Baby and Child Care,* he felt compelled to raise a small red flag over "excessive" masturbation. Dr. Spock didn't see the problem as sexual. Kids who can't keep their hands out of their pants "are usually tense or worried children," he wrote. "They are not nervous because they are masturbating; they are masturbating because they are nervous."[20] The parents' job was to find and respond to the source of anxiety, not to stop the diddling. But because the good doctor did not, could not, quantify "too much" masturbation, parents were left to worry on their own.

In the 1980s, as we saw in chapter 3, self-proclaimed experts like Toni Cavanagh Johnson emerged, signaling persistent self-pleasuring as a symptom of deeper sexual pathology or even as a pathology in itself. No doubt Johnson drew on dormant, barely assuaged parental fears of self-abuse—but "expert" advice like hers also fueled those fears. A study in the mid-1980s found that while a majority of parents of three- to eleven-year-olds accepted the fact that their children masturbated, less than half wanted the kids to have a positive attitude toward self-pleasuring.[21]

No, self-abuse can't shed its stigma. Take, for example, the extraordinary collective free-association inscribed in the *Congressional Record* of September 28, 1994. That was the session in which Republican members of the House of Representatives called for the resignation of Surgeon General Joycelyn Elders, whose transgression was to suggest, in response to a question following a speech to sex educators, that masturbation was an appropriate subject for classroom discussion. This remark, according to one congressman, was part of a social movement that was "killing the moral fiber of America" and just one symptom of a decline also manifested in reckless driving, an indecisive military policy dubbed "mission creep," and homosexuals in the Boy Scouts.[22] Still scratching her head a year later, Elders wrote a piece called "The Dreaded 'M' Word" in the online magazine nerve.com. "What other word, merely voiced," she asked, "can provide justification to fire a surgeon general—or anyone?"[23]

The Elders debacle left the U.S. government bereft of an indefatigable advocate of children's health, minors' reproductive rights, and comprehensive sexuality education, not to mention rational drug policy. But this outrageous act of censorship had the unintended speech-freeing effect of getting the M-word on prime-time television. And that sort of discussion, say sex therapists, may be key to saving a lot of people, both children and adults, a lot of grief and even delivering them a bit of happiness. Therapist and sexologist Leonore Tiefer, who spends much of her time in the consulting room repairing the damages of sexual ignorance in a culture that demands but does not teach sexual virtuosity, is a tireless promoter of masturbation. "If you're going to play Rachmaninoff," she quips, "you've got to practice your scales." Masturbation is the C-major scale of sex.

To encourage practice, should a parent or teacher remark, "Oh, you're masturbating! How nice! Let me show you a more effective method"? Opinions vary. Few advocate technical instruction. Only one woman I interviewed fondly recalled an afternoon when she was about six, during which her mother and she took off their underpants, examined their clitorises, and discussed the feelings they got from touching them. For the most part, though, American children offer hints of either shame or ignorance about masturbation: somebody has told them to hide it and shut up about it; or no one has mentioned it at all. One clue: Kids invent their own names for the practice (among the coinages I collected: *pressing* and *squishing my parts* from girls, *pulling* from a boy, and also from a girl the strangely evocative *whistling*). Another bit of evidence: After the publication of a young-adult novel in which the protagonist masturbates, the author Judy Blume received a letter from an astonished reader inquiring, Where in the world had the writer heard about *that*? The correspondent believed she was the only one who did it.

Because masturbation often starts early and is unselfconscious in the youngest children, parents do have the opportunity to casually affirm it. The baby's game of Name Your Parts lets parents point out organs of sensation ("Where's your nose? *There's* your nose! Where's your clitoris? *There's* your clitoris!"). But even toddlers deserve some privacy. "We felt that anybody exploring themselves was a very natural thing that inevitably would happen," said Jack Martin, the father of four children. But Jack and his wife, Leah, didn't put their children under surveillance. "I don't remember a single instance of seeing them at it, but I wouldn't expect to," he added. "I wouldn't expect to inquire about it."

The Martins' daughter Flora, now in her early thirties and the mother of an infant boy, benefited from the family policy of open discussion about sexuality coupled with parental respect for their children's privacy. Flora masturbated at six or seven and had orgasms starting at ten or eleven. When she was that age, a thirteen-year-old friend joined her. "We would lay around and take off our clothes," Flora recalled. Eventually, they talked technique. "She must have said, 'I do this,' and I said, 'I do that.' We even made dildos out of toilet paper and Vaseline." She recounted the story without shame or regret; in fact, she spoke with glee.

From leisurely, guiltless exploration, Flora made the first discoveries of her body and her personal tastes in pleasuring. From conversation with her friend, she learned to describe what she liked and hear what might feel good to another person. Together, the girls embarked on a course of self-knowledge and good sexual communication.

Sex Play between Children

Contrary to popular notions, veteran teachers say, today's pre-schoolers are no more interested in sex than preschoolers of the past few decades (when there was less television), though there's some evidence that toddlers who go to school play at sex more than those who don't go to school.[24] My own hypothesis on this last point: Day-care kids have more opportunities for partners and are generally more worldly than their stay-at-home peers; and because they are more exposed to the scrutiny of adults, their behavior is reported more frequently. In any case, the researchers who discovered the greater-than-average activity found no ill effects.[25]

Still, these facts present a problem for teachers: Perhaps more than parents, they witness children's sex play. What, if anything, should they do? Turning a blind eye to the behavior, as the Martins did, could get a nursery or elementary school teacher in trouble. Calling too much attention to it could embarrass a child and get the educator in trouble. The play need not even involve explicitly sexual touch to pose a dilemma. One teacher told me that she had been reprimanded by an administrator for not intervening when a group of four- and five-year-olds enacted childbirth with a doll in the "house" corner of her nursery school room. She thought it was an excellent game, in fact, and, because one child had seen her baby sister being born, impressively accurate. But her student teacher was disturbed (apparently too disturbed to talk to the older teacher about it) and, after a little boy reached between the spread legs of a little girl, complained to the school's headmistress, who in turn instructed the teacher to stop such games in future. The headmistress averred that the play was harmless and might even be educative, but she feared that parents, if they found out, might react as the student teacher had. The senior teacher protested that such a situation offered a good opportunity to educate such parents, but she was overruled. She told me she wasn't sure what she would do the next, inevitable, time such a game occurred. Fifteen or twenty years ago, she added, such play would have been regarded as healthy and unremarkable.

How can adults adopt a less hysterical approach to children's sex play that is at the same time informed by advances in pedagogy, psychology, and understandings of sexual politics since the 1970s?

Stress Friendliness and Safety

When I met E. J. Bailiff in 1998, the wiry, buzz-cut, body-pierced dynamo was head teacher in the Yellow Room for four- and five-year-olds at the publicly funded Children's Liberation Daycare Center on the Lower East Side of Manhattan. Bailiff was also a student at the pioneering progressive Bank Street College, working under Jonathan Silin, an AIDS activist, early-childhood educator, and principal advocate for "making a place for pleasure."

Despite the tie-dyed name left over from the 1960s, Children's Liberation is not extraordinarily iconoclastic or progressive either in philosophy or methodology. So Bailiff struck a balance between her own more libertarian views on child sexuality and the administration's more cautious inclinations. That mix worked well, too, in respecting the diverse families and cultures represented by her charges.

She talked frankly with the children about body parts, childbirth, AIDS, and homosexuality. She hugged, kissed, and stroked them constantly. She sent the kids to the bathroom in coed groups and let them linger (when time permitted) to have a look at each other's bodies. Her rules on child-on-child touch were simple: (1) "Make sure the other person wants it, and stop if they don't"; and (2) "Let's always be safe and take care of each other's health." Very few parents objected to any of these practices in ten years of teaching, she said, attributing this acceptance at least in part to the physicality of child-raising customs in the communities of color that the school serves. But E. J. said she would do what she does even if parents were uncomfortable, because "learning about your body is a big part of learning about yourself." And, she insisted, "you cannot teach a child without touching."

To spend even a few hours with preschoolers is to verify these sentiments. Surrounded by twenty four-year-olds, one is overwhelmed with the evidence of what developmental psychologists call their sensory-motor learning style and by the fact that they not only learn but also express and react—live—deeply in their bodies. In one corner of E. J.'s room, three girls and a boy, while drawing, were singing a then-popular song and demonstrating how to "shake your booty." Sitting cross-legged in a circle, singing about a little red box, a soulful-eyed boy named Keanu spontaneously leaned over, hugged, and loudly kissed the cheek of the boy beside him. Seated or standing beside the children, an adult feels them leaning against her body, like large dogs; in turn, it is hard not to stroke their backs or hair.

"In my room, the bottom line is being a good friend, taking care of each other. And it's about learning to work things out among themselves, without me," E. J. told me. Fights were always broken up, and the children were helped to "use their words" to resolve conflicts. But outright aggression was fairly rare in the busy, sunny Yellow Room. Rather, said E. J., "There's lots of kissing and hugging because there's lots of really strong emotion all over the place." She added, laughing: "There is this one problem of them passing their snot and germs around to each other. So I do tell them, 'Not too much slobbery kissing, please.'"

Robin Leavitt, chair of the educational studies department of Illinois Wesleyan University and a scholar of the "management" of children's emotions and bodies in the preschool classroom, put it this way: "I do think children need to be supervised, so that no child is hurt or touched in a way they don't want to be. Our role as adults is protective. But I don't think for preschoolers, for example, touching each other and looking at each other when they are both willing parties is a bad thing. We think it is, because we get the idea that we're encouraging inappropriate sexuality. But children don't interpret their behavior the same way we do."

Don't Rush to "Civilize"

In its high degree of affectionate touching, E. J. Bailiff's classroom was somewhat unusual. (It's more common to female-run rooms, even in schools with no-touch policies, because women teachers have more freedom in this regard than male teachers. But male nursery school teachers are rare, and many, like Johnson, have been run off by such policies.) This is not to say, however, that the body is ignored in early-childhood education. In fact, argue Leavitt and her colleague Martha Bauman Power, while the school day is consumed with learning numbers and colors, with block play and stories, its primary goal is to "civilize" children's feelings and bodies, to make them obedient, productive, conforming, and authority-pleasing social beings.[26]

Needless to say, it's a good thing to learn to use a fork and a napkin when eating, to wipe yourself after going to the bathroom and wash your hands when you're through. But Leavitt and Power contend that school "overcivilizes" young children's bodies and often with perplexing or punitive arbitrariness. A schoolchild hears an endless litany of physical instructions: Sit cross-legged, not on your knees; don't wiggle. Keep your fingers out of your nose. Move closer; no, don't sit so close. Walk straight, don't hop. The child must adjust her bodily needs and desires not only to space but to time: Eat your crackers at snack time. Be hungry now, not later. Pee before lunch, fall asleep after, wake up two hours hence. In one article, Leavitt and Power tell of a child who cannot fall asleep during naptime and is scolded and excluded from the charmed circle of "good nappers."[27] Educators usually justify such rigidity with the argument that such behavior will be demanded in elementary school. "They say, 'Well, he'll have to sit still at a desk the first grade," Leavitt told me. "But you tell me: does it really take three years to learn to sit at a desk?"

Among the aspects of the embodied life that schools socialize, of course, is the sexual. This is done in two ways: first, by giving children information, answering their questions, or teaching them with more deliberate lessons, including programs like good touch/bad touch; and second, by responding to children's behaviors, their games of look and touch, masturbation, "dirty talk," or physical aggression. In doing so, teachers assign meanings to the ways that children live in their bodies and with the bodies of others.

As we saw in chapter 1, sex educators and developmental psychologists agree that little kids are curious—"alive with curiosity about how their bodies work, why boys and girls are different, and how babies are born and grow," as Planned Parenthood's guide to early-childhood sex ed, *Healthy Foundations,* puts it. To satisfy what they view as the child's healthy curiosity, progressive educators encourage questions by being "askable"; they supply accurate but "age-appropriate" answers; and they use the correct terminology for the body parts.[28]

These are unimpeachable practices. But informing curious minds may also be a way of avoiding children's bodies and their disturbing desires. Larry Constantine, a psychologist whose work on children's sexual experiences has been among the most enlightening (and controversial) of the last few decades, has suggested that a fear of children's sexuality shapes sex education. Lessons lean toward a "cognitive" rather than an experiential approach, he argued, which renders them largely ineffective in getting any message across at all. A four-year-old is a concrete thinker, Constantine pointed out. Like everyone else, she connects what she's told with what she already knows. But what she knows is literal, hands-on. So in her mind the mother's "egg" looks like the egg she had for breakfast (of conception, one child said, "The mommy has the egg and the daddy has the thing to crack it"). Masturbation and bodily pleasures, on the other hand, are common childhood experiences. "The latter sensual aspects are, of course, the ones omitted from most sex education in favor of the former, more intellectual, matters," wrote Constantine.[29]

In other words, schools teach plenty of lessons about the body but they are mostly disciplinary, scary, or intellectual ones. "There's lots of talk about sex in preschool, mostly about dangerous sex and where babies come from. There may even be anatomically correct dolls" or a mother doll that gives birth to a baby doll, said Hawaii's Joseph Tobin. "Schools are not exactly prudish in that way. What's missing—and this is where the left and right wing come together—is pleasure."

Be Circumspect When Naming "Sex"

To Tobin, the preschool teacher walks a precarious line between acknowledging the sexual aspects of certain childhood feelings and behaviors and refraining from the imposition of sexual meanings on things children do that resemble adult sex but may not be experienced that way by the child. "In one way it's good to say sex play is *sex* play," Tobin explained. "There is something that kids do which is the same as what adults do, which is about the body and desire. On the other hand, you don't want children's sexuality to be understood by projecting adult desires onto it." As Leavitt said, children don't always interpret their behavior as adults do.

The adult rush to name and judge can come to an ironic end. "Our terror about sex actually 'sexualizes' behaviors that aren't sexual," said Tobin. At the same time, if adults fear so much that nonerotic touch might be construed as erotic, they shy away from holding or caressing children, especially as they get older. That deprives the children of sensual touch and teaches them to refrain from it as they enter adulthood. In this way, kids learn to associate touch *only* with sex, to the point where they may seek sex early when what they really want is emotional and bodily intimacy. As adults, they may become unable to express love and intimacy except sexually.[30]

Respect Children's Knowledge

Children need help learning to control their bodily impulses and negotiate consent, the same way they must learn to share toys, follow the rules of a game, refrain from hitting, and express compassion. But we don't need to interpret for children everything about touch, because they already have their own, perfectly legitimate ideas. "We need to get over this idea that kids are empty and need to be filled with the wisdom of adults," said Jonathan Silin, of Bank Street College.

Illustrating this principle, educator Sue Montfort related the story of a three-year-old boy in a day-care class. "This little guy said he was going to marry so-and-so, a little girl in the class." Oh yes? the teacher inquired, leaving room for him to elaborate. "First I'm going to kiss her, then lay her down on my cot, take off her diaper, and put her in big-girl pants," the child explained. The teacher might have become upset when the boy got to the part about taking off her diapers; she might have interpreted his idea of touching the other child's naked body as sexual, even perverse. Instead, she let him tell his story his own way—and understood it his way. "To him, that was the ritual of marriage," which "meant being older, being a grown-up"—just like being toilet-trained. Commented Montfort: "It could be so helpful if adults would just listen to the understanding and knowledge children already have and come to them where they are."

Not imposing meanings on children's sensual play doesn't mean never telling them what we think of it, as long as we're not telling a kid he's possessed by the devil or will get warts on his hands if he touches his penis. Children need adult affirmation of the emotions and sensations we would call sexual excitement. They need names for pleasurable touching that do not convey shame and that communicate positive feelings about the sensations those touches elicit. What name can we assign to desire, arousal, physical comfort, or thrill without importing too many grown-up meanings? "A step in the right direction," answered Tobin, "is to call it pleasure."

In the realm of the senses, children are experts. I asked E. J. Bailiff if she does anything in particular to encourage the kids to use their eyes, ears, noses, and tongues. "Look at them," she answered, waving her arm over the multitude. One girl was proudly displaying the purple paint she had just mixed, another was making a face at the sour plum she was tasting; a boy was elegantly trailing his hand through the brownish liquid in the water table. E. J.'s expression asked, "Do I really have to do anything?"

Respect Children's Privacy

It's no mean task to socialize sexuality without prohibiting it, to condone and even celebrate a child's appetites without intrusively participating in their gratification. A way of balancing these imperatives, rarely mentioned, is to do nothing. In fact, much of sex education implicitly, if unwittingly, rejects the child's right to be left alone.

Here is a typical example, from a page of SIECUS's Web site that is designed to help parents make decisions about dealing with their children's sexuality. The page presents situations, then invites parents to ask themselves questions, and suggests the implied meanings and possible outcomes of those choices. "You walk into your five-year-old son's bedroom and find him and his friend Johnny with their pants off," reads one item. "They are looking at and touching each other's penises." Why are they doing this? Because they are curious, curiosity sometimes extends to touching, and touching feels good, SIECUS explains. How should a parent respond? Scolding and banishing the friend only convey blame (and don't stop the behavior; the kids will probably do it again, but hide better). Best, SIECUS implies, is to acknowledge the children's curiosity, tell them to put their clothes back on, because "bodies are private," then invite them to look at some instructional pictures with you. Ignoring the behavior is counterproductive, the page suggests.

The messages about privacy here are complex. On one hand, "bodies are private" implies that consenting children should not share their physical selves with each other. If sexual pleasure is acceptable, masturbation is the only acceptable form of pleasure-getting, but masturbation should be done in bed or in the bathroom, privately. A crucial element in this and most other such scenarios though, is not what the parent happens to observe but the fact that she observes it at all. Mom is presumed to be free to enter a child's room without knocking (wouldn't the door be closed if the kids were touching each other's penises?); she feels free to comment on what she sees. Why not advise the mother to say "Excuse me" and leave the room? That a child might deserve privacy *from adults* is not considered.

I asked Tobin what he thought of the often-prescribed practice of commenting on a child's masturbation, while reminding her or him that such things are private. "I distrust those impulses," he answered, quick to add that adults should not do the opposite and condemn the behavior, either. He suggested that adults might let sex remain a little shadowy, without making it bad or confusing. "Shedding light or rationality on [sexuality] isn't always the best thing. After all, the ideal sexual life of an adult isn't always about being open." Why should it be for a kid?

Perhaps the best reaction to young children's consensual fondling is no reaction at all. At school, that means providing a safe, friendly, nonviolent, orderly environment and then *backing off*. "The best [preschool] teachers aim at a kind of conscious not-doing," said Tobin. "Of course, they are active in their classrooms, but when it comes to desire and its gratification, they mostly want to get out of the way of a child's experience of the world and itself." The same could surely be said of parents at home. Concluded Tobin, "Children need room for transgression away from adults' eyes and without adult commentary."

Outercourse: Pleasure and Safety

Remember those first sexual experiences? Maybe you did it in the back seat of a car, in the local cemetery, or in your own bed—until the sound of the key in the lock had you scrambling for your other sock and splashing water on your flushed face. You were awkward as hell, you hadn't a clue about what to do, maybe you never had an orgasm or you suffered "blue balls" too many times (yes, girls, it's real). But those hours of kissing and touching, plus hours of slumping in your seat during history class and longing for more kissing and touching, made those early sexual experiences exquisite. "We had no place to go, we never knew when we'd be able to do it. We never had oral sex, we never had intercourse. We never even got to take all our clothes off!" a male friend who graduated high school in 1971 told me about his first high school love affair. "But it was some of the hottest sex of my life."

Memory may soft-pedal anxiety and pain, smooth over frustration and coercion; nostalgia heightens romance, excitement, and satisfaction. Indeed, some readers of this passage, especially men, did not concur *at all*. One estimated that maybe "one in 300,000" would agree that awkward teen sex was lovely. In his own life, this man put it in a category with other "ghastly" trials of adolescence, including "playing football, having zits, and eating my mother's cooking." A sex therapist reminded me that sexual "*knowledge, not ignorance, improves sexual satisfaction.*"

Points taken. Still, there was something about those sessions with your pants tangled around your knees—beyond sex's newness, beyond anticipation, beyond the feeling of transgression—that made them great. There was an upside to being clueless about the "right" way to go about it, particularly if, for you, "home base" was off-limits. You were not sprinting down a narrow, well-trod home stretch to slide into it. You didn't have a goal. You were just exploring your bodies and each other.

Sex therapists use the term *outercourse* for the infinite collection of acts that can be done with the body to create sensual and sexual pleasure but that do not include penetration.[31] But outercourse doesn't even have to include two bodies touching. Writing a letter or having phone sex can be outercourse, and so is masturbation. Most important, as Marty Klein and Riki Robbins point out in *Let Me Count the Ways: Discovering Great Sex without Intercourse,* outercourse is a different way of thinking about sex. Although much of it might look like what we call foreplay, it's not a preparation for the Main Event. Indeed, it does not even assume that intercourse is going to happen. Without a prescribed beginning, middle, or end, write Klein and Robbins, "ultimately, outercourse is the vehicle for humans writing a new sexual narrative."[32]

Information on various sexual practices can be found in sources from gURL.com to *The Joys of Sex.* These can be available for children and teens to peruse in private. The benefits of outercourse include enhanced communication, sexual equality, pleasure, and safety. If young lovers get used to nonpenetrative pleasures as "normal" sex from the start, they may avoid much of the sexual misery that afflicts so many American adults.

Outercourse's Benefits: Enhanced Communication

Outercourse necessitates communication and therefore increases the likelihood of consent. Because outercourse doesn't proceed in a prescribed order, neither partner can predict what the other will come up with or what they might come up with together. They simply can't make love without communication, either in bed or out. This enhances self-exploration and intimacy, mutual knowledge and affection. "You can have successful intercourse with a stranger," writes sex therapist Tiefer, "but you have to like someone to enjoy petting. Because the physical sensations are less intense, much of the reward must come from closeness."[33] Paying attention to each other's verbal and physical cues and checking in regularly to find out how the other is doing almost guarantee full consent from both partners at each juncture.

But the elements of outercourse don't need to be discovered in the context of a sexual relationship at all. Rob Yaeger, Minneapolis sex educator and Safer Sex Slut, encourages kids to talk in detail with a trusted friend about every sexual thing they might imagine liking. There's just one ground rule: "You have to promise not to say, 'That is so *sick!*'"

Sexual Equality

Because outercourse breaks down gender roles, it is a boon to sexual equality. Obviously, males and females have different genital equipages, which rev up and cool down at different rates and work differently along the way. And—a major element in how people feel about sex—some of us have the body that carries the baby, some of us don't. But technology, from birth control to the sex-change operation, largely mitigates the sexual differences and thoroughly disarranges the social arrangements once wrought by biology. Modern life, in which women fight fires and men diaper babies, wipes out most of the rest of the differences, if we let it.

Take intercourse out of the picture, and the sex differences that were left in the bedroom can be swept out too. If they remain, it's just for fun or for old times' sake. For those who want it to, though, outercourse returns lovers to what Freud called polymorphous perversity—the infantile state of full-body sensuality, in which various body parts don't enjoy greater or lesser respect or greater or lesser capacity for pleasure. Male, female, or transgendered, we all have mouths, necks, toes, anuses, brains, and nerve endings. We all have hearts, voices, and souls.

When people stop playing by the familiar rules, they can feel anxious—or free. The inexperienced teenage boy doesn't have to "perform"; his penis doesn't have to "work" at the right moment. The girl doesn't have to be "ready" for penetration. The heterosexual couple doesn't even have to think about chasing that chimera, the simultaneous orgasm during intercourse. Freed from the gender roles of initiator and responder (or resister), doer and done-to, penetrator and penetrated, a couple can play with all the roles. They may begin to discover a new kind of sexual equality.

Dismantling the intercourse model also undermines the presumption of heterosexuality (which is only one reason you don't hear the fundamentalist Christian marriage counselors prescribing outercourse). Boys can do what girls do and girls do what boys do in heterosexual outercourse. The result: As some gay blade once put it, there's no sex act gay people do that straight people do not also do (except maybe have orgasms listening to Judy Garland).

Increased Pleasure

In an essay called "Bring Back the Kid Stuff," Tiefer wrote, "The skin is the largest sex organ, yet many of us have learned to regard as sexual only a tiny percentage of the available acreage."[34] Odd that we should do that. Which of us would propose an overnight hiking trip in the backyard?

The pleasures of outercourse go beyond the number of inches of body that can be involved. In fact, outercourse is more dependent on that other largest sex organ, the brain; it is limited more by the flexibility of the mind than of the limbs. Fantasies may be verbally shared or not; in either case they can greatly heat up the sexual experience, with or without another person. Outercourse can also make use of any extracorporeal accouterment the participants can think of, as long as it's safe, practical, and comfortable for everyone involved: whipped cream or whips, stuffed bears or bubble bath, MTV, *Star Wars,* or porno tapes. Preteens and teens can whisper sweet nothings and talk dirty or create Web sites in each other's honor. Klein and Robbins suggest that breathing together is a way to connect with a partner and increase the spiritual experience of sexuality.

Finally, a happy paradox: While outercourse eliminates the forced march toward intercourse, it increases the probability of orgasm for women. Many women, and most teenage girls, don't get enough touching, kissing, or time to feel ready for intercourse, much less have an orgasm that way. And then, once it's "over" (that is, the guy comes), they've missed their chance. Because of the physical arrangement of the female sex organs, intercourse isn't usually the most effective way to climax anyhow. As for boys and men, although they are "supposed" to enjoy intercourse more than anything else, many like to orgasm in other ways too. Changing the means by which the two partners climax also can relax gender roles and abet sexual equality.

More Safety

Certainly some would argue that teaching kids all this fancy stuff will turn them on so much they will want to do nothing but have sex. And this will push them into intercourse even faster.

Experience suggests otherwise. In Europe, for instance, some sex education actually includes lessons in the varieties of sexual expression (a friend told me about viewing a Swedish film that suggested more pleasurable techniques of touching). In much of Western Europe, teens initiate intercourse at about the same age as here.[35] Adult couples who learn to enjoy nonintercourse pleasures tend not to have intercourse every time they make love.

Outercourse is safer sex, and the skills it teaches make intercourse, if it happens, safer too. If a young couple is having enough pleasure without intercourse, they can postpone that decision indefinitely. In the meantime, many kinds of outercourse are virtually without risk of pregnancy or STD and HIV transmission (oral and anal sex can pass certain viruses and bacteria, however, and unprotected anal intercourse poses the highest risk of HIV transmission, so condoms are recommended for these practices). Much of outercourse—mutual masturbation, bathing together, kissing—is 100 percent risk-free.

The skills of communication and invention and the spirit of mutuality that outercourse nurtures can make intercourse safer, when and if a young couple decides to take that step. Young people who are used to thinking and talking about sex and who learn to be aware of themselves and their partners are far more likely to approach intercourse consciously, with advance planning, and with the express and considered desire of both partners. This is a far cry from sex that "just happens," with an STD or a baby "just happening" as a result. With planning, condoms and lubrication will be purchased; a safe place and an unhurried time selected. The first time, and other times after that, can be more satisfying physically and emotionally and far safer.[36]

11. Community

Risk, Identity, and Love in the Age of AIDS

[I]n the communities most at risk . . . [s]afer sex became a means of negotiating sex and love, of building a respect for self and others, in a climate of risk and fear. . . . Safer sex . . . can be taken as symbolic of a wider need for a sense of caring responsibility that extends from sexual behavior to all aspects of social life.
—**Jeffrey Weeks**, *Invented Moralities* (1995)

"But what about AIDS?" The question arises immediately, almost every time I hazard the opinion that sex is not harmful to minors. Often it is not a question at all but a kind of preemptive statement: as long as there is AIDS, there cannot be adolescent sex. In 1981, when only gay men and their friends knew about the incipient epidemic, "chastity education" was a laughingstock. But as soon as HIV hit the cover of *Newsweek,* not far behind was the remarkable popular consensus that no-sex was the best thing to teach and the best thing for teens to practice. Just when mass public education about transmission, condoms, and nonpenetrative forms of sex was most crucial, AIDS became the rationale for not talking about sex. "The right wing's demand to 'teach' abstinence created the next generation's paradox," wrote Cindy Patton in her searing *Fatal Advice: How Safe-Sex Education Went Wrong.* "[E]quating 'no sex' and safe sex suggests that no sex is safe."[1]

That paradox did not yield mass abstention. Sex continued more or less unabated, but instead of safely, many youths did it ignorant of the difference between those acts that abetted HIV transmission, those that were relatively safer, and those that virtually precluded transmission. And exactly as the militant AIDS activist group ACT-UP warned, silence has equaled death. By the mid-1990s, a young person was being infected with HIV every hour of every day.[2] And while AIDS deaths dropped in the general U.S. population,[3] the disease became the leading cause of mortality for people ages twenty-five to forty-four, many of whom had likely contracted the virus in their teens.[4]

If abstinence is not the key, what is? Public-health experts have long observed that the populations hit hardest by AIDS overlap in predictable ways with those otherwise afflicted by poor health, education, or housing—and a poor standing in America's social hierarchies. Infection rates have fallen dramatically among adult men who have sex with men, especially white, middle-class, out gay men.[5] Nevertheless, it was estimated in the 1990s that 20 to 30 percent of gay youths would be infected by their thirtieth birthday.[6] Of all HIV-infected American youths in 1998, 63 percent were black.[7] And a survey of young, gay men of color conducted in six major cities by the National Centers for Disease Control from 1998 to 2000 revealed an even more astonishing figure: almost a third of gay black men in their twenties are HIV-positive.[8]

People in extremis, as usual, are at more extreme risk. Runaway teens show infection rates as high as 10 percent.[9] Half of New York City's people with HIV in the 1990s were intravenous drug users,[10] many of whom were young and marginally housed or employed.

These patterns are even more baldly visible globally. For instance, as the disease has ravaged Africa and steadily crept over South Asia, the United Nations reports that the near-total sexual, social, and economic abjection of women in those regions is translating into catastrophic rates of HIV infection and AIDS deaths among them.[11] The 1997 International AIDS Conference had predicted such dire developments. "Social norms and structural factors" exert a major impact on the spread and containment of the epidemic, the conferees concluded, advising policymakers to start paying more attention to such factors.[12]

Risk, in other words, is like sex itself: it is made up of acts that are given meaning and relative gravity by social context. Without basic changes in the most encompassing of those contexts (those "structural factors" such as economic, racial, and gender inequality), the AIDS plague will not end. Stagnant social structures are the reason the relatively wealthy, middle-class, urban, gay white male populations of the United States were able to stem the spread of the disease relatively quickly in the 1980s and why today many sero-positive men in those communities are living longer, healthier lives with the help of expensive drugs and medical care. It's also why the same thing has not happened among poor people of color, women, and drug addicts in America and Eastern Europe. In Africa, countries already decimated by war and famine now watch their populations stagger while international lawyers adjudicate their "rights" to buy cheaper generic versions of exorbitantly expensive AIDS drugs patented in the global North.[13]

The good news is that social norms even within these stubborn structures can change—if people feel it's in their interest to change and if what they're changing to isn't vastly more onerous than what they are used to doing. The failure of abstinence education may prove less about the intransigence of young people's mores (these can turn on an advertiser-flipped coin) than about the plain fact that sex is more appealing than abstinence. Abstaining promises a definite negative (you don't have sex, and you don't get pregnant or sick) in place of a positive linked only to a possible negative (you do have sex, and you may not get pregnant or sick).

The norm of safe sex has taken hold most firmly where it has represented not a wholesale reversal of already established norms but rather a variation on those norms. Some early gay AIDS activists such as Larry Kramer and Michelangelo Signorile have since repented of their earlier sexual libertarianism and indicted the "promiscuity" of gay men for their own demise. But other activist-intellectuals such as Douglas Crimp and Jeffrey Weeks argue far more persuasively that the inventive public sexual culture that defined the liberationist gay community also provided the motherlode of techniques from which safe sex was mined and the sexual frankness and intimate networks that got the word out. Similarly, AIDS-prevention workers in distressed communities have adopted the strategy of "harm reduction": they don't try to make drug addicts stop using before getting help, for instance (though they offer treatment when possible). Instead, they promote needle sterilization and clean-needle exchange programs so that intravenous users won't share dirty needles, one of the main transmitters of HIV.

Successful AIDS prevention, then, must be based on at least two principles: It must recognize the urgency of the problem of HIV and the exigencies, both personal and structural, of the people it is targeting. And it must respect their social norms: their identities, values, and desires, expressed in the relationships between individuals and within communities.

To witness sexuality education and HIV prevention where these principles are taken intelligently, creatively, and passionately to heart, I traveled in the spring of 1998 to Minneapolis and St. Paul, Minnesota, where the imperiled yet flourishing communities of gay, lesbian, bisexual, and homeless youths are the recipients of some extraordinary adult care and attention.[14]

As communities go, the Twin Cities are hardly the worst place to be young, gay, homeless, or at risk of dropping out, having a baby, getting HIV, or otherwise losing your way. A slow-moving, leafy metropolis of manageable size, with a history of progressive politics and philanthropy, a well-funded network of social service agencies, a university that has done groundbreaking work on sexuality and AIDS, and a cottage industry of "recovery" facilities, the Twin Cities are also blessed with a committed cadre of gay and lesbian public-health and youth workers. These people are determined to make growing up gay happier and safer for this generation than it was for theirs.

Not everything is perfect in the Twin Cities, of course. There aren't enough beds for homeless kids, for instance. As elsewhere, some of the neediest clients slip through the cracks: by definition runaways and street kids are fliers by night. The majority of youth and AIDS professionals in the Twin Cities are male, white, educated, healthy, and handsome, whereas many of their clients meet few of the above descriptions. State policymakers don't always appear to be on the same page as the workers on the ground. For instance, during the snack break of a student-taught HIV-prevention class run by a drop-in agency for homeless youth called Project Off-streets, the young staffer told me her program was about to lose its funding. Why? Because youth AIDS cases were diminishing in the Twin Cities. "Well duh-uh," commented the frustrated worker. "Maybe prevention is working."

If AIDS prevention is working, why is it? How are the strategies developed over twenty years by progressive grassroots gay and lesbian organizers and public-health educators being applied? What lessons can we take from the Twin Cities about sex and safe-sex education as part of young people's lives?

Meet people where they are: Identity and exigency

Out-of-the-closet gay youths have one thing going for them. Whereas abstinence-only sex education gives straight kids the message that sex is not a seminal part of adolescence, when a kid announces his identity in sexual terms, the people around him have no choice but to deal with him as a sexual person. That's both a blessing and a curse.

Coming out can give a kid a secure affiliation, a way to fit into the scheme of things. But the evil twin of affiliation is conformity, and, as we saw in chapter 9, the rigidly homophobic monoculture of the average high school hallway dictates that "queers" be punished—that they be reminded continually that they don't fit anywhere in the scheme. Some states, with Minnesota in the lead, have instituted legal antiharassment policies and student-faculty gay-straight alliances throughout the public schools. Nevertheless, facing ostracism and violence, gay students drop out at high rates.

Family life can be awful for a homosexual child, too. Youth who come out meet with parental grief, confusion, denial, or rage so hot that, for everyone involved, the prospect of the child eating from Dumpsters and sleeping under bridges may be preferable to coexisting under the same roof. "My brother says to my mom, 'You have a faggot-ass son,'" said Stephen Graham, a twenty-year-old African American gay activist, recalling his early teens. He was speaking at a sexuality-education conference for teachers run by the young denizens of District 202, Minneapolis's drop-in center run "by and for gay, lesbian, bi, and transgendered youth." "My mom just said to me, 'I can't agree with it. I can't love you.'" Stephen's pastor also branded him a sinner and banished him from the church. The boy ended up in state institutions, in squats, and crashing at friends' places throughout much of his adolescence.

Family hostility, in fact, is a leading cause of homelessness among gay youth. Of 150 youngsters surveyed in 1997 at District 202, 40 percent said they had been homeless at some time.[15] In cities nationwide, 25 to 40 percent of homeless youth identify themselves as gay or lesbian.[16] And what they do when they leave home isn't always the safest things. "Parents' abandonment or overt rejection of homosexual adolescents is partially responsible for the dramatic rise of teen male prostitution in the United States," wrote adolescent public-health doctors Martha Sturdevant and Gary Remafedi in a review of the special health needs of homosexual youth.[17] If you're fourteen and can't get a worker's permit or even a driver's license, sex is one of the few services you've got to offer on the labor market. "This may be the most politically unsavvy thing I can say," averred Paul Thoemke, Offstreets' gay lesbian bisexual transsexual (GLBT) case manager. "But I sometimes think the greatest risk for these kids is their families."

It is hardly surprising that among gay and lesbian youth drug and alcohol use is high,[18] and while getting high does not cause people to take risks, people tend to do a number of dangerous and self-destructive things at the same time.[19] Despair plus disinhibition can equal death, as the disproportionate number of gay and lesbian kids in the suicide statistics suggests.[20]

A gay identity can present other, less obvious troubles in growing up and shaping a self. A straight kid's straightness does not box his identity in; he is straight, yes, but mostly he's seen as African American or Filipino or Jewish, a jock or a gangsta or a nerd. But a gay kid is defined by what he is not: he is not straight. That makes it hard even for a securely gay or lesbian teen to express his or her individuality. "Coming out gives kids the freedom to express and explore their sexuality," said Ed Kegle, a youth worker at District 202. "But it's also limiting, because that's the only way other people see you, as 'that little fag' or 'that little dyke.'" A sixteen-year-old lesbian activist summed up the dilemma: "I love being queer," she told me, running a hand through her cherry-red crew cut. "But sometimes I just wanna be Jenny, not Queer Jenny."

Many kids may feel that a gay identity describes them no more accurately than the names they inherited from the communities that expelled them. In one study of seventh- to twelfth-graders in Minneapolis, more than 10 percent said they were unsure of their sexual orientation.[21] "I meet a lot more kids who say they're bi, or just 'sexual,' not homo or hetero," said Rob Yaeger, the high-wattage risk-reduction educator for the community-based Minnesota AIDS Project and member of the Safer Sex Sluts introduced in an earlier chapter. Courie Parker, a District 202 youth who identifies herself as bisexual, described her orientation this way: "There are the consonants and the vowels—*a, e, i, o, u,* and sometimes *y.* That's me: *sometimes y.*'"

The dangers of coming out and teens' disinclination to join one sexual "team" or another can flummox those who are trying to deliver culturally specific or community-based safe-sex education to them. This is especially true when the adults, like those in Minneapolis, come from strongly gay-identified politics, social circles, and even career paths. One way everyone seems to have dealt with this fluidity of identity is to classify *it* as an "identity," too. In the lengthening train of labels attached to "queer" youth, GLBTQ, the Q stands not for "queer" but for "questioning." In a sense, it's a description that could fit almost every teenager.

Of course, sexuality is not the only way that people identify themselves. Even if their parents may sometimes regard them as foundlings, queer youngsters are not born in some independent offshore Queer Nation and imported to Boston's Italian American South Side or Utah's Mormon Salt Lake City. Nor do all kids reject their religious or ethnic communities of origin, even when some people in those communities reject them. The best safe-sex education takes into account the complex interplay of identities and loyalties in any given person or group.

In the African American community of north Minneapolis, a group of young women and men calling themselves the Check Yo'self Crew got started producing one poster with the slogans "Check yo'self before you wreck yo'self," "Educate your mind, protect your body," and "No parachute, no jump" emblazoned over a photo of a bunch of hip-looking black kids. After their poster won an award, they got grants to put up six billboards of the same image and message, and then they hunkered down in the neighborhood, channeling gangs' energy into HIV peer education and establishing a free condom source on every block. A similar project was later undertaken in a Latino community in town.

Some of the smartest and most moving culturally specific HIV/AIDS youth work in the Twin Cities is masterminded by the Minnesota American Indian Task Force. Its director is Sharon Day, a forty-six-year-old Ojibwa Indian, out lesbian, mother of two, and custodial grandmother of one. "We need to understand what has allowed us native people to survive since time began," Day told me in a voice as soft and tough as chamois. Her theater work began with that and related questions. "If the birth rate is an indication of the frequency of the sex act," she reasoned, Native Americans' high birth rate "shows we haven't gotten so depressed that we've lost that ability to be sexual. Why is that?" Western psychological models don't explain it. Even if parents are alcoholic or otherwise "dysfunctional," Native American children like herself have survived intact by gleaning intimacy and security from the extended family and the wider community. In directing the task force's youth theater troupe, which travels to community centers, schools, and reservations statewide, doing AIDS-awareness plays, Day said, "We are trying to recapture those traditions and expressions that have kept our people emotionally and sexually healthy."

My Grandmother's Love, written by Day in collaboration with the young actors, is one part family soap opera, one part Native American vision quest, one part safe-sex agit-prop skit. It opens with four boys beating one large drum and chanting the traditional men's songs in their high children's voices. Then it moves to short reminiscences about grandmothers, whose photos are projected onto a large screen. "She's a good cook, her hair is all black, no gray," one boy says. "She's a basic grandma." The main story concerns a gay college boy (played by an androgynous fourteen-year-old girl) who returns home to tell his family he is HIV-positive. "You little faggot!" the father explodes, pounding his fist on the kitchen table. Scared and depressed, the young man withdraws. But he is sustained, and finally restored, by his grandmother's unconditional love and a dream-vision of running to safety. In the final scene, the group chants his vision—"I have been to the brink, to the rim of the canyon. / I've looked over the edge. / It's not so scary to me anymore"—and asks the audience to pray for the ill. Family, spirituality, community, said Day: "This is what has enabled native people to survive, gay or straight."

By the same token, Day knows that as much as sex education must focus on specific cultural beliefs and practices, it must also be catholic enough to accommodate young people who fall victim to those same beliefs and practices. Stephen Graham, the gay boy rejected by his pastor, for instance, was lucky to find another African American church whose dogma and liturgy resembled his old congregation's, with the major difference that this one embraced him, sexuality and all. Other gay youth have felt driven more radically from their faith communities by antagonism toward homosexuality, so they've had to find other sources to satisfy their spiritual needs. In the 1997 District 202 survey, almost every respondent filled in the blank under religious affiliation. But the largest single group called themselves Pagan.

Don't box people in: The "risk-group" fallacy

Identities are multiple. Their facets sometimes harmonize; at other times they are dissonant. In AIDS prevention, the challenge is to find people where they affiliate and speak to their sense of belonging for the purpose of instilling and reinforcing safe-sex values and habits. But the construction of categories can also be perilous. Indeed, the error (some say the fatal error) of AIDS prevention over the past two decades has been its strategy of labeling groups of people, not as potentially powerful allies in fighting the disease, but as collections of mutually antagonistic virus-carrying harm-spreaders, or "risk groups."

The first decade of public-health AIDS education told us there were two kinds of people in the world of AIDS. The "high-risk groups" included gay men, Haitian immigrants, and intravenous drug users and their sex partners and babies. These people used to be called AIDS victims but were actually thought of as AIDS victimizers. In the "low- or no-risk groups" were suburban teens, heterosexuals, white Yuppies— as Patton put it, the people who qualified as bona fide "citizens." Prevention for the "low-risk" folks meant avoiding the poisonous populations, first, by steering clear of people who looked suspicious and, second, by practicing "partner selection": interrogating potential partners for their possible inclusion or interaction with "high-risk" persons and rejecting those who might be "unsafe" lovers.[22] Teens did not have to perform this discretionary process. They were instructed to say no to everyone.

The concept of the risk group helped neither presumptive group. The people supposedly inside it were either stigmatized (and neglected by policymakers) for their allegedly self-destructive lifestyles or ignored. Some of those relegated to this status used it as a powerful political motivator: ACT-UP emerged from gay men's rage at being excluded as legitimate recipients of health care resources. For others, however, being branded "at risk" only induced fatalism. The idea that one is likely to die simply by virtue of being a certain kind of person does not concentrate the mind wonderfully on life-saving strategies. And for already hurt people, this new denigration only compounded hopelessness. "Individuals who have been at high risk," like kids who have been abused, lived on the streets, or turned tricks, "are likely to see themselves as at risk of getting HIV," said Gary Remafedi, director of the University of Minnesota's Youth & AIDS Project. "Or they'll say, 'I'm gay. It's inevitable I'm gonna die. So what?'" According to Jeffrey Escoffier, a New York public educator, sociologist, and AIDS activist, research shows that gay men who learn that all gay-associated sex, including fellatio, is equally fatal come to believe they are doomed, so they engage in more of the riskiest behaviors. In one San Francisco survey of seventeen- to nineteen-year-old men who have sex with men, 28 percent had recently had unprotected anal sex, the behavior carrying the highest risk for HIV transmission;[23] in a six-city study of young gay men of color, almost half had done so in the preceding six months.[24]

For people both "inside" and "outside," however, the risk-group theory had a profound flaw: *there is no such thing as a discrete social-sexual population.* No group is an island; all risk is shared, potentially, with a limitless universe of partners. While in America most people travel in social ruts, apart from other races and classes, not even the most insular, cautious people always stay in those ruts. Drug users don't congregate only in crack houses; they also frequent trendy nightclubs. And a man who has unprotected sex with a seropositive teenage hustler in a downtown city park may have sex the next day with a guy he knows from a neighborhood bar, and that guy will have sex with his middle-class suburban wife the next.

One way to circumvent the hazards of the risk-group assumption, while being realistic about the fact that it's been drummed into everybody's head, is to use it to get people's attention, then redirect their thinking. Rather than choosing or rejecting certain people or "kinds" of people, specific *behaviors* can be rejected. As a pamphlet displayed with a couple dozen others on District 202's wall put it: "Being Young and Gay does NOT have to mean being at Risk for HIV & AIDS. . . . But being unsafe does."

Taking a kernel of wisdom from the "risk-group" concept—that individuals within certain social or sexual groups may more commonly engage in behaviors that can transmit HIV—and tempering it with the understanding of the fluidity of communities and individual diversity within them, AIDS-prevention professionals have lately conceived the notion of "target populations." These comprise not people who are "by nature" risk-prone but those who live in situations of high risk, say, in a neighborhood or social circle a large number of whose members are seropositive. Most important, educators identify these populations by sexual behavior: not by how they dress, where they drink, or what they call themselves, but by what acts they do. MSM, for example, is HIV/AIDS shorthand for "men who have sex with men," a category that takes in both the Puerto Rican husband and father who lives in upper Manhattan but occasionally goes to a bar in the Bronx and has sex with a man and the teenage Anglo who dies his hair green and marches in the Castro Street Gay Pride parade in a goatee and tutu.

In Minneapolis, I watched numerous AIDS-ed workers in various settings, from off-the-cuff conversations in a scruffy city park to the makeshift stage in a Native American cultural center, from a peer-run class in a high school for returning dropouts to sex- and AIDS-ed sessions at District 202. In all of these, instructors started with the acts they believed their students might engage in, making these broadest determinations by the group's sexual or age identity or perhaps its religious or ethnic affiliation. But they assumed nothing about the specifics of any individual's predilections. A lesbian group at District 202 discussed the use of a square of latex called a dental dam that can be laid over a partner's vagina before performing cunnilingus. At the center's conference for teachers, a quick safe-sex rap by the twenty-year-old peer educator Toyin Adebanjo reminded the audience not to forget such youth-specific contaminated-blood risks as body piercing and tattooing. At the same time, the woman addressing the young lesbians talked about contraceptive and safe-sex precautions for penile-vaginal intercourse. And a youth worker addressing fifteen-year-olds did not neglect information on the HIV-transmission risks of breast feeding.

Gary Remafedi, who educates young gay men, described the balance of the main message, identity, and personal taste this way: "One message is, 'Always use condoms while you're fucking.' But that assumes that every gay man fucks. So the other message is, 'Fucking is not a fundamental part of being a gay man. Not everyone likes it. And everyone can enjoy safe sex behavior that is not intercourse.'"

Respect people's choices as rational

A fair number of the youngsters who find their way to Offstreets, District 202, or Remafedi's program at the university either regularly or occasionally turn to prostitution to get by. In the risk-benefit calculus of life on the street, sex is both a plus and a minus.[25]

"Survival sex"—sex in trade for a bed, a shower, or a pair of shoes—may also offer some personal rewards, such as adult companionship and affirmation. And like other adult-minor sex, it is not always an interaction of utter abjection on the young person's side. "A lot of the youth don't see survival sex as prostitution," said Ludfi Noor, the easygoing director of Offstreets' HIV education. Added Gonne (pronounced "Honnah") Asser, a young outreach worker, "This youth was talking the other day, saying, 'I was going to clubs and getting lucky. Older people wanted to have sex with me.'" Of the here-today-gone-tomorrow relationships between youngsters and adults, she added, "It can be a relationship that lasts a week, but to the kid, it's still a relationship."

Of course, prostitution without even that rudimentary relationship poses its own risks. Working girls (and boys) have long adopted their own health and safety practices, notably condom use. Among homeless youth, it appears that when the trick is a stranger, condom use is also the rule.[26] No educator should underestimate a young person's ability to make informed decisions about sex. To make informed decisions, though, people need information, and some AIDS experts argue that what they need is the kind of detailed information about risk that is available throughout most of Europe but that U.S. health departments are reluctant to give out. Rather than listing acts as either safe or unsafe, period, so-called relative-risk data disseminated in Paris or Berlin tell you that such-and-such behavior has led to HIV transmission in a particular number of known cases in this or that country, or that findings about this other behavior are still inconclusive. Armed with such data, people can make choices about their sex lives in the same way they craft the rest of their lives: by weighing desires and rewards against dangers and unwanted consequences.

That said, there are a lot of reasons not to put on a rubber if you're a young person selling or bartering sex. Sex without a condom demands a higher price than sex with one, so taking a higher risk per trick in order to turn fewer tricks overall may feel like a reasonable business decision. (Other considerations go into the equation, too: receiving fellatio, a fairly common act of male prostitution, is of extremely low risk to the receptor. For a young woman in heterosexual sex, the opposite is true: as the giver of oral sex and the receiver of vaginal intercourse, she takes practically all the risk of HIV and other STD transmission.)[27]

A homeless kid turning a trick may not protect himself or herself for some subtler and sadder reasons as well. Such youngsters typically have been the victims of inordinate violence; "more than half have been physically abused, more than one-third, sexually abused, more than one-third beaten by an intimate partner during the last year," said a report of Minneapolis's gay, lesbian, bisexual, and transgender homeless youth conducted by the Wilder Research Center in 1996.[28] About once a week, said Paul Thoemke, a girl comes into Offstreets and says she's been raped. For people who have been treated with routine cruelty, particularly by their "loved" ones, self-care can be a foreign concept. "A lot of women and girls don't see sex as a source of pleasure or their bodies as something they have control over," noted Beth Zemsky, a lesbian AIDS educator who works on gay and lesbian student issues at the University of Minnesota. Ine Vanwesenbeeck, in a study of sexual power and powerlessness among Dutch prostitutes and other young women, found that those who capitulated to johns' demands that they forgo a condom were more often younger, drug users, and immigrants and "had experienced more victimization, both in childhood and in adult life, both on and off the job." Once they'd become known as "risk takers," they were "most often visited by recalcitrant condom users."[29]

AIDS prevention for the street kids of the Twin Cities, then, means more than pressing a bundle of condoms into a hustler's tight jeans pocket. "So many of the youth I work with have been treated in such a disrespectful way, they can't respect themselves," said Youth & AIDS Project caseworker Jerry Terrell. "A third of the people I see are suicidal, a fifth are actively using chemicals, and then for the homeless youth, there's no tomorrow; everything is today. The main thing is helping them to imagine that there is a future and beginning to get a toehold in whatever that might be. HIV is at the end of a long line of other issues."

Those issues are both emotional and material. When the Wilder researchers queried homeless youth on what would really make a difference in their lives, their sights usually focused somewhere between hand and mouth. Several suggested access to a free washing machine. "I can wear dirty clothes, pants, shirts, and stuff," said one girl. "As long as I can have clean underwear, I'm okay." Under such circumstances, safe sex can be a rather abstract and distant notion. "'Safety' means finding a bed tonight," explained Amber Hollibaugh, former head of the Lesbian AIDS Project at GMHC in

New York. "Putting on a condom is not exactly the Number One priority."[30]

Still, risk taking should not be considered a symptom of pathology, as it so often is among teachers, adolescent psychologists, and public-health professionals. Instead, said Jeffrey Escoffier: "People are also doing a rational assessment of their environments. They tally the odds." On the street, kids know their lives are by definition unsafe, that they can't eliminate all risk. So the task is to figure out the route of greatest reward—financial, practical, emotional—with the least endangerment along the way. It is the job of prevention workers to understand that calculus, too, and help young people incrementally refigure the emotional and material factors so that they can make more self-protective decisions in their sexual behavior and stick to them. In "sex education" with his young hustlers, Jerry Terrell told me, "most of what I do is not about sexuality."

Rethink all assumptions: Pleasure, love, and trust

Street kids are not another species. Even for them, sex is not all work, exploitation, or pain. "Sex is nice, it's intimate, it's fun, it doesn't cost anything," Project Offstreets' Thoemke said, in answer to my question about the role of pleasure in his clients' lives. "These kids, not having close relationships with their families, or if they were abused, sex was a really awful thing. To find sex as a pleasure, that's so great." He grumbled at the relentless Lutheran-ness of the bureaucrats who check up on his agency. "They come in, and they're appalled that we have condoms available at our front door or the kids are watching cartoons or smoking cigarettes." Homeless kids carry all the responsibilities of adult independence, he reasoned. Why not get a few of the perquisites? He paused. "But sex is the easiest thing in the world. It's love that's hard to find."

The personality structures and circumstances of disenfranchised youths vex the already difficult search for love. On one hand, as abused or rejected children, they are desperate to love, to plunge into trusting. On the other, as abused or rejected children–turned–street rats, they are trained in mistrust, and touchy, sometimes paranoid. They want stability and monogamy, yet they are also hot to try out their sexuality, sometimes with many partners (these last two contradictory desires are often split by gender, with girls and women rushing to the altar, so to speak, and boys and men reveling in sexual novelty, variety, and quantity). On balance, though, homeless boys and girls want what everyone wants, Thoemke insists: love *and* sex, plus a measure of security—"a permanent partner and not to worry about how the bills will get paid."

Love? A permanent partner? Regular bill paying? These wishes would bring sunshine to the hearts of the bureaucrats at Offstreets' door or to the abstinence-until-marriage campaigners, who claim that a committed relationship is the best and only prophylactic against AIDS. But the fact is, love is no fortress against sexual risk. One of the biggest paradoxes of HIV prevention is that love—not just careless love, but also love that is desperately coveted and conscientiously nurtured—may compound the dangers of sex. Contrary to the propaganda that advertises the perils of the backroom or the bathhouse, *people, both gay and straight, are more likely to have unsafe sex inside a committed, loving relationship than in casual encounters.*[31] Trust, conceived in the way we currently conceive it, can be "a risky practice."[32]

"One of the most striking and consistent findings of behavioral research on gay men is that high-risk sex is more frequently reported with someone described as a 'regular partner or lover,'" wrote the British medical sociologist Graham Hart. In a study of 677 men, Hart and his colleagues found that "unprotected intercourse . . . was a way of expressing the love and commitment to a shared life that the men felt."[33] Sarah Phillips's survey of heterosexual adolescents' condom use came to similar conclusions: "[B]oth young men and women who claimed to be in love with their partners were significantly more likely to agree to sexual intercourse without a condom than were those who reported that they were not in love."[34] The certainty that the other person is perfectly monogamous is viewed, by people of all classes, as an automatic right conferred in loving that person. "Once I'm married, that's *it*," declared Keisha, a seventeen-year-old Minneapolis peer educator, ramming a firm fist into her hip and raising an instructing finger to face height. "If he brings me home AIDS, then I have a right to kill him." If the implicit agreement of Keisha's marriage is that her husband knows he'll be "killed" if he admits to having been unfaithful—and therefore feels he can't tell her—then he may end up killing her too, only more slowly.

Although many definitions of trust cross gender lines, those that do not tend to put women at a disadvantage. "There was a strong shared understanding that 'steady' relationships are based on trust," wrote the psychologist Carla Willig, paraphrasing the conclusions of some researchers who interviewed inner-city young women. "At the same time [the women] identified a tendency to define a relationship as 'steady' in order to justify sex. Since discontinuation of condom use can signify increasing commitment to a relationship, condom use within 'steady' relationships is difficult to maintain." Among a group of Canadian college students, "for women [the implicit compact between committed lovers] meant trusting that one's partner would disclose relevant information, and for men it meant trusting that one's partner had nothing to disclose. As a result, women found it very difficult to request condom use from partners whom they knew well, but ironically, 'they were most able to protect themselves from all three dangers—pregnancy, disease, and emotional hurt—in casual encounters.'"[35] The prejudice that respectable girls are nonsexual (except with the current partner), moreover, makes safe sex additionally difficult for young women. Planned HIV prevention can give a girl a bad reputation, sex educator Rob Yaeger said. "Girls say, 'If I pull out a condom, he'll think I'm a slut.'" Because women are far more likely to contract HIV from a male partner than vice versa, and young women's vaginal linings are more fragile than mature women's and therefore additionally infection-prone, these gendered assumptions endanger young women disproportionately.

For many people, simply bringing up the subject of protection is so threatening to trust that trust requires absolute censorship. Some of the people Willig interviewed went so far as to say that requiring long-term couples to start talking about or, worse, using condoms would mean an irreparable rent in the social fabric. "I mean there's got to be some sort of element of trust somewhere," said a young man named John, "unless life as we know it ain't gonna happen."[36]

True love is monogamous, trust depends on monogamy and monogamy on trust, and trust is the cornerstone of love: unfortunately, from the point of view of the sexually transmitted virus, this formulation is heavy with potential dangers. First, although statistics vary widely depending on the surveyor, the way the questions are asked, and the sexuality of the subjects, at least a significant number of married and committed couples stray at least once, at least a third of teens do,[37] and even youths who are monogamous are only serially so. Meanwhile, fewer than 60 percent of sexually active adolescent boys who use only condoms say they use them every time.[38]

Yet many of these people predicate their relationship on unerr-
ing fidelity. That sets up an untenable dilemma: the confession of a
lapse fatally threatens the relationship, but keeping a secret fatally
threatens both the person and his or her beloved. Carla Willig's in-
formant John accepted that maintaining a societal and personal
contract of trusting silence might mean the sacrifice of a few "innocent victims" whose partners committed crimes of omission.[39] Is
the symbolic and moral risk of abandoning loving trust "as we
know it" really greater than the risk of rampaging HIV infection?
Federally funded abstinence-only education says yes, by teaching,
contrary to evidence, that the only safe sex is within a "traditional" committed (read unquestionably monogamous) heterosexual
marriage.

Fortunately, some independent AIDS educators are going whole-
heartedly in the other direction. "I tell them, *love is not the answer,*"
said Rob Yaeger. "Love will not protect you. The virus doesn't care
if you're in love, if you're married. It doesn't care what your favorite song is." And it doesn't care what your favorite song says
love is, either. Given the urgent historical circumstances, a policy of
confession and forgiveness when a partner strays from intended
monogamy might be *more* loving than censorship enforced by the
expectation of rage and rejection. But such ways of relating require
less dependency, less jealousy, less unwavering confidence in the
other person's ability and willingness to take care of you, and at the
same time, more personal maturity, flexibility, independence, and
self-esteem, and more altruism from both partners.

Aside from altruism, these emotions are different from the ones
we are used to associating with love. Nevertheless, it is these qualities and values, not the blind faith of "true" love and the hound
dog's acuity for "risky" partners, that we need to be nurturing
in kids.

Cultivate the best values. Create brave new communities

Plenty of the teens who flow through the agencies where I hung out
in Minneapolis and St. Paul are notoriously tough cases. It's hard to
get them back to the clinic for a follow-up visit, much less to a GED
class or job-training program. District 202 youth volunteer Courie
Parker, who has been homeless herself, explained why homeless
kids drift further and further from "normalizing," adult-overseen
institutions such as school and work. "You can't plug in an alarm
clock under a bridge," she said simply.

But exclusion from the mainstream can also engender tight affiliation, and as history has shown for blacks, women, gays, and the disabled, collective survival is the first step toward the creation of a resistant community identity. Homeless youth form scruffy mutual-aid societies, tight little tribes that scavenge food or locate shelter for each other, often moving about with a brace of equally disenfranchised dogs. To the Offstreets kids, group cohesiveness is everything, said Thoemke. "They always want to say 'we.' If we could harness that good energy, we'd have a powerful community."

During the early years of gay liberation, despised communities harnessed the energy of the hatred directed at them and transformed it into pride—for instance, appropriating as flags of distinction the derogatory terms *dyke, faggot,* and *queer.* When the AIDS epidemic hit them, gay men and women turned that energy toward aggressive political confrontation that, for all its outward rage, was fueled by love, both fraternal and erotic. "The AIDS crisis, in all its frightening impact, bearing the burden of fear of disease and death in the wake of pleasure and desire, seems to many to embody the downside of the transformation of sexuality in recent years, a warning of the dangers of things 'going too far,'" wrote the British social critic Jeffrey Weeks. "Yet in many of the responses to it we can see something else: a quickening of humanity, the engagement of solidarity, and the broadening of the meanings of love, love in the face of death."[40]

Self-love and self-esteem are necessary to practicing safe sex. But this history speaks of love that goes beyond the self and even beyond the beloved. This is *communal* love, a kind of modern agape, based in shared pride of identity and collective self-defense and practiced within circles of personal friendship and desire. *Love and loyalty, the same feelings that can discourage safe sex, can also motivate it.* People care about their communities even when their communities are hostile to them, and they put on a condom with that caring in mind. "When people are asked why they practice safe sex," said Jeffrey Escoffier, "one of the main reasons they give is altruism." He cited a study of gay Latino men, done by the Rafael Diaz Center for AIDS Prevention Studies in San Francisco. "The most common response was, 'There are people who count on me.'" Escoffier noted that the people who depend on those men were not necessarily part of any gay community but rather family members, friends, and neighbors in their Latino communities of origin. What this study and others uncovered, he said, was "a high level of integration even into a community that they feel ambivalent about.

"A lot of [HIV] prevention aims at self-interest," he concluded. "That's a mistake."

America has made many grievous mistakes in trying to protect its children from the dangers of sex. Underlying these errors is fear. Some is "good" fear, that they will be sickened or traumatized, will lose their direction, their ambition, their sense of self. But much is fear of eros, to which we attribute anarchic, obliterating power—the power to destroy individuals and civilization itself.

Yet eros is not a wild animal prowling outside the civilizing meanings we assign it, beyond the moralities with which we govern it. We create eros for ourselves and for our children; it is we who teach our young the meanings and moralities of sex. In the age of AIDS, we must invent new iterations of the best old values, creating new expressions of love, trust, loyalty, and mutual protection. Inspired and sheltered by the values of caring, young people can discover their sexual power without dominating or diminishing others; they can find romance without surrendering self-protection. They can arrive at the divine oblivion of sex consciously, with responsibility, forethought, and consent.

While laboring to vanquish AIDS and the conditions that abet it, we must remember what we were taught by the gay and lesbian heroes of one of modern sexuality's most terrible epochs. The infinite gifts of the erotic can empower people and unite communities. The embrace of pleasure can be the greatest defense against peril.

Epilogue

Morality

In 1999 a team of social scientists at the University of Washington in Seattle reported their discovery of a groundbreaking method for preventing adolescent violence and other "risk behaviors," including early sexual intercourse. They enrolled a group of first-graders attending some of the city's toughest schools in a "test program" that lasted throughout the elementary years. These children were treated with respect, encouraged to cooperate with one another and with their teachers, rewarded for their accomplishments, given a quiet place to do their homework, and taught how to say no without endangering their friendships or social status. By the sixth grade, the participants were far less likely than kids at "comparable schools with no special intervention" to have committed a violent act or started drinking heavily, engaged in intercourse or been involved in a pregnancy.[1]

A friend and I have a name for this kind of research, which marshals lots of scientific methodology and statistics (and usually money) to demonstrate what is already patently obvious to almost everyone. We call it "Studies Show, People Who Are Happy Smile More."

And yet in the last decade of the second millennium, at a time when social-science funding was tight, these scholars felt called upon to design a major study and procure six years of grants to demonstrate that children who are treated with respect and appreciation, given space to think, and helped to compromise while also standing up for their beliefs will do better in life. These points were not obvious enough to enough people. In fact, to me, the more disturbing aspect of the study was the part that was not reported. If attention to these basic needs constituted "special intervention," what were the children in the control group subjected to all those years? If you have spent any time in a school lately, you will know the depressing answer: ordinary "education."

Perhaps we adults could use a little values clarification. Which is what, in closing, I would like to do.

Hardly a day goes by when one of our nation's leaders does not stand before a camera, dab a tear from the corner of his eye, and deliver a little paean to Our Nation's Children. But truth be told, the United States is not a child-friendly place. For one thing, though we might love each child separately, in the aggregate the younger generation does not win much esteem from its elders. In 1997, the public-interest research group Public Agenda asked adults what came to mind when they thought of children and teens. A majority of the respondents snatched at the words *undisciplined, rude, spoiled,* and *wild.* The older the kids, the more frequently cited were these characterizations.[2]

We say we love our children. But, as a disgruntled boyfriend once told me, love isn't a feeling, it's an act. And America acts as if it does not love its children. The United States lags far behind other industrialized nations in many indicators of child well-being and behind some nonindustrialized ones as well. In this, the only developed nation that does not provide health care to all its citizens, 11.3 million children age eighteen and under are uninsured, and that number is growing by 3,000 a day. In part because of this health-care crisis, a fifth of American mothers get no prenatal care, which predisposes their children to many chronic health problems. Twenty industrialized nations surpass us in preventing infant mortality, according to the Children's Defense Fund,[3] and the percentage of children who die before the age of five is the same in this fabulously rich country as it is in Cuba, a desperately poor country.[4]

Many families' lives were not improved by American history's longest boom. The coming recession will hurt them most. Large numbers of the poor worked during those fat years, yet the lowest fifth of wage earners saw their incomes drop from 1970s levels, and the poverty rate has stuck stubbornly around 12 percent for decades, according to the Bureau of Labor Statistics and the Census Bureau. "Welfare reform"—the federal Social Security Act of 1997 and the new regulations instituted by the states in its wake—appears to be worsening life for the poorest Americans. One study in 1999 found that the poorest 20 percent of families lost an average of $577 a year, and the poorest 10 percent more than $800. As state agencies erected more obstacles to obtaining food stamps, fewer poor and working-poor families applied for them. By 2001, soup kitchens were reporting the longest lines they'd ever seen at their doors.[5] In the month after September 11, when eighty thousand New Yorkers lost their jobs, calls to the city's hunger hotlines tripled.[6]

While the image of hungry, crying babies makes the most effective propaganda, there's evidence that welfare reform might be hurting teens even more than smaller kids. Studies show that elementary school children whose parents are in programs that encourage employment and continue to offer financial assistance do better at school and get into less trouble than poor children whose parents aren't undergoing such regimens. But, said the director of Chicago's Joint Center for Poverty Research, "for adolescents there's a different story." Teens in such families spend even less time than usual under adult supervision. So they smoke, drink and misbehave more, and their health and school achievement decline.[7]

These studies compare poor children with other poor children and teens. But the fact is, at six or sixteen, simply being a child predisposes a person to poverty in America: almost twice as many children as adults are poor,[8] and one in six American children is poor (12.1 million in 1990), including more than one in three black or Hispanic children.[9] Poverty is the single greatest "risk factor" for most every life-smashing condition a kid might be at risk for, save perhaps compulsive shopping. Among these are sexual risks, including unwanted pregnancy and too-early motherhood, AIDS, and sexual abuse.

Not only is child abuse related to poverty, poverty *is* child abuse. David Gil, a Brandeis University social policy professor and lifelong child advocate, put it eloquently. "Children are abused and their development tends to be stunted as a result of a broad range of perfectly legitimate social policies and public practices which cause, permit, and perpetuate poverty, inadequate nutrition, physical and mental ill-health, unemployment, substandard housing and neighborhoods, polluted and dangerous environments, schooling devoid of meaningful education, widespread lack of opportunities, and despair," he wrote. "The massive abuse and destruction of children is a by-product of the normal workings of our established social order and its political, economic, and cultural institutions."[10] It is wrong to single out sexual abuse as the worst harm to children, Gil told me, when child abuse is business as usual.

I am not saying we should worry about inadequate nutrition and substandard housing *instead* of worrying about sex. Or even that if everyone were well fed and well housed, all the sexual troubles in the world would go away (though a lot would). Rather, I am saying that these things are connected: the way we organize our economic lives and the way we conduct our sexual lives and teach our children to conduct theirs are connected in more profound ways than the linear correlations described above. They have to do with the same basic values.

A friend discussing the relative scariness of horror movies on a trip to Bali some years ago named *Jaws* the scariest, while his Balinese acquaintance voted for *The Exorcist*. "How could that be," my friend asked, "when you live surrounded by shark-invested waters?" "Oh, sharks," said the Balinese, flicking his hand dismissively. "Everyone knows a shark hardly ever eats a person. But possession by spirits—*that* happens all the time!"

Historically, we have tended to categorize problems as sharks (material) or spirits (moral)—disease or sin; underfunded schools or lack of academic standards; tight job market or personal sloth. According to that same Public Agenda report, "Americans define the children's issue as predominantly moral in nature, not one of money or health." Accordingly, their chosen solutions were on the order of character building, not situation bettering. Among those cited, more government money for health care and childcare ranked eleventh out of twelve, with increased welfare spending last. Higher up the list were nighttime curfews for minors (number four) and tougher punishment for those who commit crimes (number seven).

While improving the quality of U.S. education was first on the list, and presidential candidates seem to have been campaigning on it for the last two decades, the federal Department of Education is virtually an empty shell, and given the chance, Congress has been unwilling even to spend the dollars needed to fix the roofs of America's decrepit school buildings. Washington's proposed remedies for the hellacious state of public education—private-school vouchers and standardized testing—don't signal a commitment from this "education president" any more robust than that demonstrated by the last one, his dad. George W. Bush isn't likely to reverse the trends: The United States, which a half century ago was a world leader in high school graduation, widely regarded as a person's first step toward economic self-sufficiency, lagged in the 1990s behind Finland, Norway, Poland, South Korea, the Czech Republic, France, Germany, Canada, and Ireland.[11] And only half of American youth spent even a year in college.[12]

Those Public Agenda respondents had it wrong. You can't separate the sharks from the spirits. Money and health are moral issues, and where public policy is concerned, you put your money where your moral commitment is. That's why the only money the federal government has ever spent on sex education has been to teach chastity. And why, during more than a decade of death and community devastation, no U.S. president even mentioned AIDS, much less committed funds to attack it (Bill Clinton was the first).

The money-morality link operates in the area of personal character as well. It's not an accident that the people who end up in prison, having committed crimes both violent and nonviolent, are poor people, and many of them are also illiterate.[13] "Fulfilled people don't hurt other people," David Gil said. "People who have their material, emotional, and spiritual needs met are generally very nice, likable people. People whose needs are blocked and whose development is blocked, their constructive energy is transformed. This can be expressed through domestic violence, sexual abuse, street crime, insanity, self-destruction, suicide—all these things are variations on the theme of destructive energy. The question is, what social conditions cause people not to develop?" Or, put the other way around, what social conditions cause people to develop to their highest potential, intellectually, emotionally, spiritually, and sexually?

Social conditions are shaped by moral priorities. So, the question becomes: What values would make a world that's good for children to grow up in?

Not "family values," either the orthodox religious version set forth by the Christian Coalition or the secular-consumerist one promoted by every breakfast cereal advertisement on television. Needless to say, the family is extraordinarily important to children's welfare. It may take a village to raise a child, but most children go home and sleep in a bed in a house with a family; the family buys the Nikes and puts the Chicken McNuggets on the table.

On the other hand, when you get down to cases, "family values" is another way of saying "privatization," which means a withdrawal of public—that is, shared—financial responsibility to the community. A featured and enthusiastically received speaker at almost every convention of the groups regarded as the "moral" or religious camp of the conservative movement, such as Concerned Women for America, is the indefatigable Grover Norquist, head of Americans for Tax Reform. ATR's goal is to abolish the Internal Revenue Service and establish a flat tax so that you and Bill Gates would pay at the same rate, and in the utopian future, presumably, you'd pay no taxes at all. At the conferences, after Norquist speaks, somebody usually stands up to ridicule the slogan "It takes a village to raise a child." "It doesn't take a village!" she proclaims. "It takes a family!" Wild applause. What does this mean? The village be damned? Without the communal bank account—the national treasury, now threatened by massive tax cuts to corporations and the rich—that's what would happen to our villages, and our families and children with them.[14]

"Family values" will not make the world safe for children and surely not sexually safe. For starters, most child abuse happens inside the family. And if economic security and a sense of shared responsibility by all adults for all children are among the requisites of sexual safety, "family values" endanger children at home and everywhere else.

As I have said, it is out in the world, as much as in the home, that children learn to be friends, workers, and lovers. Therefore, parents who care about what happens to their kids need to stop seeing themselves exclusively as Jennifer's mom or Jamal's dad. Mom and Dad are also firefighters, Web site designers, doctors, shopkeepers, and corporate executives; they are neighbors, school board members, and voters. Mom and Dad are *citizens,* and if they want their children safe, they must behave as such, which means looking out for the other children in the village too. And that goes further than making sure the tax dollars flow equitably to all children.

We also need to start seeing children as citizens. Twenty-five years ago, the child development sage Gisele Konopka identified nine basic requirements for children to grow up happy and healthy. Along with such personal essentials as kids' need to experiment with identities and roles, she named "the need to participate as citizens." Indeed, she put it first on her list. "A sense of belonging" and "a feeling of accountability to others" were among the nine too. But responsibility and duty weren't all that children needed, said Konopka. Also crucial were the experiences that would "cultivate the capacity to enjoy life."[15]

When we are ready to invite children into the community as fully participating citizens, I believe we will also respect them as people not so different from ourselves. That will be the moment at which we respect their sexual autonomy and agency and realize that one way to help them cultivate the capacity to enjoy life is to educate their capacity for sexual joy.

Sex is a moral issue, but the teaching of "sexual values" is a redundancy. The same things that make you a solid member of your third-grade class—cooperation, respect, integrity—also make you a considerate lover, a consistent safe-sex practitioner, a person able to say yes or no to sex and honor the consent of a partner. If we want children to protect themselves yet accommodate others, feel pride in their individuality yet tolerate difference, if we want them to balance spontaneity and caution, freedom and responsibility, these are the capacities and values that apply to all realms of their private and public lives, with sexuality no greater or lesser a realm.

That said, you do not learn everything you need to know in kindergarten. Ethical questions get more complicated as you grow up; crucial moral priorities compete, such as the imperative to protect children versus the value of respecting their choices. For our part, then, to be moral about children's sexuality is to balance those priorities: not only to guard their bodies and souls from harm, but to embrace the profound rewards of opening the boundaries of the self through intimacy and shared pleasure. To be moral about children and their sexuality is to realign our idea of what promotes their best interests and what truly imperils them.

In a lush and mysterious photograph by Sally Mann, a naked three- or four-year-old, draped loosely in a blanket, dozes on a deck above a muddy river. Her face is lax, her mouth ajar, her pale body languid. Onto the bank below, a small alligator crawls.

Looking more closely at the photo, however, one sees that the alligator is not real. It is a blown-up plastic float, its teeth and claws printed on. The mist off the river obscures its cartoon shape, makes it look fierce and mobile. The photograph is entitled "The Alligator's Approach."

What is the alligator? A pedophile with the child's fragrance in his nostrils? A Hollywood mogul concocting the commercial sex that will invade her fantasies? Is it pregnancy or AIDS, poverty or homelessness? Which are the people and conditions that can hunt the child's flesh and devour its spirit? Which are the bags of air, the mass-produced masquerades of danger? The line between perils real and illusory is not always crisp. As we have seen, a make-believe monster can terrify and tear as effectively as a real one. Yet if we are to guide children wisely as they navigate the waters of desire and violence, we need to know the difference.

What will impede a child as she steps into the currents? The hierarchies of race, gender, and beauty that make her doubt herself and despise others who are different. The economic and social inequities that close down her horizons before she is tall enough to gaze out beyond them. The sexual shame and ignorance that lead to dissatisfaction at best, catastrophe at worst.

And what will buoy a child? Knowledge and pride in her body, freedom for her feelings, adult respect for her intelligence, will, and privacy. Good food and a secure kitchen in which to eat it, green space, libraries filled with books and computers, family and friends with the time and means to love her without hurting her. A community that cares for its smaller, weaker members as much as it lionizes its aggressive and successful, that celebrates happiness as much as it routs out malevolence.

Alligators lurk at the bottom of every child's sleep. Peril is inevitable in childhood, and adults' greatest pain may be the powerlessness to prevent it. But as children move out into the world, protecting them from sex will not protect them from those dangers that have little to do with sex but may ultimately make sex dangerous.

Sex is not harmful to children. It is a vehicle to self-knowledge, love, healing, creativity, adventure, and intense feelings of aliveness. There are many ways even the smallest children can partake of it. Our moral obligation to the next generation is to make a world in which every child can partake safely, a world in which the needs and desires of every child—for accomplishment, connection, meaning, and pleasure—can be marvelously fulfilled.

Afterword

A month before the April 2002 publication of *Harmful to Minors*, in the middle of the Catholic Church's sex abuse scandal, I received a call from a reporter for a syndicated news service. His story focused on academics who were questioning the orthodoxy that every sexual experience between a minor and an adult is unwanted by the former, traumatic, and permanently damaging. A friend had referred the reporter to me, thinking that my academic-press book could use a little free publicity.

Although I began by informing the reporter that only a small portion of my book is about sex between adults and minors, I told him I agreed with researchers who believe the term "abuse" had become so broad as to be virtually useless. Fortunately, research was creating a more nuanced picture of the "victims" and their experiences; for instance, it was making distinctions between being raped nightly by a father and groped once by a stranger at the pool. Even the same act does not feel the same to everyone, I said. Some children or teens are traumatized, others unmoved, and some say they initiated the sex and enjoyed it.

"Could a priest and a boy conceivably have a positive sexual experience together?" the reporter asked.

"Conceivably? Absolutely it's conceivable," I answered, "because the data tell us that some kids report such relationships as positive." I cited a large meta-analysis of the abuse literature by Temple University psychologist Bruce Rind and two colleagues, published in the *Psychological Bulletin* of the American Psychological Association, which found that not all minor-adult sex is traumatic at the time nor leads to long-term harm; boys were likely to call the experiences neutral or positive, girls negative or abusive. The researchers stressed that their work was not meant to exonerate anyone. Rather, they hoped that isolating the factors that render such sexual events painful for the child or troubling long into adulthood could help in tailoring more effective therapies.

I knew I was treading on dangerous turf when I praised Rind. In 1997, he was the target of conservative radio talk show host "Dr." Laura Schlesinger and Judith Reisman, a prominent right-wing activist against pornography, sex education, and sex research, who has made a career of discrediting pioneer sexologist Alfred Kinsey. An anti-homosexual group had objected to Rind's study and gotten in touch with Dr. Laura. She denounced him repeatedly on the air as an apologist for pedophilia and soon was joined by a coalition of Christian conservative organizations. They in turn found support from a group of therapists who specialize in the aftereffects of sexual abuse and whose work is based on the axiom that all child-adult sex leads to adult psychopathology; more controversially, many also believe that a troubled patient is likely to have sexual abuse in her past, even if she doesn't remember it and therefore needs the therapist's help in "recovering memories." Dr. Laura and her friends eventually persuaded Congress to censure the APA for publishing work that suggested sexual abuse was not always harmful. Rather than defend its scientific peer-review process, the APA issued a *mea culpa* and vowed to vet politically sensitive material more carefully in the future. Dr. Laura's victorious legions looked for other infidels to subdue.

They found me. A few days after the interview with the syndicate's reporter, his story ran in the Web edition of the *Minneapolis Star-Tribune*, my publisher's hometown paper, under the headline, "University of Minnesota Press Book Challenges Demonization of Pedophilia." I was quoted this way: "[Levine] said the pedophilia among Roman Catholic priests is complicated to analyze, because it's almost always secret, considered forbidden and involves an authority figure. She added, however, that, 'yes, conceivably, absolutely' a boy's sexual experience with a priest could be positive."

Although *Harmful to Minors* discusses pedophiles hardly at all, overnight I became the author of "the pedophilia book." Although the book doesn't condone, much less promote, child molesting, that was suddenly its reputation.

Within days, the University of Minnesota Press was inundated with calls. Half were demanding that the press's management resign and *Harmful to Minors*—and maybe its author—be burned. The rest were from producers from talk shows. My publicist in New York was playing off requests from *The Today Show* against *Good Morning America* and Fox's Greta Van Susteren. The AM-radio shock jocks were the most numerous and persistent. "My host is very fair, very intelligent," one from Los Angeles told me. With the sensitivity of an eagle a mile downwind of a field mouse, he could sniff his prey through the phone line. When he realized he was stalking an egghead, he added, "She's an NPR type."

She wasn't.

"So, Judith, do you have any children?" the host asked, a few minutes into the interview.

"No, no children." I confessed, followed by a petition for indulgence: "I have a niece and nephew."

"Do you touch your niece and nephew?"

"Of course I touch them."

"And how do you touch them?"

I could feel where this was going, but was powerless to escape. "I hug and kiss them, I stroke their hair, I rub their backs."

"And at what age would you say it was appropriate to start touching your niece and nephew in order to initiate them into sex?"

I gulped, then declared, "Never, never!" But it sounded feeble. She'd already asked me when I stopped beating my wife.

I hung up the phone and dialed my publicist, Katie. "Tell the next person who calls that Judith is unavailable," I said. "It's the second night of Passover, and she's out eating Christian children."

A few minutes later, a friend phoned in from her car: "Hey Judith! I just heard Dr. Laura denouncing you on the radio. Congratulations!"

So, Dr. Laura was the force behind my sudden fame. I'd soon learn that she had been alerted by Judith Reisman, who also called Robert Knight, with whom she'd worked at the Christian-conservative Family Research Council. He was now at a sister organization,

Concerned Women for America. In the mid-1990s, CWA had run a massive campaign against America's flagship advocate of mainstream comprehensive sexuality education, the Sex Information & Education Council of the U.S., generating 30,000 letters to Congress calling SIECUS and its sex-ed guides "blatant promoters of promiscuity, pornography, abortion, pedophilia, and incest." Now Dr. Laura had uncovered another member of "the pro-pedophile lobby."

I started to weep. It was late, but I called Katie again. My voice was little: "I'm cooked."

Katie answered with the un-flak-like candor I would grow to love. "You're right. It's pretty bad." She put me on hold to decline several invitations from other AM talk-radio shows. When she returned, she'd regained her professional pluck. "Don't worry," she said. "We'll spin it."

The good news was the book would get tons of publicity. Within the next two months, it was covered by scores of media outlets, from the Lancaster, PA, *New Era* to the *New York Times*, the gay and lesbian out.com to the neo-Nazi Jeff's Archives, WNBC Radio to college stations in rural Wisconsin. The bad news was that most of the publicity was about a book I didn't write.

Never mind what *Harmful to Minors* is about, though. Most of my critics didn't read it. And even those who did, and took it seriously, felt obliged to lead their stories with the allegation that is was an apologia for sexual abuse, "the most controversial book of the year." Spending up to 12 hours a day being interviewed, I just could not spin the story back to sanity.

In these stories, my "critics" got equal time. These were always the same few. Knight led the charge. Although he hadn't read the book, he pronounced it an "evil tome." Reisman made more secular, if no less satanic, associations. She had not read the book either, she told one major daily, but she didn't have to. She averred that she hadn't read *Mein Kampf* and she knew what was in it. I thought of writing a letter to the editor noting a small evidentiary difference between that book's author and myself: I had not yet invaded Poland.

As in the Rind attack, politicians got into the act. Republican House Majority Leader Tom DeLay introduced a resolution calling on former Surgeon General Joycelyn Elders to remove her preface from the book (unsurprisingly, Dr. Elders felt no inclination to oblige the conservative members of Congress). A New York City Councilman from Queens introduced his own resolution denouncing the book. But it was local politicians in the Press's home state who had the greatest effect and reaped the greatest benefit. Minnesota House Majority Leader Tim Pawlenty, who was also vying for the GOP's gubernatorial nomination, condemned *Harmful to Minors* as "disgusting," and "an endorsement of child molestation." He got more than 50 legislators to demand that the University suppress the book's publication. With alerts on the Christian Right Web sites, hundreds of e-mails and calls poured into the Press's office supporting this demand. None of these people had read the book, which was not yet available. When a protest at the university president's house drew only a few participants, its organizer, the lone member of his own political party, undertook a hunger strike (reliable sources observed him drinking a canned protein shake, after which I called him my dieting striker).

For some of my attackers, though, ordinary political activism did not suffice. In the heat of that cool spring month, I received a death threat. A university policewoman told me that her colleagues were doing all they could to track down the owner of the hotmail account. But the writer was too far away and appeared too disorganized to carry out any promises. His missive, originating in the aptly named Escondido, California, was addressed to "that woman who wrote the book" and e-mailed in care of the Press. Not to fret, the officer assured me. This was a "benign death threat."

In the end, the University administration yielded to the legislature's pressure and instituted an outside review of the University of Minnesota Press's editorial practices. The review was more than vindicating: UMP's standards were found to equal those at other university presses and in some instances were deemed "more rigorous than most." But the effects of the attack are likely to linger anyway. Just as the American Psychological Association's surrender emboldened Bruce Rind's attackers to go after me, the University of Minnesota's acquiescence in my case is likely to encourage other smear campaigns and censorship threats.[1] Commercial publishers, who shied away from the book on the first round, will only be more squeamish about similarly controversial titles. The Christian conservative organizations, whose public profiles had lately flattened, enjoyed a momentary spike of attention. And Tim Pawlenty's career soared. He was elected governor of Minnesota in 2002, from which office he is over-seeing massive cuts to the state's higher-education budget.

When asked to explain the "firestorm of controversy" (as every-one called it) around *Harmful to Minors,* I always answered that the book was about the American hysteria over children's sexuality and this attack was an example of the same hysteria.

But *hysteria* is the wrong word. Hysteria—irrational fear, panic, exaggerated rage—surely moved many of the letter-writers and my would-be assassin. But hysteria implies something more anarchic and unconsciously motivated than what happened to me, or to Rind or SIECUS, or before us to sex researchers, educators, and advo-cates from Margaret Sanger to Alfred Kinsey to Joycelyn Elders—indeed, from the original modern proponent of "normalizing" chil-dren's sexuality, Sigmund Freud, to the public school teacher who utters the word *clitoris* in a seventh-grade classroom.

What happened to us all was more deliberate, orchestrated, and sophisticated than hysteria. We were the targets of a campaign pros-ecuted by sexual ideologues and political opportunists for whom the incitement of hysteria is only one tactic. I knew the histories of these campaigns—*Harmful to Minors* tells them. But every book publication teaches the author something she didn't learn in writing the book. My lesson, as the object of what I'd written about, was an intimate knowledge of the way anti-sex campaigns work.

Distortion

Here's how Sean Hannity of Fox News' TV mudslinger *Hannity & Colmes* quoted *Harmful to Minors*: "We relish our erotic attraction to children."

This is what *Harmful to Minors* says: "We relish our erotic at-traction to children, says [literary critic James] Kincaid.... But we also find that attraction abhorrent." Not only does the book exten-sively discuss this contradiction, I was quoting somebody else.

In a petition for the suppression of *Harmful to Minors* to Minnesota's then-governor, Jesse Ventura, Jim Hughes of Survivors And Victims Empowered (SAVE) wrote: "Levine's previous work provides us a clue to her pro-pedophile thinking...She describes men this way: *Men's sexuality is mean and violent, and men so powerful that they can 'reach WITHIN women to...construct us from the in-side out.' Satan-like, men possess women, making their wicked fan-*

tasies and desires women's own. A woman who has sex with a man, therefore, does so against her will, 'even if she does not feel forced.'"

Actually, this passage, from my first book, *My Enemy, My Love*, is a quotation from someone else too. The characterization of men's sexuality comes from the propaganda of a group called Women Against Sex, which I describe as representing "the most extreme edge of an already marginal politics." I also call them "nutty."

Selective quotation, exaggeration, and outright lies are time-honored tactics of the Right. Judith Reisman has long circulated the calumny that Alfred Kinsey conducted sexual experiments on infants at his institute; she offers no substantiation. Focus on the Family routinely refers to sex-ed curricula as "pornography." For decades, sex-ed opponents have broadcast rumors of teachers disrobing in the classroom and children molding genitals out of clay. In *Talk About Sex*, sociologist Janice M. Irvine calls these "depravity narratives," tales that strain credibility one by one, but in great enough numbers stir suspicion that something *like* them must be true. Would I actually molest my niece and nephew? A listener might dismiss that insinuation as too extreme. But a person *like me* who wrote a book *like that* might do something almost as bad—such as condoning molestation.

In the past, such stories were reproduced in right-wing publications and at public meetings, on radio and television. The Internet only multiplies the speed and reach of this dissemination. By June, 2002, a Google search for the term "Judith Levine abuse" yielded more than 7,400 matches, most resembling the second one on the screen: "BOUNDLESS — EXCUSING CHILD ABUSE...One of the apostles of this movement, Judith Levine..."

In an already combustible atmosphere of sexual panic, distortions and lies raise the temperature and throw in the match. Voilà, a "firestorm of controversy."

Guilt by Association, or Sexual McCarthyism

The charge against me was not only that I am an advocate of pedophilia, but that I am part of an organized and increasingly influential "pro-pedophile lobby," whose aim is "normalizing" child abuse. One clue to my membership was that citation of Bruce Rind. Another was the author of the book's forward, Joycelyn Elders. You may remember Elders' pro-pedophilic crime. She told an audience of sex educators that masturbation would be an appropriate topic of sex-ed classroom discussion; this inspired the Republican House of Representatives in 1994 to demand her resignation. Knight, on Concerned Women's Web site, described the events this way: "Elders was fired by Bill Clinton shortly after she began a campaign to teach children to masturbate."

The pro-pedophile lobby allegedly has been around for a long time. In a *U.S. News & World Report* column rebuking me, John Leo recalled his own prescience in uncovering the conspiracy. "Back in 1981, an astute writer at *Time* magazine (that would be me) noticed that pro- pedophilia arguments were catching on among some sex researchers and counselors, [psychologist] Larry Constantine, [sex researchers] Wardell Pomeroy, and Alfred Kinsey," he wrote, leading up to my own connections to the lobby. "*Harmful to Minors* has a foreword by former Surgeon General Joycelyn Elders, so don't say you weren't warned." *Washington Times* writer Robert Stacy McCain contributed a catalogue of my "pedophile sources" to the Web site of Concerned Women. "Yes, Virginia," he wrote. "There is a pedophile movement, and Judith Levine's book is part of it."

But pedophiles and their lobbyists were not bad enough for some, so worse co-conspirators were proposed. While Reisman linked me to Hitler, a NewsCorridor columnist named Gregory J. Hand located me at the other end of the political spectrum, as a "bisexual Marxist Jewess," apparently part of the international Jewish conspiracy that not only controls the banks and the press, but also is "promoting adult-child sex." McCain's Concerned Women piece offered this bit of commentary: "A Google search reveals that [Levine] has described herself as a 'red-diaper baby'—that is, the child of Communist Party activists—and a socialist herself, who has written that she is 'allergic to religion.' Very interesting, but not a word of it in the *New York Times* or *USA Today*." This revelation, along with the writer's insinuation that the press was covering it up, evoked a charming bit of nostalgia. The John Birch Society and Christian Crusade in the 1960s called the Republican Quaker founding president of SIECUS, Mary Calderone, and her colleagues "atheists" and "one-worlders," a code word for communists. They also frequently pointed out how many sex educators and sexologists were Jews (who were also suspected of traitorous sentiments) and declared that together these people were softening up America's youth for conversion by the godless Reds. When the "red-diaper" comment came up at the end of a long phone interview, I broke the news to McCain: "I hate to tell you, Rob, but the Communist Party's position on sex was about as progressive as the Catholic Church's."

Marginalization

The claim about Rind, Elders, SIECUS, and me is not only that we have a political agenda, but that it is a radical one held by a small minority. Even sympathetic reporters played up this alleged eccentricity. "Their theories are explosive," read the blurb of an even-handed piece in the *LA Times*. "A handful of maverick[s]..." Don Feder in the *Boston Herald* repeated the claim that sex educators, and I as their fellow traveler (see Guilt by Association), are libertines and hedonists: "Levine thinks we interfere with the primary mission of sex educators – teaching kids that whatever feels good by definition is good." Actually, sex-ed has always been an eminently moderate project, since its inception teaching kids to wait until marriage. Moreover, in survey after survey, upwards of 80 percent of American parents say they want comprehensive sexuality education of the kind Feder decries.

Another rhetorical tactic is to quote something that would sound reasonable to most people and call it perverted. Among "Levine's bizarre theories" that Knight kept invoking was the "theory" that children are sexual from birth and, left to their own devices, will probably engage in masturbation and sex play. This "bizarre theory" is explicitly accepted by every reputable developmental psychologist and anthropologist in the industrialized world and implicitly by most everyone else in the world.

While the object of an attack is portrayed as a wild-eyed radical, the critics are described as reasonable, and legion. "In *Harmful to Minors: The Perils of Protecting Children From Sex,* its author, Judith Levine, says parents should recognize their children as sexual beings and that in some instances, sex between adults and minors may actually be a good thing," Greta Van Susteren introduced me on her show, misrepresenting the book. She added: "As you may expect this has parents around the country in a uproar."

The "critics" also appear to be politically unaffiliated. In the *New York Times*, Knight was identified as a fellow of the Heritage Foundation, not as "the Heritage Foundation, a conservative think tank," its own self-description. Only rarely in the scores of articles mentioning Concerned Women for America was the organization identified as it identifies itself: one that "seeks to instill Biblical principles in public policy at all levels." During the time I was featured on CWA's home page, so was a campaign to halt the teaching of "the lie of evolution" in public schools and an indictment of the Bush Administration's "homosexual agenda," evidenced by its hiring of a few members of the gay Log Cabin Republicans. Without such details, Concerned Women for America sounds moderate and matronly, another League of Women Voters.

The point of pushing someone to the margins is not only to discredit her in others' eyes, but to mobilize her own shame, even fear. And it works. Feeling despised as an outsider, one grasps at mainstream status.

Not married? *I've been in a relationship for eleven years!*

Have suspiciously short hair and don't wear skirts? *My partner is a man!*

No children? *Wait, wait! I'm a doting aunt!*

Sexual McCarthyism works with marginalization to discourage solidarity among the accused. In order to secure the credentials of normalcy, to remain in the safe precincts of what anthropologist Gayle Rubin describes as the "systems of sexual stigma," the targeted person distances herself from those who are even further out on the edges. The sex education community, already reeling from the Right's pummeling, declined to come to my aid. Thus divided and conquered, it's not unusual for victims of an attack to blame each other, rather than the real source of their pain. One prominent sex educator wrote me, "You should think about the harm you've done to sexuality education by dragging us into your pedophile thing."

But when called a pervert, one often goes further than not helping others accused of perversion. Ashamed, one wins respectability by expressing disgust for the "real" perverts. "What do you think of NAMBLA?" I was often asked. That's the North American Man Boy Love Association, an advocacy/support group for men with intergenerational sexual desires. "I think they're creeps," I replied to one interviewer. But I am angry at myself for doing that. NAMBLA is a tiny, ineffectual group, exercising its right to free speech; it doesn't advocate criminal activity. Already utterly despised, NAMBLA's members don't need me trashing them, too.

Naming names of the "true" subversive gains the witness immunity from prosecution. This is how McCarthyism works—until, of course, someone names your name.

Anti-Intellectualism

"The road to hell is paved with academic studies," wrote the *Boston Herald*'s Feder. In the Right's demonology, "academics" are players at the seashore, tossing abstractions back and forth like beach balls, as if all ideas were light, happy, and harmless. A number of well-designed studies led me to find it "conceivable" that sex between a priest and a boy could be a positive experience for both, I told the syndicated reporter. Such data are a good place to start, I implied, because they are neutral and objective.

But if the wrong kind of sex at the wrong time inevitably wreaks unparalleled harm, as my critics contend, then such idle conceiving might itself be harmful, because it might weaken a crucially important social taboo and lead to more sexual abuse. This is the principle behind all censorship: that bad ideas lead to bad acts. To the Family Research Council, no datum is neutral. All are charged with moral freight. Knowledge is propaganda. Indeed, the indictment of both pornography and sexuality education is that they work as advertisements, users manuals for sex.

There is something to this argument. The Right understands that science and art are ideological. They know that ideas matter. Indeed, Gayle Rubin—hardly a Christian conservative—viewed Kinsey's neutrality toward everything we now call "queer" as a step toward tolerance of sexual difference; she praised him for it. Of course, tolerance of sexual difference is what the Right abhors. They call it "defining deviancy down."

Lately, the Right has started to appropriate "science" to its own ends—for instance, changing the name of Christian creationism to "creation science" and circulating long-discredited studies that link abortion to breast cancer. Such tactics play on Americans' faith in scientific expertise. But Americans simultaneously worship and mistrust experts, especially outside the hard scientists. For many, the only unassailable expertise is gleaned from personal experience, and from emotion uninfected by reason.

Thus, the daytime TV talk shows always invite, as foils to the ivory-tower expert with the university press book, a "real person" –

a parent, a teen, or best of all, a "victim." This person is presumed to be a source of down-home wisdom and pain, as if the expert might not also be a parent or the victim of a painful experience.

Here, from a monitoring service's synopsis of Fox's *Good Day Live*:

"Visual - Newsfile. Judith Levine argues that children of all ages are sexual beings. She says they should be free to seek out pleasure with consenting peers.

Jillian talks about this. She was molested as child. She wants to punch these people in the face. NAMBLA is a group that advocates sex between men and boys. Jillian is [a] huge Howard Stern fan. She flew American Airlines and loves the women on there."

I don't mean to ridicule Jillian, whoever she is, but rather to point out the way in which her experience of abuse gives her authority, far more than someone like me, who only studies abuse.

Terror

Terrorists have replaced pedophiles in our nightmares as the inscrutable, obsessive, and endlessly proliferating cultists of perverse aggression. But the political psychology surrounding the two phenomena is similar. Repression cannot operate without fear. If there isn't enough danger, it must be exaggerated or invented. Yellow alert to red alert; predator to sexually violent predator—the boogeyman can be as scary as anyone wants him to be. As *Harmful to Minors* shows, how he becomes scary in the public imagination is a complex process, engaging the sometimes-antagonistic efforts of authoritarians and well-meaning healers, political ideologues and media sensationalists.

Sexual peril is real, just as terrorism is real. But the kind of "protection" that is mobilized by fear, the kind that purports to keep the young safe by locking them in their rooms, ignorant and scared to death—policies like abstinence-only education—will not protect them. Like the U.S.A. PATRIOT Act, such policies offer only illusory security, because they do nothing to stop the wellsprings of danger. Ironically or intentionally, those wellsprings are the very ignorance and terror we're instilling in kids, whereas the means of their self-defense are knowledge and courage, as well as rights and respect, political and sexual citizenship.

Such "security" imperils something else we cannot afford to destroy: freedom. For in sex or in democracy, freedom is not a luxury;

it is constitutive. We need to balance respect for young people's sexual freedom with adults' obligation to protect them. In dangerous times, we must discern which dangers threaten us for real, in the form of a virus, a rapist, or a flaming jetliner, and which are of our own making.

Notes

Foreword

1. These statistics appear in *The Surgeon General's Call to Action to Promote Sexual Health and Responsible Sexual Behavior,* a publication of the U.S. Public Health Service and the Department of Health and Human Services (Rockville, Md.: DHEW Publications, 2001).

2. Recent reports by the Kaiser Family Foundation state that in interviews 98 percent of parents thought sex education should include information about sexually transmitted diseases; 97 percent thought it should talk about abstinence; 90 percent said birth control should be discussed; and 85 percent said it should teach kids how to use condoms. The following two reports of the Kaiser Family Foundation provide this information: "The AIDS Epidemic at 20 Years: The View from America," *A National Survey of Americans and HIV/AIDS* (June 2001), and "Sex Education in America: A Series of National Surveys of Students, Parents, Teachers, and Principals" (September 2000).

3. Ralph J. Di Clemente, "Preventing Sexually Transmitted Infections among Adolescents: A Clash of Ideology and Science (Editorial)," *Journal of the American Medical Association* 279, no. 19 (20 May 1998): 1574–75.

4. Ira L. Reiss and Harriet M. Reiss, *Solving America's Sexual Crisis* (Amherst: Prometheus Books, 1997). My two immediate predecessors as Surgeon General, Antonia Novello and C. Everett Koop, had called for sex education and advocated the use of condoms. The call to action of our present Surgeon General, Dr. David Satcher, would also appear to be supportive.

Introduction

1. Whereas the assets of the richest 20 percent of Americans can keep them afloat for about two years without a paycheck (at the same level of spending) most of the middle class are able to last just over two months. The poorest 20 percent can't make it a day. Doug Henwood, "Wealth Report," *Nation* (April 9, 2001): 8.

2. Lauren Berlant, *The Queen of America Goes to Washington City* (Durham, N.C.: Duke University Press, 1997), 3.

3. Hillary Rodham Clinton, "Doing the Best for Our Kids," *Newsweek,* special issue, spring/summer 1997.

4. The average age at which girls show signs of puberty is just under nine for African American and just after ten for white American girls. Susan Gilbert, "Early Puberty Onset Seems Prevalent," *New York Times,* April 9, 1997. In 1990, the median age of first marriage for women was twenty-five; for men, it was twenty-seven. Sally C. Clarke, "National Center for Health Statistics Advance Report of Final Marriage Statistics, 1989 and 1990," *Monthly Vital Statistics Report* 43, no. 12 S1 (July 14, 1995).

5. This is true even when the groups are comparable in terms of family income, neighborhood, and so on. "Teen Sex and Pregnancy," Alan Guttmacher Institute report, September 1999; "Adolescent Sexual Behavior: I. Demographics" and "Adolescent Behavior: II. Socio-Psychological Factors," Advocates for Youth reports, Washington, D.C., 1997.

6. Kristin Luker, *Dubious Conceptions: The Politics of Teenage Pregnancy* (Cambridge, Mass.: Harvard University Press, 1996), 89.

7. A more recent dip is being seen among boys but not among girls. "Trends in Sexual Risk Behaviors among High School Students—U.S. 1991–97," *Morbidity and Mortality Weekly Report* 47 (September 18, 1998): 749–52.

8. "Teen Sex and Pregnancy," Alan Guttmacher Institute.

9. Luker, *Dubious Conceptions,* 9.

10. National Health and Social Life Survey of 1994. Freya L. Sonenstein et al., *Involving Males in Preventing Teen Pregnancy* (Washington, D.C.: Urban Institute, 1997), 16.

11. Lucinda Franks, "The Sex Lives of Your Children," *Talk* (February 2000): 104.

12. Diane di Mauro, *Sexuality Research in the United States: An Assessment of the Social and Behavioral Sciences,* pamphlet (New York: Social Science Research Council, 1995). Since Alfred Kinsey's research in the 1940s and 1950s, the only major comprehensive large-scale national behavioral study was conducted by Edward Laumann et al. at the University of Chicago and published as *The Social Organization of Sexuality: Sexual Practices in the United States* (Chicago: University of Chicago Press,

1994). This study, initially planned to be much larger, was repeatedly stymied by conservative political interference in its funding.

13. "Research Critical to Protecting Young People from Disease Blocked by Congress," Advocates for Youth press release, December 19, 2000, www.advocatesforyouth.org/news/press/121900.htm.

14. "Most Adults in the United States Who Have Multiple Sexual Partners Do Not Use Condoms Consistently," *Family Planning Perspectives* 26 (January/February 1994): 42–43.

15. See, e.g., Sarah Blaffer Hrdy, *Mother Nature: A History of Mothers, Infants, and Natural Selection* (New York: Pantheon, 1999).

16. Phillipe Ariès, *Centuries of Childhood: A Social History of Family Life* (New York: Vintage Books, 1962).

17. J. H. Plumb, "The New World of Children in 18th-Century England," *Past and Present* 67 (1975): 66.

18. Quoted in Alan Prout and Allison James, "A New Paradigm for the Sociology of Childhood?" in *Constructing and Reconstructing Childhood*, ed. Allison James and Alan Prout (London: Falmer, 1990), 17.

19. Karin Calvert, *Children in the House: The Material Culture of Early Childhood, 1600–1900* (Boston: Northeastern University Press, 1992).

20. Marina Warner, "Little Angels, Little Monsters," in her *Six Myths of Our Time* (New York: Vintage Books, 1994).

21. James R. Kincaid, *Child-Loving: The Erotic Child and Victorian Culture* (New York: Routledge, 1992).

22. Philip J. Greven, "Family Structure in Seventeenth-Century Andover, Massachusetts," *William and Mary Quarterly*, 3d series, 23 (1966): 234–56. In any period "the most sensitive register of maturity is the age at marriage," wrote Greven. It could be argued that this is no longer true. However, the *legal* age of marriage may be read as a register of ideologies that define *immaturity*. In America, though that age has ranged from as young as twelve, it was not until the late Progressive Era that policymakers perceived a "child marriage problem," and the legal marriage age crept into the midteens in a number of states. Kristie Lindenmeyer, "Adolescent Pregnancy in the 20th Century U.S.," paper delivered at the Carleton Conference on the History of the Family, Ottawa, May 15, 1997.

23. Deborah Gray White, *Ar'n't I a Woman? Female Slaves in the Plantation South* (New York: W. W. Norton and Co., 1985), 106.

24. John D'Emilio and Estelle B. Freedman, *Intimate Matters: A History of Sexuality in America* (New York: Harper and Row, 1988), 12–14, 43.

25. G. Stanley Hall, *Adolescence: Its Psychology and Its Relations to Anthropology, Sociology, Sex, Crime, Religion and Education* (New York: D. Appleton, 1904).

26. Kincaid, *Child Loving*, 126–27.

27. Warner, "Little Angels, Little Monsters," 55–56.

28. Susheela Singh and Jacqueline E. Darroch, "Adolescent Pregnancy

and Childbearing: Levels and Trends in Developed Countries," Alan Guttmacher Institute report, February 2000.

29. A summary of many studies found an average prevalence for non-
sexual dating violence of 22 percent among high school students and 32
percent among college students. D. B. Sugarman and G. T. Hotaling, "Dating Violence: Prevalence, Context, and Risk Markers," in M. A. Pirog-Good
and J. E. Stets, eds., *Violence in Dating Relationships* (New York: Praeger,
1989), 3–32. One study showed that teenage girls were almost three times
more likely to suffer a beating at the hands of a date than were teenage
males. M. O'Keefe and C. Treister, "Victims of Dating Violence among
High School Students," *Violence against Women* 4 (1998): 193–228.

30. SIECUS, *SHOP (School Health Opportunities and Progress) Talk
Bulletin* 4, no. 1 (March 19, 1999).

31. Bill Alexander, "Adolescent HIV Rates Soar; Government Piddles,"
Youth Today (March/April 1997): 29.

32. They were down 44 percent in the first six months of 1997 compared
with 1996. Lawrence K. Altman, "AIDS Deaths Drop 48% in New York,"
New York Times, February 3, 1998, A1.

33. These people probably contracted HIV in their teens. Philip J. Hilts,
"AIDS Deaths Continue to Rise in 25–44 Age Group, U.S. Says," *New
York Times,* January 16, 1996, A22.

34. *Annie E. Casey Foundation Annual Report 1997* (Baltimore: Annie E.
Casey Foundation, 1997).

35. "Facts about Adolescents and HIV/AIDS," Centers for Disease Control and Prevention report, Atlanta, Ga., March 1998.

36. Lawrence K. Altman, "Study in 6 Cities Finds HIV in 30% of Young
Black Gays," *New York Times,* February 6, 2001.

1. Censorship

1. People for the American Way, *Attacks on the Freedom to Learn*
(Washington, D.C.: People for the American Way, 1996).

2. Marc Silver, with Katherine T. Beddingfield and Kenan Pollack,
"Sex, Violence and the Tube," *U.S. News and World Report* (September
1993): 76–79.

3. Susan N. Wilson, "Who's Afraid of the Big Bad Word?" *Censorship
News,* National Coalition Against Censorship (winter 1996): 5.

4. Jane D Brown, "Sexuality and the Mass Media: An Overview,"
SIECUS Reports 24, no. 10 (April/May 1996): 3–5.

5. I borrow this term from Agnes Repellier, "The Repeal of Reticence,"
Atlantic, March 1914, 207–304.

6. The term *hypermediated* was coined by Henry Jenkins, of the Massachusetts Institute of Technology.

7. Quoted in Judith H. Dobrzynski, "A Popular Couple Charged into

the Future of Art, but in Opposite Directions," *New York Times*, September 2, 1997.

8. "Child's Eye View," *New York Times*, December 31, 1997.

9. Sherry Turkle, *Life on the Screen: Identity in the Age of the Internet* (New York: Simon and Schuster, 1995), 26.

10. Roy Porter, "Forbidden Pleasures: Enlightenment Literature of Sexual Advice," in *Solitary Pleasures: The Historical, Literary, and Artistic Discourses of Autoeroticism*, ed. Paula Bennett and Vernon A. Rosario II (New York: Routledge, 1995), 81.

11. New York Society for the Prevention of Cruelty to Children, *Fifteenth Annual Report*, Case 39,591 (New York: the society, 1890), 15–16.

12. Repellier, "The Repeal of Reticence."

13. Ira S. Wile, "The Sexual Problems of Adolescents," *Journal of Social Hygiene* 20, no. 9 (December 1934): 439–40.

14. Bernard Weintraub, "Fun for the Whole Family," *New York Times*, July 22, 1997.

15. Samuel S. Janus and Barbara E. Bess, "Latency: Fact or Fiction?" *American Journal of Psychoanalysis* 36, no. 4 (1976): 345–46.

16. Right-wing fundamentalist Christians are today's firmest articulators of the view from Genesis, that philandering with worldly experience can lead to no good. One of their conspiracy narratives dates the fall of American civilization to the takeover of Harvard University by Unitarians, the country's preeminent educational institution hijacked by its preeminent doubters. Conservative opposition to sex education, similarly, is always connected with opposition to other forms of moral questioning and intellectual exploration at school, from values clarification to creative spelling.

17. See Roger Shattuck's *Forbidden Knowledge: From Prometheus to Pornography* (New York: St. Martin's Press, 1996) for an interesting exploration of this conflict.

18. Nicole Wise, "A Curious Time," *Parenting*, March 1994, 110.

19. Janice Irvine, "Cultural Differences and Adolescent Sexualities," in *Sexual Cultures and the Construction of Adolescent Identities*, ed. Janice Irvine (Philadelphia: Temple University Press, 1994), 21.

20. Interview with Leonore Tiefer, May 1996.

21. This is still true in many non-Western cultures and Western ethnic subcultures, which is why HIV/AIDS workers have coined the term "men who have sex with men," or MSM, to reach people who don't identify as gay but may still engage in so-called gay sex.

22. Anne C. Bernstein, *Flight of the Stork: What Children Think (and When) about Sex and Family Building*, rev. ed. (Indianapolis: Perspectives Press, 1994), 31.

23. Elizabeth Kolbert, "Americans Despair of Popular Culture," *New York Times*, August 20, 1995, 23.

24. Marjorie Heins, INDECENCY: *The Great American Debate over Sex, Children, Free Speech, and Dirty Words,* Andy Warhol Foundation for the Visual Arts, Monograph Paper #7, 1997, 4.

25. While the courts have often balked at censorship of books and films, because presumably a child could be kept from seeing them, they have upheld "safe-harbor" restrictions in numerous cases involving radio and television broadcasting. A landmark decision came in 1978, when the New York listener-supported Pacifica radio station WBAI aired the comedian George Carlin's baroque exegesis of the "Seven Filthy Words" that the Federal Communications Commission prohibited from the airwaves: *shit, piss, fuck, cunt, cocksucker, motherfucker,* and *tits.* The FCC imposed sanctions on Pacifica, which appealed the decision to the Supreme Court. There, the justices ruled that the FCC could punish Pacifica, not because the content was legally obscene, but because it broadcast the words at a time when minors were likely to be listening. Heins, INDECENCY, 11.

26. Barbara Miner, "Internet Filtering: Beware the Cybercensors," *Rethinking Schools* (summer 1998): 11.

27. *Butler v. Michigan,* 352 U.S. 383–84 (1957).

28. Janelle Brown, "Another Defeat for 'Kiddie Porn' Law," salon.com, June 23, 2000.

29. *Report of the Commission on Obscenity and Pornography* (Washington, D.C.: Lockhart commission, 1970), 23–27.

30. Mary R. Murrin and D. R. Laws, "The Influence of Pornography on Sexual Crimes," in *Handbook of Sexual Assault,* ed. W. L. Marshall, D. R. Laws, and H. E. Barbaree (New York: Plenum Press, 1990), 83–84.

31. David E. Nutter and Mary E. Kearns, "Patterns of Exposure to Sexually Explicit Material among Sex Offenders, Child Molesters, and Controls," *Journal of Sex and Martial Therapy* 19 (spring 1993): 73–85.

32. See John Money, *Love Maps: Clinical Concepts of Sexual/Erotic Health and Pathology, Paraphilia and Gender Transposition, Childhood, Adolescence and Maturity* (New York: Irving Publishers, 1986); Irene Diamond, "Pornography and Repression: A Reconsideration," *Signs* (summer 1989): 689; David Futrelle, "Shameful Pleasures," *In These Times* (March 7, 1994): 17.

33. Marjorie Heins, *Sex, Sin, and Blasphemy: A Guide to America's Censorship Wars* (New York: New Press, 1993).

34. Edward de Grazia, *Girls Lean Back Everywhere: The Law of Obscenity and the Assualt on Genius* (New York: Vintage Books, 1993): 541n, 551–61.

35. U.S. Department of Justice, *Report of the Surgeon General's Workshop on Pornography and Public Health* (Washington, D.C.: Government Printing Office, 1986), 344.

36. Sources in Massachusetts identify this "expert" as one who gave

later-discredited testimony against day-care workers accused of "satanic ritual abuse."

37. *Public Eye,* CBS-TV, October 8, 1997.

38. *Morning Edition,* National Public Radio, September 12, 1997.

39. Declan McCullagh and Brock Meeks, "Keys to The Kingdom," *Cyberwire Dispatch,* cyberworks.com, July 3, 1996.

40. Steven Isaac, "Safe Cruising on the Info Highway," *Focus on the Family* (February 1998): 12.

41. Amy Harmon, "Parents Fear That Children Are One Click Ahead of Them," *New York Times,* May 3, 1999, A1.

42. Jon Katz, "The Rights of Kids in the Digital Age," *Wired,* July 1996. In the same spirit, Katz's cyber-news Web site, frequented by youngsters, has become journalists' main source for what kids think, and also a strong source of opposition to proposed harder Internet restrictions, following the student shootings at Columbine High in Littleton, Colorado. Two studies released in June 2001 found that most preteens and teens online can take unwanted or unsolicited online communications in their stride. Three-quarters of the youth questioned both by Crimes Against Children Research Center of the University of New Hampshire and by the Pew Internet and American Life Project said they weren't upset by posts from strangers asking to have sex or talk about it, and simply deleted or blocked them. Commented Donna Hoffman, a Vanderbilt University management professor specializing in online commerce, to the *New York Times,* it is "no surprise" that children might be approached by people looking for sex on the Net. "It's how children are educated to deal with these experiences that is important." Jon Schwartz, "Studies Detail Solicitation of Children for Sex Online," *New York Times,* June 20, 2001.

43. *Report of the Surgeon General's Workshop,* 36–38.

44. Penelope Leach, "Kids and Sex Talk," *Redbook,* October 1993, 178.

45. Neil Postman, *The Disappearance of Childhood* (New York: Vintage Books, 1994), 80.

46. Laura Megivern, "Net Controls Won't Block the Curious," *Burlington Free Press,* September 24, 1997, 2C.

47. See chapter 8 for more on good public sources of sex education.

2. Manhunt

1. This account was constructed from articles in the *Boston Herald, Boston Globe,* and *Cambridge Chronicle* between October 1997 and December 1998; also Yvonne Abraham, "Life after Death," *Boston Phoenix,* September 25, 1998, 23–30; and interviews with Boston and Cambridge residents.

2. In spite of the proliferating coverage of pedophilia and child abuse, the media frequently claim that we are inexcusably silent on the subject.

"[The pedophile] is protected not only by our ignorance of his presence, but also by our unwillingness to confront the truth," Andrew Vachss, one of the more sensationalist writers on the subject, opined in 1989, for instance.

3. Paul Okami and Amy Goldberg, "Personality Correlates of Pedophilia: Are They Reliable Indicators?" *Journal of Sex Research* 29, no. 3 (August 1992): 297–328; author's review of state laws.

4. See, e.g., Andrew Vachss, "How We Can Fight Child Abuse," *Parade Magazine*, August 20, 1989, 14.

5. A pedophile is defined as a person who has "recurrent intense sexual urges and arousing sexual fantasies involving sexual activity with a prepubescent child or children." *Diagnostic and Statistical Manual of Mental Disorders III-R* (Washington, D.C.: American Psychiatric Association, 1987).

6. Mike Smith, "Sex Offender Registry OK'd," *Journal Gazette* (Fort Wayne, Indiana), February 20, 1996.

7. Ann Landers, "There's One Cure for Child Molesters," syndicated column, August 2, 1995.

8. Debbie Nathan and Michael Snedeker, *Satan's Silence: Ritual Abuse and the Making of a Modern American Witch Hunt* (New York: Basic Books, 1996), 91.

9. Tim LaHaye and Beverly LaHaye, *Against the Tide: How to Raise Sexually Pure Kids in an "Anything-Goes" World* (Colorado Springs: Multnomah Books, 1993), 189.

10. "Improving Investigations and Protecting Victims," *Boston Herald*, May 4, 1994.

11. Richard Laliberte, "Missing Children: The Truth, the Hype, and What You Must Know," *Redbook*, February 1998, 77.

12. The death-penalty bill was defeated by one vote at the end of the 1997–98 legislative session, though the incoming Republican governor, Paul Cellucci, promised to pass it in the next term. Bob Curley, feeling used by his political handlers and used up by a life of rage, has retreated to crusade against child pornography and raise funds for child-abuse prevention programs. Abraham, "Life after Death," 30. In 2000, the Curleys brought a civil suit against the North American Man/Boy Love Association and several individuals allegedly associated with it, claiming that Jaynes was a heterosexual before reading the organization's propaganda and that his crimes were "a direct and proximate result of [its] urging, advocacy, and promoting of pedophile activity." *Barbara Curley and Robert Curley v. North American Man Boy Love Association, Best Interest Communications Inc., Verio Inc.* [and various individual defendants], U.S. District of Massachusetts (announced April 15, 2000). In April 2001, the family's lawyers filed additional charges against NAMBLA, seeking dam-

ages under the Racketeer Influenced and Corrupt Organizations Act (RICO), usually used to prosecute gangsters. The Massachusetts Chapter of the ACLU is representing NAMBLA on free-speech grounds; the Civil Liberties Union has asked the judge to dismiss the case. David Weber, "Family of Slain Cambridge Boy Wants NAMBLA Held Responsible," BostonHerald.com, April 11, 2001.

13. Laliberte, "Missing Children," 77.

14. J. M. Lawrence, "Molesters Hide Evil behind Image of the Normal Guy," *Boston Herald,* October 12, 1997, 30.

15. According to the FBI, "classic" abductions, in which a child is taken by a nonfamily member more than fifty miles from home, held overnight, and ransomed or murdered, number two hundred to three hundred annually, or 1 child in every 230,000 (as of 1997).

16. FBI statistics, phone interview, summer 1993.

17. Lieutenant Bill D'Heron points out that the case is still open. Phone interview with the lieutenant, of the Hollywood (Florida) Police Department detectives unit, December 15, 1998.

18. Laliberte, "Missing Children," 78.

19. Anna C. Salter, "Epidemiology of Child Sexual Abuse," in *The Sexual Abuse of Children: Theory and Research,* vol. 1, ed. William O'Donoghue and James H. Geer (Hillsdale, N.J.: Lawrence Erlbaum Associates, 1992), 129–130.

20. See Paul Okami, "'Slippage' in Research on Child Sexual Abuse: Science as Social Advocacy," in *The Handbook of Forensic Sexology: Biomedical and Criminological Perspectives,* ed. James J. Krivacska and John Money (Amherst, N.Y.: Prometheus Books, 1994), 559–75.

21. Quoted in Bruce Selcraig, "Chasing Computer Perverts," *Penthouse,* February 1996, 51.

22. More than eight times more people were incarcerated for low-level sex offenses in 1992 than in 1980. Bureau of Justice Statistics, "Correctional Populations in the United States," report, Washington, D.C., 1992, 53.

23. Federal Bureau of Investigation, "Uniform Crime Reports: Crime in the U.S.," report, Washington, D.C., 1993, 217.

24. Okami and Goldberg, "Personality Correlates," 317–20. The article is an excellent review of the literature.

25. In one study, fewer than a fifth of pedophiles interviewed said they desired genital sex, whereas another fifth wanted "non-sexual, platonic friendships." Glenn D. Wilson and David N. Cox, *The Child-Lovers: A Study of Paedophiles in Society* (London: Peter Owen), 35.

26. Okami and Goldberg, "Personality Correlates," 297–328. A study of the members of a British pedophile organization found that "the majority [of subjects] showed no sign of clinically significant psychopathy or

thought disorder." Wilson and Cox, *The Child Lovers,* 122–23. Even the commonly held belief that a molested child will grow up to be a molester is exaggerated: studies find that about a third do, which means that as many as two-thirds do not. Joan Kaufman and Edward Zigler, "Do Abused Children Become Abusive Parents?" *American Journal of Orthopsychiatry* 57, no. 2 (1987): 186–92. The degree of social anxiety that pedophiles exhibit may be a result, not a cause, of the intense hatred and ostracism they experience, say a number of observers, including psychologists Theo Sandfort and Larry Constantine.

27. Wilson and Cox *(The Child-Lovers)* add a caveat to Money's comment about erotophobia in the families of paraphilics. They note that just about everyone describes his or her parents as repressive about sex.

28. There was no proof of a sexual relationship between the two men. Nor was there any of a general propensity toward child molesting in the Sicari family, although police inferred one from the conviction of Salvi's sixteen-year-old brother in a sexual encounter with a ten-year-old boy. The gay historian Allan Bérubé suggested that the crime fit another stereotype and piqued another fear: that the child molester's prey is not only a boy but a white boy (author conversation with Bérubé).

29. Margaret A. Alexander, "Quasi-Meta-Analysis II, Oshkosh Correctional Institution," State of Wisconsin Department of Corrections/Oshkosh Correctional Institution report, Oshkosh, 1994; Lita Furby et al., "Sex Offender Recidivism: A Review," *Psychological Bulletin* 3 (1989); R. Karl Hanson and Monique T. Bussière, "Predictors of Sexual Offender Recidivism: A Meta-Analysis," Department of Solicitor General of Canada, *Journal of Consulting and Clinical Psychology* 66, no. 2 (1996).

30. These numbers are inflated by reoffenses by adult rapists. In her metanalysis of seventy-nine studies encompassing almost eleven thousand subjects, Oshkosh (Wisconsin) Correctional Institution clinical director Margaret Alexander reconfirmed the fact that men who rape adult women are the most intransigent, with about a fifth striking again whether they undergo a treatment program in prison or not. But men arrested for having sex with children are usually overcome with shame and remorse; they want to stop. For them, good treatment has made a great difference: Since 1943, an average of 11 percent of "child molesters" who were treated in jails, hospitals, and outpatient clinics found their way back to prison, compared with 32 percent of those who took part in no treatment. Margaret A. Alexander, "Sexual Offender Treatment Efficacy Revisited," State of Wisconsin Department of Corrections/Oshkosh Correctional Institution report, Oshkosh, May 1998. There's also evidence that better treatment is increasingly successful. Before 1980, recidivism among treated sex offenders was almost 30 percent; after 1980, it dropped to 8.4 percent. Eric

Lotke, "Sex Offenders: Does Treatment Work?" National Center for Institutions and Alternatives report, Washington, D.C., 1996, 5.

31. James R. Kincaid, *Child-Loving: The Erotic Child and Victorian
Culture* (New York: Routledge, 1992); and James R. Kincaid, *Erotic In-
nocence: The Culture of Child-Molesting* (Durham, N.C.: Duke University
Press, 1998).

32. Judith Lewis Herman, *Father-Daughter Incest* (Cambridge, Mass.:
Harvard University Press, 1981).

33. *National Incidence Studies of Child Abuse and Neglect,* vol. 2
(Washington, D.C.: Department of Health and Human Services, 1993).

34. Ellen Bass and Laura Davis, *The Courage to Heal: A Guide for
Women Survivors of Child Sexual Abuse* (New York: Harper Perennial,
1988): 22.

35. Richard Ofshe and Ethan Watters, *Making Monsters: False Memories, Psychotherapy, and Sexual Hysteria* (New York: Scribner's, 1994),
65–67. In fact, any catalogue of symptoms is suspect. "Psychological evidence suggests that it is impossible to tease out a set of symptoms that are
related to sexual abuse but are never seen in victims of other types of
abuse." Elizabeth Wilson, "Not in This House: Incest, Denial, and Doubt
in the Middle-Class Family," *Yale Journal of Criticism* 8 (1995): 51.
Wilson's conclusion, drawn from examinations of the *Diagnostic and
Statistical Manual of Mental Disorders,* is supported by a thorough review
of the abuse literature by Bruce Rind at the University of Pennsylvania, as
well as Paul Okami and others. Such careful work is in the minority. The
complete confounding of data has led to huge inflations of the statistics,
which are commonly repeated by journalists. In the 1980s, estimates of
women abused as children ranged as high as 62 percent. S. D. Peters, G. E.
Wyatt, and D. Finkelhor, "Prevalence," in *A Source Book on Sexual
Abuse,* ed. David Finkelhor (Beverly Hills, Calif.: Sage Publishers, 1986),
75–93.

36. This estimation is drawn from the hundreds of articles I've read in
writing about child abuse.

37. U.S. Department of Health and Human Services, *Third National Incidence Study of Child Abuse and Neglect* (Washington, D.C., 1993); 3–3.

38. Judith Lewis Herman, D. Russell, and K. Trocki, "Long-Term Effects of Incestuous Abuse in Childhood," *American Journal of Psychiatry*
143, no. 10 (1986): 1293–96.

39. "By far the largest group of defendants [in child pornography cases]
seems to be white males between 30 and 50 who are interested in teenage
boys, usually between 14 and 17," concluded Bruce Selcraig, a government investigator of child pornography during the 1980s who went online
in 1996 as a journalist to review the situation. Selcraig, "Chasing Computer

Perverts," 53. The same is true of the majority of men in jail for consensual sex with girls or boys: their partners are teenagers. I conclude this from my own surveys over the past ten years of journalism, police sources, and defense attorneys.

40. Jennifer Allen, "The Danger Years," *Life,* July 1995, 48.

41. Lawrence, "Molesters Hide Evil," 31.

42. As quoted by Harry Hendrick, "Constructions and Reconstructions of British Childhood: An Interpretive Survey, 1800 to the Present," in *Constructing and Reconstructing Childhood,* ed. Allison James and Alan Prout (London: Falmer Press, 1990), 42.

43. Judith R. Walkowitz, *City of Dreadful Delight: Narratives of Sexual Danger in Late-Victorian London* (Chicago: University of Chicago Press, 1992).

44. The reports of the New York Society for the Prevention of Cruelty to Children, for instance, frequently described the alleged exploiters of children in vicious and often confused ethnic stereotypes. Italian "padrones" who traffic variously in child labor, entertainment, and flesh are ubiquitous. A "rabbi" who runs a beer-bottle and cigarette-strewn gambling den behind a bogus "bird store" is characterized, incongruously, by his "little Chinese ways of enticement." Society for the Prevention of Cruelty to Children, *Sixteenth Annual Report* (New York, 1891), 23.

45. See, e.g., Walkowitz, *City of Dreadful Delight*; Ellen Carol DuBois and Linda Gordon, "Seeking Ecstasy on the Battlefield," in *Pleasure and Danger: Exploring Female Sexuality,* ed. Carole Vance (London: Pandora Press, 1989); Kathy Peiss, *Cheap Amusements: Working Women and Leisure in Turn-of-the-Century New York* (Philadelphia: Temple University Press, 1987); Christine Stansell, *City of Women: Sex and Class in New York, 1789–1860* (Champaign: University of Illinois Press, 1987); and Ruth C. Rosen, *The Lost Sisterhood: Prostitution in America, 1900–1918* (Baltimore: Johns Hopkins University Press, 1983), for a fuller picture of turn-of-the-century urban prostitution.

46. Walkowitz, *City of Dreadful Delight,* 81–120.

47. Judith R. Walkowitz, *Prostitution and Victorian Society: Women, Class, and the State* (Cambridge: Cambridge University Press, 1980): 17.

48. DuBois and Gordon, "Seeking Ecstasy on the Battlefield," 33.

49. Walkowitz, *City of Dreadful Delight,* 82.

50. John D'Emilio and Estelle Freedman, *Intimate Matters: A History of Sexuality in America* (New York: Harper and Row, 1988), 153.

51. Estelle Freedman, "'Uncontrolled Desires': The Response to the Sexual Psychopath, 1920–1960," *Journal of American History* 71, no. 1 (1987): 83–106.

52. D'Emilio and Freedman, *Intimate Matters,* 260–61.

53. Allan Bérubé, *Coming Out under Fire: The History of Gay Men and Women in World War II* (New York: Macmillan, 1990).

54. As quoted by George Chauncey Jr., "The Postwar Sex Crime Panic," in *True Stories from the American Past,* ed. William Graebner (New York: McGraw Hill, 1993), 162.

55. Freedman, "'Uncontrolled Desires.'"

56. Chauncey, "Postwar Sex Crimes," 160–78.

57. Freedman, "'Uncontrolled Desires,'" 92.

58. Freedman, "'Uncontrolled Desires,'" 84.

59. Chauncey, "Postwar Sex Crimes," 160–74.

60. Heidi Handman and Peter Brennan, *Sex Handbook: Information and Help for Minors* (New York: Putnam, 1974).

61. Lawrence Stanley, "The Child Porn Myth," *Cardozo Arts and Entertainment Law Journal* 7 (1989): 295–358.

62. U.S. House Committee on the Judiciary, *Sexual Exploitation of Children: Hearings before the Subcommittee on Crime,* 95th Congress, first session, 1977, 42–48. See also, Judianne Densen-Gerber and Stephen F. Hutchinson, "Sexual and Commercial Exploitation of Children: Legislative Responses and Treatment Challenges," *Child Abuse and Neglect* 3 (1979): 61–66.

63. "'Child Sex' Cop Transferred," *Bay Area Reporter,* March 18, 1982, 8.

64. U.S. House Judiciary Committee, *Sexual Exploitation of Children,* 48.

65. Stanley, "The Child Porn Myth," 313.

66. Joel Best, "Dark Figures and Child Victims: Statistical Claims about Missing Children," in *Images of Issues: Typifying Contemporary Social Problems,* ed. Joel Best (New York: Aldine de Gruyter, 1989), 21–37.

67. Stanley, "The Child Porn Myth," 313.

68. Lucy Komisar, "The Mysterious Mistress of Odyssey House," *New York Magazine,* November 1979, 43–50. The charges were not indictably substantiated, but they were enough to exile Densen-Gerber from Odyssey House and, for a time, social service altogether. In 1998, she was running Applied Resources Corporation in Bridgeport, Connecticut.

69. "'Child Sex' Cop Transferred."

70. See Nathan and Snedeker, *Satan's Silence.* Nathan was for a long time the only journalist in America who published skeptical investigations of "satanic ritual abuse." Later, she was joined by the documentarist Ofra Bikel and others, and by the early 1990s, their painstaking reporting began to turn some opinion around.

71. Daniel Goleman, "Proof Lacking in Ritual Abuse by Satanists," *New York Times,* October 31, 1994.

72. The charges were brought by the adopted daughter of a zealous police chief, and, as in Salem, the people who objected to what looked to them like a widening witch-hunt, found themselves accused. The defendants were disproportionately poor, uneducated, and in several cases mentally disabled, and no defendant without a private attorney was acquitted. Kathryn Lyons, *Witch Hunt: A True Story of Social Hysteria and Abused Justice* (New York: Avon, 1998).

73. Documented by the Justice Committee, San Diego, Calif.; Boston Coalition for Freedom of Expression, Boston, Mass.; Nathan and Snedeker *(Satan's Silence)*; and others.

74. Selcraig, "Chasing Computer Perverts," 72.

75. Seminar conducted at the University of Southern California by R. P. Tyler (reported by James R. Kincaid, author interview).

76. Lawrence A. Stanley, "The Child-Porn Myth," *Playboy,* September 1988, 41.

77. The notion of predisposition informs all sting operations: police are not allowed to entice somebody into breaking the law (that would be entrapment) unless they have evidence indicating he is likely to do so on his own. Narcotics agents commonly buy from a known dealer; occasionally an undercover cop will put herself into a position to be assaulted by a rapist whose m.o. is known.

However, the establishment of predisposition in child pornography enforcement is not so straightforward, because the enforcers' motives aren't. If the goal is to eradicate deviance and not necessarily to prevent actual crimes, as the ACLU's Marjorie Heins suggests, suspicion of deviance goes a long way toward legally establishing predisposition to criminality. The National Center for Missing and Exploited Children's manual for law enforcers suggests including in requests for search warrants a profile of what they call a "preferential child molester," accent on *preferential,* since he might want to do something he's never done.

Since the person needs to have demonstrated no greater erotic interest in children than logging onto a site where they congregate (I, in researching this chapter, could be accused of such acts), the tactic resembles setting somebody up for a drug bust not because he's actually sold or bought drugs but because he has watched the doings of the dealer next door or because he has an "addictive personality."

Once a "preference" for "child molestation" has been thus established, a search warrant stating this preference in the suspect alerts cops to the probability that a collection of illegal child pornography awaits their search. And the search fulfills their expectations: they find pictures and, whether they're pornographic or not, take them to be clues to molestation. "The photograph of a fully dressed child may not be evidence of an obscenity violation, but it could be evidence of an offender's sexual involvement with children," says the National Center's manual.

In 1995 I asked Raymond Smith, who heads the Postal Inspection Service's child pornography investigations, about his estimation that PI agents find "evidence of child molestation" in 30 percent of their searches of the homes of suspected pedophiles:

"We'll find pictures of kids—no sexual act; we don't know where these kids come from. But you get a gut feeling . . . you learn to identify it. . . . We're not finding a videotape of this guy having sex with the ten-year-old girl next door. We're not finding a picture. Just from what we see in the house and how they talk.

"When we get into these cases, many of these individuals literally confess to committing horrible acts, before they're arrested. Sometimes that is fantasy, which is not against the law. But when you have the child pornography present, combined with the fantasy, in my opinion not only are they violating the law, they also pose a serious threat to children in the community where they live. If somebody told me this man never molested before, but, man, he loves kids and I knew he was a member of NAMBLA [the North American Man/Boy Love Association, a support group–propaganda organization], I would think that person was a threat to my child. But I have no, quote, evidence that he molested."

78. *Ashcroft v. Free Speech Coalition* 795 U.S.

79. "Cynthia Stewart's Ordeal," editorials, *Nation* (May 1, 2000).

80. James R. Kincaid, "Hunting Pedophiles on the Net," salon.com, August 24, 2000.

81. A particularly harrowing account of a year-long entrapment campaign resulting in the conviction of a man who seemed to have no preexisting sexual interest in children can be found in Laura Kipnis, *Bound and Gagged: Pornography and the Politics of Fantasy in America* (New York: Grove Press, 1996).

82. Christopher Marquis, "U.S. Says It Broke Pornography Ring Featuring Youths," *New York Times,* August 9, 2001.

83. Kincaid, "Hunting Pedophiles on the Net."

84. During the U.S. Postal Inspection Service's late-1980s Project Looking Glass investigations, 5 of the 160 people indicted saved the government the effort of seeking a plea bargain by promptly committing suicide.

85. Marquis, "U.S. Says It Broke Pornography Ring Featuring Youths."

86. Susan Lehman, "Larry Matthews' 18-Month Sentence for Receiving and Transmitting Kiddie Porn Raises Difficult First Amendment Issues," salon.com, March 11, 1999. The brazenness of the putative mother's post gives it the scent of a sting operation, in my view. Frequenters of such chat

rooms, and surely criminals involved in child prostitution, are meticulously secretive, understanding that they are under constant surveillance. In the mid-1990s, lawyer Lawrence Stanley was also indicted (though not convicted) for receiving alleged child-pornographic images through the mail. He had received the pictures from a client for whom he was acting as defense counsel; they were the indictable items in the client's case, and Stanley was challenging the prosecutor's claims that the images were indeed legally pornographic.

87. Kimberly J. Mitchell, David Finkelhor, and Janis Wolak, "Risk Factors for and Impact of Online Sexual Solicitation of Youth," *Journal of the American Medical Association* 285 (June 20, 2001): 3011–14 (unpaginated online). Commenting on the study, Harrison M. Rainie, the director of a more comprehensive study called "Teenage Life Online," by the Pew Internet and American Life Project, said, "Virtually every kid we talked to knows there are some really bad things and bad people in the online world, and know that there are some good things and good people. When they get down to weighing the pluses and minuses, most kids will say the pluses pile up and the minuses are manageable." John Schwartz, "Studies Detail Solicitation of Children for Sex Online," *New York Times,* June 20, 2001.

88. Ron Martz, "Internet Spreading Child Porn, Investigators Say," *Sunday Rutland Herald,* June 28, 1998, A8.

89. "Bonfire of the Knuckleheads," *Contemporary Sexuality* 28 (April 1994): 1.

90. James Kincaid documented a dozen or so with newspaper articles, but my researches would suggest there are many more that don't make the papers. James Kincaid, "Is This Child Pornography?" salon.com, January 31, 2000.

91. Katha Pollitt, "Subject to Debate," *Nation* (December 13, 1999); "Cynthia Stewart's Ordeal"; and Cynthia Stewart and David Perrotta, "Thank You, Nation Family," letters, *Nation* (May 1, 2000).

92. Matt Golec, "Bill Would Expand Sex Offender Notification Law," *Burlington Free Press,* January 30, 2000, A1.

93. Ross E. Milloy, "Texas Judge Orders Notices Warning of Sex Offenders," *New York Times,* May 29, 2001.

94. In 1997, the first subject of the Kansas law, who had no record of violence, but rather a rap sheet of exhibitionism and mild fondling, brought his case to the U.S. Supreme Court and lost. The law was upheld. By that year, Washington, Arizona, California, Minnesota, and Wisconsin had passed similar laws.

95. Bill Andriette, "America's Sex Gulags," *Guide* (August 1997) (reprint): 1–3.

96. A 1996 review of the data by the National Center for Institutions

and Alternatives concluded that only 13 percent of former sex offenders are arrested for subsequent sex crimes. This compares with a recidivism rate of 74 percent for all criminal offenders. The NCIA estimated at this time that of 250,000 potential compliers with community registration statutes, 217,000 were "ex-offenders" or people who were not destined to commit additional crimes. National Center for Institutions and Alternatives, "Community Notification and Setting the Record Straight on Recidivism," Community Notification/NCIA/info@ncianet.org, November 8, 1996.

97. In Corpus Christi, several of the men who posted warning signs immediately had their property vandalized, two were evicted from their homes, and one attempted suicide. An intruder threatened the life of the father of one of the men, who had been arrrested for indecency with a child in 1999 "after a night of drinking ended with an encounter with a fifteen-year-old girl." Milloy, "Texas Judge Orders Notices."

98. Todd Purdum, "Registry Laws Tar Sex-Crimes Convicts with Broad Brush," *New York Times,* July 1, 1997. Later that year, California excised the names of men convicted of consensual homosexuality from the list. "Gay Exception Made to Registration Law," *New York Times,* November 11, 1997.

99. U.S. Senate Committee on Governmental Affairs, Permanent Sub committee on Investigations, "Child Pornography and Pedophilia," Report 99-537, October 6, 1986, 3.

100. Evidence suggests that statutory rape, or sex with minors, did occur at Waco. David Koresh did so with the parents' consent, because his followers believed it "was his religious duty to father 24 children by virgin mothers." Because the parents cooperated, the state did not bring charges. Dick J. Reavis, *The Ashes of Waco: An Investigation* (Syracuse, N.Y.: Syracuse University Press, 1998).

101. The number of fatalities, including the number of children among them, is hard to pin down. On James Tabor and Eugene Gallagher's "Why Waco?" Web site, a list of Branch Davidians counts seventy-two dead, including twenty-three children. The *New York Times,* reporting on the FBI's belated admission that it had fired pyrotechnic gas canisters at the compound, noted on August 26, 1999, that "about 80 people, including 24 children, were found dead after the fire." The following day, a subsequent story said "about 80 people, including 25 children." David Stout, "FBI Backs Away from Flat Denial in Waco Cult Fire," *New York Times,* August 26, 1999, A1; Stephen Labaton "Reno Admits Credibility Hurt in Waco Case," *New York Times,* August 27, 1999, A1. The Justice Department's report directly following the events said "the medical examiner found the remains of 75 individuals" but did not specify how many were children. Edward S. G. Dennis Jr., "Evaluation of the Handling of the

Branch Davidian Stand-Off in Waco, Texas, February 28 to April 19, 1993," U.S. Department of Justice report, Washington, D.C., October 8, 1993.

3. Therapy

1. The story of the Diamonds was drawn from interviews and time spent with the participants, including the family, their therapist, Phillip Kaushall, and various social-service professionals, lawyers, and others involved in their case, as well as from several thousand pages of Child Protective Services case files kept between December 1994 and late 1996, when I visited. I have changed the names of the family members, as well as the social workers and foster parents whose names appear in the case records.

2. Brian's story was constructed from interviews with the family and from San Diego police, court, and psychologists' records.

3. Shirley Leung and Stacy Milbauer, "New Hampshire Boy, 10, Charged in Rape of 2 Playmates," *Boston Globe,* August 22, 1996, A1.

4. Andy Newman, "New Jersey Court Says 12-Year-Old Must Register as a Sexual Offender," *New York Times,* April 12, 1996.

5. "Police Uncover Child Sex Ring in Small Pa. Town," Associated Press, *Burlington Free Press,* July 5, 1999.

6. See Paul Okami, "'Child Perpetrators of Sexual Abuse': The Emergence of a Problematic Deviant Category," *Journal of Sex Research* 29, no. 1 (February 1992): 109–30; and Okami, "'Slippage' in Research of Child Sexual Abuse."

7. Leonore Tiefer, "'Am I Normal?' The Question of Sex," in *Sex Is Not a Natural Act and Other Essays* (Boulder, Colo.: Westview, 1995), 10–16.

8. San Diego County Grand Jury, *Report No. 2: Families in Crisis,* February 6, 1992, 4–6.

9. Mark Sauer, "Believe the Children?" *Times Union,* August 29, 1993.

10. Toni Cavanagh Johnson, "Child Perpetrators—Children Who Molest Other Children: Preliminary Findings," *Child Abuse and Neglect* 12 (1988): 219–29.

11. Carolyn Cunningham and Kee MacFarlane, *When Children Abuse* (Brandon, Vt.: Safer Society Program, 1996), viii–ix.

12. David Gardetta, "Facing the Monster: Teenage Sex Offenders in Treatment," *LA Weekly,* January 13–19, 1995, 17.

13. Jeffrey Butts, "Offenders in Juvenile Court, 1994," *Juvenile Justice Bulletin,* U.S. Department of Justice, Office of Juvenile Justice and Delinquency Prevention, Washington, D.C., October 1996.

14. See, for instance, the literature of the Safer Society Program in Vermont.

15. Claudia Morain, "When Children Molest Children," American Medical Association *News,* January 3, 1994.

16. William N. Friedrich, "Normative Sexual Behavior in Children," *Pediatrics* 88, no. 3 (September 1991): 456–64.

17. Okami, "'Child Perpetrators of Sexual Abuse.'"

18. Okami, "'Slippage' in Research of Child Sexual Abuse," 565.

19. Toni Cavanagh Johnson, "Behaviors Related to Sex and Sexuality in Preschool Children," photocopied typescript, undated, S. Pasadena, Calif.

20. Johnson, "Child Perpetrators," 221.

21. National Clearinghouse on Child Abuse and Neglect, NCCAN Discretionary Grants FY 1991, award number 90CA1469.

22. A group of clinicians distributed the proposal at the Fourteenth Annual Conference of the Association for the Treatment of Sexual Abusers (October 11–14, 1995), trying to win additional support.

23. *The Third National Incidence Study of Child Abuse and Neglect (NIS-3)* (Washington, D.C.: U.S. Department of Health and Human Services, 1997), 2–14.

24. See, e.g., Cunningham and MacFarlane, *When Children Abuse,* ix.

25. See, e.g., David Finkelhor, *Child Sexual Abuse: New Theory and Research* (New York: Free Press, 1984); L. M. Williams and David Finkelhor, "The Characteristics of Incestuous Fathers," in ed. W. Marshall, D. R. Laws, and H. Barbaree, *The Handbook of Sexual Assault: Issues, Theories, and Treatment of the Offender* (New York: Plenum Publishing, 1989).

26. Friedrich's 1992 comparison between sexually abused and non-abused children found that abused kids act out sexually with greater frequency than other kids do, but both groups do all the same sexual things. William N. Friedrich and Patricia Grambsch, "Child Sexual Behavior Inventory: Normative and Clinical Comparison," *Psychological Assessment* 4 (1992): 303–11; Robert D. Wells et al., "Emotional, Behavioral, and Physical Symptoms Reported by Parents of Sexually Abused, Nonabused, and Allegedly Abused Prepubescent Females," *Child Abuse and Neglect* 19 (1995): 155–62. J. A. Cohen and A. P. Mannarino, "Psychological Symptoms in Sexually Abused Girls," *Child Abuse and Neglect* 12 (1988): 571–77; R. J. Weinstein et al., "Sexual and Aggressive Behavior in Girls Experiencing Child Abuse and Precocious Puberty," paper presented at the annual convention of the American Psychological Association, New Orleans, 1989.

27. Many researchers have decried the lack of systematic collection of data and their paucity on this subject. Nevertheless, all the data there are support my statement, and none contradict it. See, e.g., Friedrich, "Normative Sexual Behavior in Children"; William N. Friedrich et al., "Normative Sexual Behavior in Children: A Contemporary Sample," *Pediatrics*

101, no. 4 (April 1998), e9; William N. Friedrich, Theo G. M. Sandfort, Jacqueline Osstveen, and Peggy T. Cohen-Kettensis, "Cultural Differences in Sexual Behavior: 2–6 Year Old Dutch and American Children," *Journal of Psychology and Human Sexuality* 12, nos. 1–2 (2000): 117–29; Allie C. Kilpatrick, *Long-Range Effects of Child and Adolescent Sexual Experiences: Myths, Mores, Menaces* (Hillsdale, N.J.: Lawrence Erlbaum, 1992); Sharon Lamb and Mary Coakley, "'Normal' Childhood Sexual Play and Games: Differentiating Play from Abuse," *Child Abuse and Neglect* 17 (1993): 515–26; Floyd M. Martinson, *The Sexual Life of Children* (Westport, Conn.: Bergin and Garvey, 1994); Paul Okami, Richard Olmstead, and Paul R. Abramson, "Sexual Experiences in Early Childhood: 18-Year Longitudinal Data for the UCLA Family Lifestyles Project," *Journal of Sex Research* 34, no. 4 (1997): 339–47; Jany Rademakers, Marjoke Laan, and Cees J. Straver, "Studying Children's Sexuality from the Child's Perspective," *Journal of Psychology and Human Sexuality* 12, nos. 1–2 (2000): 49–60; and sources at note 32.

28. Friedrich et al., "Normative Sexual Behavior in Children" (1998).

29. Johnson, "Behaviors Related to Sex and Sexuality in Preschool Children."

30. J. Attenberry-Bennett, "Child Sexual Abuse: Definitions and Interventions of Parents and Professionals," Ph.D. dissertation, Department of Education, University of Virginia, 1987.

31. Okami, Olmstead, and Abramson, "Sexual Experiences in Early Childhood."

32. Evan Greenwald and Harold Leitenberg, "Long-Term Effects of Sexual Experiences with Siblings and Nonsiblings during Childhood," *Archives of Sexual Behavior* 18, no. 5 (1989): 389. Similar results were reported in Harold Leitenberg, Evan Greenwald, and Matthew J. Tarran, "The Relation between Sexual Activity among Children during Preadolescence and/or Early Adolescence and Sexual Behavior and Sexual Adjustment in Young Adulthood," *Archives of Sexual Behavior* 18, no. 4 (1989): 299 ff.

33. Martinson's informants related stories of intercourse, fellatio, and anal intercourse, as well as more "childish" practices of looking and mutual masturbation.

34. Clellan S. Ford and Frank A. Beach, *Patterns of Sexual Behavior* (New York: Harper and Row, 1951), 197, 188.

35. Cunningham and MacFarlane, *When Children Abuse*, 28.

36. Theo Sandford and Peggy Cohen-Kettensis, "Parents' Reports about Children's Sexual Behaviors," paper presented at the Twenty-first Annual Meeting of the International Academy of Sex Research, September 1995.

37. Friedrich et al., "Normative Sexual Behavior in Children" (1998).

38. Okami, "'Slippage' in Research in Child Sexual Abuse."

39. Lamb and Coakley, "'Normal' Childhood Sexual Play and Games." This finding, it should be noted, troubled the authors.

40. Martha Shirk, "Emotional Growth Programs 'Save' Teens, Stir Fears," *Youth Today* 8 (May 1999); Martha Shirk, "Kid Help or Kidnapping?" *Youth Today* 8 (June 1999).

41. Contract between offenders and parents and Sexual Treatment & Education Program and Services (STEPS), 2555 Camino Del Rio South, Ste. 101, San Diego, Calif. (last revised September 19, 1994).

42. Practices at STEPS may have changed, but, considering the literature on children who molest that has come out since, I have no reason to believe it has.

43. U.S. District Court (Vermont), Civil Action No. 2: 93-CV-383: *Robert Goldstein et al. v. Howard Dean et al.*

44. Testimony of Dr. Fred Berlin in *Goldstein et al. v. Dean et al.*

45. NCCAN Discretionary Grants, FY 1991, award no. 90CA1470.

46. Other research also strongly interrogates, and condemns, sex-specific treatment for young violent sex offenders as well. One study compared boys who had committed exceedingly brutal sex crimes with other young violent offenders and found that both groups had survived childhoods afflicted by severe violence but not by sexual abuse and that the two groups exhibited identical psychiatric and neurological disorders, including depression, auditory hallucinations, paranoia, and often "grossly abnormal EEGs" or epilepsy. "The assumption that sexually assaultive offenders differ neuropsychiatrically from other kinds of violent offenders, which has led to the establishment of specific programs for sex offenders," the researchers concluded, "must . . . be questioned in the light of our data." Dorothy Otnow Lewis, Shelley S. Shankok, and Jonathan H. Pincus, "Juvenile Male Sexual Assaulters," *American Journal of Psychiatry* 136, no. 9 (September 1979): 1194–96.

47. Gisela Bleibtreu-Ehrenberg, "Pederasty among Primitives: Institutionalized Initiation and Cultic Prostitution," in *Male Intergenerational Intimacy,* ed. Theo Sandfort, Edward Brongersma, and Alex van Naerssen (New York: Hawthorn Press, 1991), 13–30; William H. Davenport, "Adult-Child Sexual Relations in Cross-Cultural Perspective," in *The Sexual Abuse of Children: Theory and Research,* vol. 1, ed. William O'Donohue and James H. Geer (Hillsdale, N.J.: Lawrence Ehrlbaum Associates, 1992), 73–80.

48. Susan Brownmiller, *Against Our Will: Men, Women, and Rape* (New York: Simon and Schuster, 1975). In 2001, the conviction by a United Nations war-crimes tribunal of three Bosnian Serbs for the rapes of captive Muslim women and girls marked the first time in history that "sexual slavery" has been designated a crime against humanity, deemed one of the

most heinous crimes. Marlise Simons, "3 Serbs Convicted in Wartime Rapes," *New York Times*, February 23, 2001.

4. Crimes of Passion

1. Although these events received considerable press attention at the time they occurred, the people involved have returned to private life. Therefore, the names of the members of the two families and their personal acquaintances have been changed, along with their cities and state of residence. The following names are fictitious: Dylan Healy; Heather, Robert, Pauline, and Jason Kowalski; Laura and Tom Barton; June Smith; Jennifer Bordeaux; and Patrick. Of public figures, only the names of "Dylan Healy's" lawyer and the sentencing judge have been deleted. Press and court sources are in the author's possession, but notes corresponding to these sources have been omitted to prevent identification of the subjects.

2. Bob Trebilcock, "Child Molesters on the Internet: Are They in Your Home?" *Redbook*, April 1997.

3. Mary Douglas, *Purity and Danger: An Analysis of the Concepts of Polution and Taboo* (London: Ark Paperbacks, 1984), 96.

4. Brownmiller, *Against Our Will*, 29.

5. Historically U.S. law has denied the right of certain people, such as slaves and married women, to say no, and others, such as the mentally disabled, to say yes to sex, marriage, or procreation. But our ideas of what sorts of people can't say yes or no to sex often compound each other. So a teenager who got pregnant in the 1920s, for instance, was often also dubbed feeble-minded, and a disproportionate number of the adolescents forcibly sterilized under eugenic policies were also black. Kristie Lindenmeyer, "Making Adolescence," paper presented at the International Conference on the History of Childhood, Ottowa, 1997.

6. *Michael M. v. Superior Court of Sonoma County*, 450 U.S. 464 (1981).

7. The volume of publicity and punishment given Mary Kay Letourneau, thirty-five, for her relationship with a thirteen-year-old student, whose baby she bore, is an indication of the rarity of such relationships and of statutory rape prosecutions in which the adult is female and the minor male. Letourneau lost her job and her children and went to jail. But the boy insisted he still loved her and was adamant that he was not a victim. "It hurts me, it makes me more angry when people give me their pity, because I don't need it," he told the local television station. "I'm fine." The two saw each other illicitly while she was on a leave from prison, and she became pregnant again. "Boy Says He and Teacher Planned Her Pregnancy," *Seattle Post-Intelligencer*, August 22, 1997, C1; "Schoolteacher Jailed for Rape Gives Birth to Another Child," *New York Times*, October 18, 1998.

8. While there are no hard facts about the sexual orientation of perpetrator or victim, anecdotal evidence suggests that these laws are being used more aggressively to prosecute consensual sex between men and teenage boys, taking over the role of antisodomy statutes, which by 1998 had been repealed in thirty states. Legislation prohibiting sex with minors, moreover, is often written more harshly against gay sex than straight. For instance, a 1996 California law compelling chemical or surgical castration for the second offense of engaging in sex with anyone under thirteen most severely penalizes the two acts commonly associated with homosexuality—anal intercourse and oral sex—but fails to mention heterosexual vaginal intercourse with girls. The prohibition against homosexual marriage affects gay teenage boys and girls as well, since youngsters can marry in most states at an earlier age than they are legally allowed to have unmarried sex. Bill Andriette, "Life Sentences," *NAMBLA Bulletin,* June 1994, 94–95; Carey Goldberg, "Rhode Island Moves to End Sodomy Ban," *New York Times,* May 10, 1998, 12; "RE: Sexual Relations with Minor," memo from Silverstein Langer Newburgh & Brady to Lambda Legal Defense Fund, February 4, 1998; Bill Andriette, "Barbarism California Style," *Guide,* October 1996, 9–10.

9. Kristin Anderson Moore, Anne K. Driscoll, and Laura Duberstein Lindberg, *A Statistical Portrait of Adolescent Sex, Contraception, and Childbearing,* pamphlet (Washington, D.C.: National Campaign to Prevent Teen Pregnancy, 1998), 11, 13.

10. The characterizations of Dylan's condition come from his lawyer, Laura Barton, and Dylan himself.

11. Sharon G. Elstein and Noy Davis, "Sexual Relations between Adult Males and Young Teen Girls: Exploring the Legal and Social Responses," American Bar Association report, Washington, D.C., 1997, 26.

12. Elstein and Davis, "Sexual Relations between Adult Males and Young Teen Girls," 5.

13. Elstein and Davis, "Sexual Relations between Adult Males and Young Teen Girls," 26.

14. Lynn M. Phillips, "Recasting Consent: Agency and Victimization in Adult-Teen Relationships," in *New Versions of Victims: Feminists Struggle with the Concept,* ed. Sharon Lamb (New York: New York University Press, 1999), 93. A local Planned Parenthood chapter funded the study.

15. Mike A. Males, *Scapegoat Generation: America's War on Adolescents* (Monroe, Me.: Common Courage Press, 1996), 45–76.

16. Patricia Donovan, "Can Statutory Rape Laws Be Effective in Preventing Adolescent Pregnancy?" *Family Planning Perspectives* (January/February 1997).

17. Elizabeth Gleick, "Putting the Jail in Jailbait," *Time,* January 29, 1996, 33.

18. Mireya Navarro, "Teen-Age Mothers Viewed as Abused Prey of Older Men," *New York Times,* May 19, 1996.

19. Phillips, "Recasting Consent," 84.

20. Donovan, "Can Statutory Rape Laws Be Effective?" See also: "Issues in Brief: and the Welfare Reform, Marriage, and Sexual Behavior," Alan Guttmacher Institute report, 2000; Kristin Luker, *Dubious Conceptions: The Politics of Teenage Pregnancy* (Cambridge, Mass.: Harvard University Press, 1996).

21. Although teen pregnancy rates have declined to their lowest levels since the 1970s, experts attribute the change not to any crackdown on adult-teen sex but to increased contraception use, particularly condoms and long-lasting implants, by teenage women. Ayesha Rook, "Teen Pregnancy Down to 1970s Levels," *Youth Today,* November 1998, 7. Mike Males, original discoverer of the connection between adult-teen sex and teen pregnancy, has reviewed California's records and expressed regrets to me that the data have been used so punitively. He also admits that any implication of a direct causal relationship might have been ill advised on his part. Interviews 1998 and 1999.

22. Elstein and Davis, "Sexual Relations between Adult Males and Young Teen Girls," 11.

23. Matt Lait, "Orange County Teen Wedding Policy Raises Stir," *Los Angeles Times,* Orange County Edition, September 2, 1996, A1. Public-health researcher Laura Lindberg found that such liaisons are not as unstable as some may think. When she checked in with fifteen- to seventeen-year-old mothers with older partners thirty months after their babies' births, she found the couples were still close and still together. Laura Duberstein Lindberg et al., "Age Differences between Minors Who Give Birth and Their Adult Partners," *Family Planning Perspectives* 20 (March/April 1997): 20.

24. Brandon Bailey, "Teen Moms Question Governor's Proposal," *San Jose Mercury News,* January 14, 1996, 1B.

25. James Brooke, "An Old Law Chastises Pregnant Teen-Agers," *New York Times,* October 28, 1996, A10.

26. Mary E. Odem, *Delinquent Daughters: Protecting and Policing Adolescent Female Sexuality in the United States, 1885–1920* (Chapel Hill: University of North Carolina Press, 1995), 5.

27. Like today, boys were afforded much greater license to play as they wished, especially if they were employed (though they also had to deliver their wages to the family cookie jar). Also like today, when a family did bring a son before the authorities on sex charges, it was usually for molesting younger sisters or stepsisters or, in a few cases, for suspected homosexuality. Odem, *Delinquent Daughters,* 178. Historian Ruth Alexander found similarly unsatisfactory outcomes for families in the cases she

tracked from New York State in the 1930s and 1940s. When accusing parents found out that the mandatory sentence for sexual misconduct was three years, most were shocked. So while their girls were locked away in Bedford Hills, several hours' trip north of New York City, mothers inundated the wardens with letters pleading for reduced sentences and more humane treatment of their daughters. Interview with Alexander, July 1998.

28. Steven Schlossman and Stephanie Wallach, "The Crime of Precocious Sexuality: Female Juvenile Delinquency in the Progressive Era," *Harvard Educational Review* 48 (1978): 65–95.

29. Luker, *Dubious Conceptions*, 30, 212.

30. Interviews with Ricki Solinger and Ruth Alexander, July 1998.

31. Odem, *Delinquent Daughters*, 188.

32. The 1995 National Survey of Family Growth found that 43.1 percent of girls lost their virginity with a partner one to two years older, 26.8 percent with someone three to four years older, and 11.8 percent with a person five or more years older. The average teen girl's male lover is three years older than she. Moore, Driscoll, and Lindberg, "A Statistical Portrait of Adolescent Sex," 13. See also: Sharon Thompson, *Going All the Way* (New York: Hill and Wang, 1995), 217, 322.

33. Security classifications are in many cases similar to mandatory sentencing laws, which designate certain categories of crime (sex offenses and drug offenses among them) as more "dangerous," even if they are not more violent, than other crimes.

34. Divorce filings in author's possession. Not identified here to protect privacy.

35. National Center on Child Abuse and Neglect, *Federal Register,* part 2 (Washington, D.C.: U.S. Department of Health and Human Services, January 23, 1978), 3244.

36. Frank Bruni, "In an Age of Consent, Defining Abuse by Adults," *New York Times,* November 9, 1997, "Week in Review," 3.

37. Allie C. Kilpatrick, *Long-Range Effects of Child and Adolescent Sexual Experiences: Myths, Mores, Menaces* (Hillsdale, N.J.: Lawrence Erlbaum Associates, 1992).

38. Kilpatrick, *Long-Range Effects of Child and Adolescent Sexual Experiences,* 58, 90.

39. Letter, *NAMBLA Bulletin,* June 1994.

40. William E. Prendergast, *Sexual Abuse of Children and Adolescents* (New York: Continuum Publishing Co., 1996), 26.

41. Bruce Rind and Philip Tromovitch, "A Meta-analytic review of findings from national samples on Psychological Correlates of Child Sexual Abuse," *Journal of Sex Research* (1997): 237–55.

42. Author interview with Lynn Phillips, January 1998.

43. Thompson, *Going All the Way*, 215–44.

44. I also asked the prominent sexologist and therapist Leonore Tiefer about these relationships. She said: "You have to take into account the subjectivity and the realm of experience of each individual young person. You can't explain this stuff with universals—with sociobiology or sociology. The power issues are not wiped out" by individual explanations, however; "they are complicated." Tiefer gave the example of Monica Lewinsky. "On one hand, you could say she's powerful: she got the leader of the free world to desire her. On the other, there is a certain powerlessness and displacement of ambition" onto the sexual conquest.

45. Phillips, "Recasting Consent," 87.

46. Martin J. Costello, *Hating the Sin, Loving the Sinner: The Minneapolis Children's Theatre Company Adolescent Sexual Abuse Prosecutions* (New York: Garland, 1991), 8–13.

47. Elstein and Davis, "Sexual Relations between Adult Men and Young Teen Girls," 19.

48. Most states allow youngsters to drive, and even to marry, before they may have unmarried sexual intercourse. In Massachusetts at this writing, a person can marry at twelve, but if someone who is not her husband inserts his finger into her vagina when she is fifteen, even with her express consent, he can be charged with statutory rape. Under a section of the state's legal code entitled "Crimes against Chastity, etc.," taking a picture of her naked seventeen-year-old buttocks will earn the photographer up to twenty years in prison. *Massachusetts Family Law*, Section 354 (1990); *Massachusetts Criminal Law*, Section 12: 16 (1992); *Massachusetts General Laws*, Section 373: 29A.

49. In 1993 in New Mexico it was thirteen; by 1998, it was seventeen; in Maine it went from fourteen to eighteen in the same years. "The Geography of Desire," *Details* (June 1993). See also Elstein and Davis, "Sexual Relations between Adult Males and Young Teen Girls." For a continual update of age of consent throughout the world, consult www.ageofconsent.com.

50. Males, *Scapegoat Generation*, 71.

51. David T. Evans, *Sexual Citizenship: The Material Construction of Sexualities* (London: Routledge, 1993), 215.

5. No-Sex Education

1. Joyce Purnick, "Where Chastity Is Not Virtuous," *New York Times*, May 25, 1981, A14.

2. My suspicion is the word *abstinence* migrated into sex ed from the hugely popular movement of twelve-step anti-"addiction" programs based on the model of Alcoholics Anonymous, which preached that only com-

plete renunciation and daily recommitment could bring a bad habit under control.

3. *Guidelines for Comprehensive Sexuality Education* (New York: Sex Information and Education Council of the U.S., 1994), 1.

4. Social Security Act, Title V, Section 510 (1997), Maternal and Child Health Bureau, U.S. Department of Health and Human Services.

5. David J. Landry, Lisa Kaeser, and Cory L. Richards, "Abstinence Promotion and the Provision of Information about Contraception in Public School District Sexuality Education Policies," *Family Planning Perspectives* 31, no. 6 (November/December 1999): 280–86; Kaiser Family Foundation, "Most Secondary Schools Take a More Comprehensive Approach to Sex Education," press release, December 14, 1999.

6. "Changes in Sexuality Education from 1988–1999," SEICUS, *SHOP Talk Bulletin* 5, no. 16 (October 13, 2000).

7. Diana Jean Schemo, "Survey Finds Parents Favor More Detailed Sex Education," *New York Times,* October 4, 2000, A1.

8. Joyce Purnick, "Welfare Bill: Legislating Morality?" *New York Times,* August 19, 1996, "Metro Matters," B1.

9. Patricia Campbell, *Sex Education Books for Young Adults 1892–1979* (New York: R. R. Bowker Co., 1979), viii.

10. F. Valentine, "Education in Sexual Subjects," *New York Medical Journal* 83 (1906): 276–78.

11. Benjamin C. Gruenberg, *High Schools and Sex Education: A Manual of Suggestions of Education Related to Sex* (Washington, D.C.: U.S. Public Health Service and U.S. Bureau of Education, 1922), 95.

12. Evelyn Duvall, *Facts of Life and Love for Teenagers,* as quoted in Campbell, *Sex Education Books for Young Adults,* 87.

13. Mary S. Calderone, "A Distinguished Doctor Talks to Vassar College Freshmen about Love and Sex," *Redbook,* February 1964 (reprint).

14. *Sex Education: Conditioning for Immorality,* filmstrip, John Birch Society, released around 1969 (n.d.).

15. Handman and Brennan, *Sex Handbook,* 170.

16. Sol Gordon, *You: The Psychology of Surviving and Enhancing Your Social Life, Love Life, Sex Life, School Life, Home Life, Work Life, Emotional Life, Creative Life, Spiritual Life, Style of Life Life* (New York: Times Books, 1975).

17. In 1972, worried that young single women's kids would end up on the dole, Congress required all welfare departments to offer birth control services to minors. The Supreme Court ruled in *Carey v. Population Services International* (1977) that teens had a privacy right to purchase contraception; in 1977 and 1979, when Congress reauthorized Title X of the Public Health Services Act of 1970, providing health care to the poor,

it singled out adolescents as a specific group in need of contraceptive services. In 1978, partly in reaction to the Guttmacher Report, Senator Edward Kennedy's Adolescent Health Services and Pregnancy Prevention and Care Act set up the Office of Adolescent Pregnancy Programs at the Department of Health, Education, and Welfare (later Health and Human Services). Its mandate was to administer "comprehensive [reproductive] services" to teens (Luker, *Dubious Conceptions*, 69). On the books, the government seemed to care about the reproductive and social health of teenagers, but the budget belied real commitment. No new funds were slated for the younger Title X clients, who would number as many as half the visitors to some birth control clinics in coming years. The Kennedy program, proposed at fifty million dollars in the first year, got only one million dollars; in its third and final year, it reached just ten million dollars and extended grants to fewer than three dozen programs nationwide.

18. Guttmacher Report, quoted in Constance A. Nathanson, *Dangerous Passages: The Social Control of Sexuality in Women's Adolescence* (Philadelphia: Temple University Press, 1991), 47.

19. The history of family planning and concomitant legislation before the Adolescent Family Life Act draws from Nathanson, *Dangerous Passages*; Rosalind Pollack Petchesky, *Abortion and Women's Choice: The State, Sexuality, and Reproductive Freedom*, rev. ed. (Boston: Northeastern University Press, 1990); and Luker, *Dubious Conceptions*, as well as interviews with birth control professionals, lawyers, and women's movement activists from the 1970s and 1980s.

20. Alan Guttmacher Institute, *Sex and America's Teenagers* (New York: the institute, 1994), 58. Luker notes that many are also discouraged at school or already dropouts and that motherhood does not diminish such a young woman's standard of living: they are poor when they have children, and they stay poor (Luker, *Dubious Conceptions*, 106–8). Sociologist Arline Geronimus had argued that for some young women early childbearing is a rational choice, the best of several not-so-great options. A girl can stay in school and take advantage of school-based day care; families more readily help young mothers with babysitting and financial support than older ones; and, when Junior heads off to kindergarten, a younger mom has plenty of years to recover missed opportunities. Besides, for the young women "at risk," babies add love, meaning, and structure to otherwise fairly stripped-down lives. Arline T. Geronimus and Sanders Korenman, "The Socioeconomic Consequences of Teen Childbearing Reconsidered," *Quarterly Journal of Economics* (November 1992): 1187–214. Teenage men, especially those who are alienated from school and pessimistic about their work prospects, feel just as affirmed by fatherhood as their girlfriends do by motherhood. William Marsigho and Constance L. Shehan, "Adolescent Males' Abortion At-

titudes: Data from a National Survey," *Family Planning Perspectives* 25 (July/August 1993): 163.

21. This number represented about 50 percent of the fifteen- to nineteen-year-olds, the same percentage who are now sexually active. Alan Guttmacher Institute, *Eleven Million Teenagers: What Can Be Done about the Epidemic of Adolescent Pregnancies in the United States* (New York: Planned Parenthood Federation on America, 1976), 9–11.

22. Nathanson, *Dangerous Passages,* 60.

23. Luker, *Dubious Conceptions,* 8.

24. For surgeon general, Reagan nominated Everett Koop, who had appeared in an anti-abortion propaganda video standing in a field of dead fetuses. But Koop turned out not to be the antichoice puppet the Right to Life had hoped for. Keeping his views on abortion to himself, he became a tireless crusader for frank AIDS education. Richard Schweiker, also staunchly antichoice and not too hot for a federal role in education or welfare either, was appointed secretary of Health, Education, and Welfare. To run that department's three-year-old Office of Adolescent Pregnancy Programs, the administration recruited Marjory Mecklenberg, a Minnesota Right to Life activist widely regarded as an unqualified hard-liner for "family values" and against nonmarital sex, which seemed to be a prerequisite for top positions in that office. It would later be occupied by Jo Ann Gasper, whose column in *Conservative Digest* attacked "homosexuals and other perverts" and "antifamily forces"; by Nabers Cabaniss, a favorite of far-right senators Denton, Jesse Helms, and Henry Hyde who at thirty boasted that she was the oldest virgin in Washington, D.C.; and by Cabaniss's erstwhile boyfriend William Reynolds "Ren" Archer III, who as a bachelor confided to a reporter that he had had sex once but didn't much like it.

25. "Block-granting" Title X into the Maternal and Child Health Bureau had been proposed during the Nixon administration too but failed.

26. African American communities had always kept such babies close to home. And by 1981, as birth mothers began to come forward and express the pain and coercion of their decisions and adopted children started looking for those birth mothers, white girls were also thinking twice about relinquishing maternal rights. Ricki Solinger, *Wake Up Little Susie* (New York: Routledge, 1992).

27. *Kendrick v. Bowen* (Civil A. No. 83-3175), "Federal Supplement," 1548. Patricia Donovan, "The Adolescent Family Life Act and the Promotion of Religious Doctrine," *Family Planning Perspectives* 4, no. 4 (September/October 1984): 222.

28. The anti-ERA Illinois Committee on the Status of Women received grants of over $600,000 to develop and evaluate the workbook *Sex Respect* (ACLU "Kendrick I," List of Grantees), authored by former Catholic

schoolteacher and anti-abortion activist Colleen Kelly Mast, and another $350,000 for *Facing Reality*, the workbook of its companion curriculum (*Teaching Fear: The Religious Right's Campaign against Sexuality Education* [Washington, D.C.: People for the American Way, June 1994], 10). *Sex Respect* was denounced for its inaccuracies and omissions, ridiculed for its sloganeering ("Pet Your Dog, Not Your Date"), and scorned for its anti-sexual moralism ("There's no way to have premarital sex without hurting someone"). Yet in 1988 the U.S. Department of Education put the curriculum on its list of recommended AIDS education videos, replacing one by the Red Cross. The next year, after former committee vice-president, then state representative Penny Pullen sponsored legislation requiring abstinence education in Illinois public schools, Sex Respect was awarded state contracts worth more than $700,000 (*Teaching Fear*, 10).

29. This figure has also been cited for the number of school districts employing any abstinence-only curriculum. "States Slow to Take U.S. Aid to Teach Sexual Abstinence," *New York Times*, May 8, 1997, 22.

30. During that time, the average grant for other organizations the size of Teen-Aid or Respect Inc. was less than half of Teen-Aid's and less than a third of Respect's. Department of Health and Human Services, Public Health Service, "Adolescent Family Life Demonstration Grants Amounts Awarded 1982–1996," Office of Adolescent Pregnancy Prevention document, Washington, D.C., 1996. Teen-Aid did not use the free startup money to reduce its prices to future customers. In Duval County, Florida, one of the people who sued in the mid-1990s to stop the schools from teaching Teen-Aid's "Me, My World, My Future" because of its inaccuracies and its biases against abortion, women and girls, gays, and "any kind of family that isn't mommy, daddy, and children" said, "The new curriculum [is] going to save the school system huge amounts of money. [With Teen-Aid], we had to buy $100,000 worth of supplies a year." "In Duval County, Florida: Reflecting on a Legal Battle for Comprehensive Sexuality Education," *SIECUS Reports* 24, no. 6, (August/September 1996), 5.

31. *Teaching Fear*, 11.

32. The statistics available at the time from the institute were that about 780,000, or 39 percent, of 2 million then-fourteen-year-old girls would have at least one pregnancy in their teen years; 420,000 would give birth; 300,000 would have abortions.

33. U.S. Senate, Jeremiah Denton, *Adolescent Family Life*, S. Rept. 97-161, July 8, 1981, 2; emphasis added.

34. "To Attack the Problems of Adolescent Sexuality," *New York Times*, June 15, 1981, A22.

35. "To Attack the Problems of Adolescent Sexuality."

36. A few years earlier, the Family Protection Act (H.R. 7955), a blueprint of the Right's agenda to come and also cosponsored by Hatch, pro-

posed defunding all state protections of children and women independent of their fathers and husbands, including child-abuse and domestic-abuse programs. It did not pass.

37. Bernard Weinraub, "Reagan Aide Backs Birth-Aid Education," *New York Times,* June 24, 1981, C12.

38. A SIECUS–Advocates for Children Survey in 1999 found that 70 percent opposed the federal abstinence-only standards and thought they were unrealistic in light of kids' actual sexual behavior. SIECUS, *SHOP Talk Bulletin* 4 (June 11, 1999).

39. "State Sexuality and HIV/STD Education Regulations," National Abortion Rights Action League fact sheet, February 1997.

40. "Sex Education That Teaches Abstinence Wins Support," Associated Press, *New York Times,* July 23, 1997.

41. "Between the Lines: States' Implementation of the Federal Government's Section 510(b) Abstinence Education Program in Fiscal Year 1998," SIECUS report, Washington, D.C., 1999.

42. Six in ten believe that sexual intercourse in the teen years was always wrong, and nine out of ten wanted their kids to be taught about abstinence at school. Yet eight in ten also wanted them to learn about contraception and preventing sexually transmitted diseases. SIECUS, *SHOP Talk Bulletin* 4 (June 11, 1999).

43. "Adolescent Sexual Health in Europe & the U.S.—Why the Difference?" 2d ed., Advocates for Youth report, Washington, D.C., 2000.

44. Douglas Kirby, "No Easy Answers: Research Findings on Programs to Reduce Teen Pregnancy," National Campaign to Prevent Teen Pregnancy report, Washington, D.C., 1997.

45. Marl W. Roosa and F. Scott Christopher, "An Evaluation of an Abstinence-Only Adolescent Pregnancy Prevention Program: Is 'Just Say No' Enough?" *Family Relations* 39 (January 1990): 68–72.

46. John B. Jemmott III, Loretta Sweet Jemmott, and Geoffrey T. Fong, "Abstinence and Safer Sex: HIV Risk-Reduction Interventions for African American Adolescents," *Journal of the American Medical Association* 279, no. 19 (May 20, 1998): 1529–36.

47. Ralph J. DiClemente, Editorial: "Preventing Sexually Transmitted Infections among Adolescents," *Journal of the American Medical Association* 279, no. 19 (May 20, 1998).

48. National Institutes of Health Consensus Development Conference Statement, *Interventions to Prevent HIV Risk Behaviors,* February 11–13, 1997 (Bethesda, Md.: NIH), 15.

49. Ron Haskins and Carol Statuto Bevan, "Implementing the Abstinence Education Provision of the Welfare Reform Legislation," U.S. House of Representatives memo, November 8, 1996, 1.

50. Haskins and Bevan, "Implementing the Abstinence Education Provision," 8–9.

51. "Changes in Sexuality Education from 1988–1999."

52. Victor Strasburger, *Getting Your Kids to Say "No" in the '90s When You Said "Yes" in the '60s* (New York: Simon and Schuster, 1993), 87–88.

53. Sol Gordon and Judith Gordon, *Raising a Child Conservatively in a Sexually Permissive World* (New York: Simon and Schuster, 1989), 101.

54. Peter C. Scales and Martha R. Roper, "Challenges to Sexuality Education in the Schools," in *The Sexuality Education Challenge: Promoting Healthy Sexuality in Young People,* ed. Judy C. Drolet and Kay Clark (Santa Cruz, Calif.: ETR Associates, 1994), 79.

55. Colleen Kelly Mast, *Sex Respect: Parent-Teacher Guide* (Bradley, Ill.: Respect Inc., n.d.), 45.

56. Other educators have pointed out the implicit inaccuracy of the impression these slides leave: unfortunately, one of the most common STDs, chlamydia, is asymptomatic.

57. *Teaching Fear,* 8.

58. Medical Institute for Sexual Health, *National Guidelines for Sexuality and Character Education* (Austin, Tex.: Medical Institute for Sexual Health, 1996), 82.

59. Saint Augustine, *Confessions* (Oxford: Oxford University Press, 1991), 24–25.

60. Medical Institute for Sexual Health, "National Guidelines," 89.

61. "HIV: You Can Live without It!" (Spokane, Wash.: Teen-Aid, Inc., 1998), 33.

62. Margaret Atwood, *The Handmaid's Tale* (New York: Houghton Mifflin, 1986), 24.

63. Scales and Roper, "Challenges to Sexuality Education," 70.

64. Irving R. Dickman, *Winning the Battle for Sex Education,* pamphlet (New York: SIECUS, 1982); Debra Haffner and Diane de Mauro, *Winning the Battle: Developing Support for Sexuality and HIV/AIDS Education,* pamphlet (New York: SIECUS, 1991); *Teaching Fear.*

65. The ad ran in the *New York Times,* April 22, 1997, the *Los Angeles Times,* April 28, 1997, as well as the West Coast editions of *Time, Newsweek,* and *People* during that month.

66. "Trends in Sexual Risk Behaviors among High School Students— U.S. 1991–97," *Morbidity and Mortality Weekly Report* 47 (September 18, 1998): 749–52. Teens may be doing better than adults. "Most Adults in the United States Who Have Multiple Sexual Partners Do Not Use Condoms Consistently," *Family Planning Perspectives* 26 (January/February 1994): 42–43.

67. Susheela Singh and Jacqueline E. Darroch, "Adolescent Pregnancy and Childbearing: Levels and Trends in the Developed Countries," *Family Planning Perspectives* 32 (2000): 14–23. The government recorded the

lowest number of teen pregnancies in 1997: 94.3 per thousand women ages fifteen to nineteen, a drop of 19 percent since 1991. Most of those pregnancies are among eighteen- and nineteen-year-old women. In 1999, the U.S. teen birth rate hit its lowest level since recording began in 1940. Of every thousand teenage women, 4.96 gave birth. Centers for Disease Control and Prevention National Center for Health Statistics, *National Vital Statistics Report* 4, no. 4 (2001).

68. About three-quarters of girls use a method the first time; as many as two-thirds of teens say they use condoms regularly—three times the rate in 1970. Long-acting birth control injections and implants have also gained popularity among teens. "Why Is Teenage Pregnancy Declining? The Roles of Abstinence, Sexual Activity and Contraceptive Use," Alan Guttmacher Institute Occasional Report, 1999. The National Campaign to Prevent Teen Pregnancy asked teens themselves the main reason they thought teen pregnancies had dropped in the last decade. Of 1,002 youths surveyed, 37.9 percent named worry about AIDS and other STDs; 24 percent credited a greater availability of birth control; and 14.9 percent said the decline was due to more attention to the issue. Only 5.2 percent named "changing morals and values," and 3.7 percent said, "Fewer teens have sex." *With One Voice: American Adults and Teens Sound Off about Teen Pregnancy* (Washington, D.C.: National Campaign to Prevent Teen Pregnancy, 2001).

69. Singh and Darroch, "Adolescent Pregnancy and Childbearing."

70. "Teen Pregnancy 'Virtually Eliminated' in the Netherlands," Reuters Health/London news story (accessed through Medscape), March 2, 2001.

71. "United States and the Russian Federation Lead the Developed World in Teenage Pregnancy Rates," Alan Guttmacher Institute press release, February 24, 2000.

72. J. Mauldon and K. Luker, "The Effects of Contraceptive Education on Method Use at First Intercourse," *Family Planning Perspectives* (January/ February 1996): 19.

73. J. C. Abma et al., "Fertility, Family Planning, and Women's Health: New Data from the 1995 National Survey of Family Growth," *Vital Health Statistics* 23, no. 19 (1997).

74. Peggy Brick et al., *The New Positive Images: Teaching Abstinence, Contraception and Sexual Health* (Hackensack, N.J.: Planned Parenthood of Greater Northern New Jersey, 1996), 31.

75. Peter Bearman, paper presented at Planned Parenthood New York City's conference Adolescent Sexual Health: New Data and Implications for Services and Programs, October 26, 1998; Diana Jean Schemo, "Virginity Pledges by Teenagers Can Be Highly Effective, Federal Study Finds," *New York Times*, January 4, 2001.

76. Lantier, "Do Abstinence Lessons Lessen Sex?"

77. "Trends in Sexual Risk Behaviors among High School Students—

United States 1991–1997," *Morbidity and Mortality Weekly Reports* 47 (September 18, 1998): 749–52.

78. Abma et al., "Fertility, Family Planning, and Women's Health."

79. It is important to point out that, in spite of these declines, nearly two-thirds of teen births resulted from unintended pregnancies. Abma et al., "Fertility, Family Planning, and Women's Health."

80. "Adolescent Sexual Health in the U.S. and Europe—Why the Difference?" Advocates for Youth fact sheet, Washington, D.C., 2000.

81. Schemo, "Virginity Pledges by Teenagers."

82. It is impossible to find a forthright statement that abstinence-plus education meaningfully delays teen sexual intercourse. Its evaluators have been able to find out only that, for instance, if you want to delay intercourse, you should start classes before kids start "experimenting with sexual behaviors." And all studies show that sex ed does not encourage earlier intercourse. J. J. Frost and J. D. Forrest, "Understanding the Impact of Effective Teenage Pregnancy Prevention Programs," *Family Planning Perspectives* 27 (1995): 188–96; D. Kirby et al., "School Based Programs to Reduce Sexual Risk Behaviors: A Review of Effectiveness," *Public Health Reports* 190 (1997): 339–60; A. Grunseit and S. Kippax, *Effects of Sex Education on Young People's Sexual Behavior* (Geneva: World Health Organization, 1993).

83. S. Zabin and M. B. Hirsch, *Evaluation of Pregnancy Prevention Programs in the School Context* (Lexington, Mass.: D.C. Heath/Lexington Books, 1988); Institute of Medicine, *The Best Intentions: Unintended Pregnancy and Well-Being of Children and Families* (Washington, D.C.: National Academy Press, 1995).

6. Compulsory Motherhood

1. This law, the first gate to open in the gradual spilling away of federally protected abortion rights, was reauthorized in every subsequent Congress; its constitutionality was upheld three times. In 1993, after a long battle, it was "liberalized" to add exceptions for rape and incest. But while the government paid for a third of abortions from 1973 to 1977, it now pays for almost none. Marlene Gerber Fried, "Abortion in the U.S.: Barriers to Access," *Reproductive Health Matters* 9 (May 1997): 37–45.

2. Ellen Frankfort and Frances Kissling, *Rosie: Investigation of a Wrongful Death* (New York: Dial Press, 1979).

3. "Who Decides? A State-by-State Review of Abortion and Reproductive Rights," 10th ed., National Abortion Rights Action League report, Washington, D.C., 2001.

4. By the 1990s, more than 80 percent of clinics were regularly picketed by anti-abortion activists. Ann Cronin, "Abortion: The Rate vs. the Debate," *New York Times*, February 25, 1997, "Week in Review," 4.

5. The agency reported at least fifteen bombings and arson attacks at clinics each year from 1993 through 1995, seven in 1996, and one in Atlanta in 1997 that injured six people. Rick Bragg, "Abortion Clinic Hit by 2 Bombs; Six Are Injured," *New York Times,* January 17, 1997.

6. Jim Yardley and David Rohde, "Abortion Doctor in Buffalo Slain; Sniper Attack Fits Violent Pattern," *New York Times,* October 25, 1998, A1.

7. Alan Guttmacher Institute, "Into a New World: Young Women's Sexual and Reproductive Lives," *Executive Summary* (New York: the institute, 1988).

8. Women ages eighteen to twenty-four are about twice as likely to have abortions as women in the general population. Stanley K. Henshaw and Kathryn Kost, "Abortion Patients in 1994–1995: Characteristics and Contraceptive Use," *Family Planning Perspectives* 28 (1996): 140–47, 158.

9. Robert Pear, "Provision on Youth Health Insurance Would Sharply Limit Access to Abortion," *New York Times,* July 3, 1997.

10. About twenty-six million have legal abortions yearly, and an estimated twenty million have illegal ones, ending about half of all unplanned pregnancies. *Alan Guttmacher Institute News,* January 21, 1999.

11. Estimated rates ran from one in ten to almost one in two, and among Kinsey's unmarried informants, 90 percent of those who got pregnant procured abortions. Lawrence Lader, *Abortion* (New York: Bobbs-Merrill, 1966), 64–74; Kristin Luker, *Abortion and the Politics of Motherhood* (Berkeley: University of California Press, 1984), 48–49; Brett Harvey, *The Fifties: A Women's Oral History* (New York: Harper Collins, 1993), 24.

12. "Abortion Common among All Women Even Those Thought to Oppose Abortion," Alan Guttmacher Institute press release, 1996.

13. Cronin, "Abortion: The Rate vs. the Debate."

14. In a New York Times–CBS poll in 1998, half of respondents thought abortion was too easy to get; as compared with 1989, fewer people felt that an interrupted career or education was an acceptable reason to get an abortion; and only 15 percent believed abortion was acceptable in the second trimester. "[P]ublic opinion has shifted notably away from general acceptance of legal abortion and toward an evolving center of gravity: a more nuanced, conditional acceptance that some call a 'permit but discourage' model." Carey Goldberg with Janet Elder, "Public Still Backs Abortion, but Wants Limits, Poll Says," *New York Times,* January 16, 1998, A1.

15. Jennifer Baumgartner, "The Pro-Choice PR Problem," *Nation* (March 5, 2001): 19–23.

16. Naomi Wolf, "Our Bodies, Our Souls: Rethinking Pro-Choice Rhetoric," *New Republic* (October 16, 1995): 26–27.

17. Janet Hadley, "The 'Awfulisation' of Abortion," paper presented to the Abortion Matters conference, Amsterdam, March 1996.

18. "Abortion Common . . . ," Guttmacher Institute.

19. *Nation* columnist Katha Pollitt is one of the few who has defended the morality of abortion.

20. See, for example, Vincent M. Rue, "The Psychological Realities of Induced Abortion," in *Post-Abortion Aftermath: A Comprehensive Consideration,* ed. Michael T. Mannion (Franklin, Wis.: Sheed and Ward, 1994). The antichoice group Operation Rescue has widely distributed Focus on the Family's pamphlet *Identifying and Overcoming Post-Abortion Syndrome,* by Teri K. and Paul C. Reisser (Colorado Springs: Focus on the Family, revised 1994).

21. "Abortion Study Finds No Long-Term Ill Effects on Emotional Well-Being," *Family Planning Perspectives* 29 (July/August 1997): 193; Jane E. Brody, "Study Disputes Abortion Trauma," *New York Times,* February 12, 1997, C8.

22. "Researchers Document Flaw in Research Linking Abortion and Breast Cancer," *Reproductive Freedom News* 20 (December 20, 1996), quoting *Journal of the National Cancer Institute* (December 4, 1996).

23. Rebecca Stone and Cynthia Waszak, "Adolescent Knowledge and Attitudes about Abortion," *Family Planning Perspectives* 24 (Narcg 1992): 53.

24. Stone and Waszak, "Adolescent Knowledge and Attitudes."

25. Connecticut, Michigan, and Rhode Island, to name three, forbade discussion of abortion as a reproductive health method; South Carolina allowed discussion of the procedure but only its negative consequences. "Sexuality Education in America: A State-by-State Review," National Abortion Rights Action League report, Washington, D.C., 1995. Under the federal abstinence-only regulations, of course, abortion may not be mentioned.

26. *Sex Respect Student Workbook,* 95.

27. On the tonsillectomy comparison, see "Safety of Abortion," National Abortion Rights Action League fact sheet, Washington, D.C., undated, received 1998; and *Review of Fear-Based Programs,* SIECUS Community Action Kit, 1994: 6. On the shot of penicillin comparison, see Margie Kelly, "Legalized Abortion: A Public Health Success Story," *Reproductive Freedom News* (June 1999): 7.

28. Girls Incorporated, *Taking Care of Business: A Sexuality Education Program for Young Teen Women Ages 15–18* (Indianapolis: Girls Inc., 1998), vol. 6, 1–6.

29. *Sex Can Wait* (Santa Cruz, Calif.: ETR Associates, 1998), 290.

30. Peggy Brick and Bill Taverner, *The New Positive Images: Teaching*

Abstinence, Contraception and Sexual Health, 3d ed. (Morristown, N.J.: Planned Parenthood of Greater Northern New Jersey, 2001).

31. After reading the curricula used in public schools, I find it a relief and inspiration to peruse the Unitarian Universalist Church's *Our Whole Lives.* Its curricula both for seventh- to ninth-graders and for older high schoolers present thorough discussions of the values debate around abortion, as well as explicit descriptions of the procedures and clear statements of abortion's safety. The tenth- to twelfth-grade text titles the section on abortion "Reproductive Rights." Pamela M. Wilson, *Our Whole Lives: Sexuality Education for Grades 7 to 9* (Boston: Unitarian Universalist Association/United Church Board for Homeland Ministries, 1999); Eva S. Goldfarb and Elizabeth M. Casparian, *Our Whole Lives: Sexuality Education for Grades 10 to 12* (Boston: Unitarian Universalist Association/United Church Board for Homeland Ministries, 1999), 199–212.

32. Alan Guttmacher Institute, "Teenage Pregnancy and the Welfare Reform Debate," *Issues in Brief* (Washington, D.C.: the institute, 1995).

33. Hector Sanchez-Flores, speaking at the Adolescent Sexual Health: New Data and Implications for Services and Programs conference, sponsored by Planned Parenthood of New York City and other organizations, October 26, 1998.

34. On metropolitan areas, see Barbara Vobejda, "Study Finds Fewer Facilities Offering Abortions," *Washington Post,* December 11, 1998, A4.

35. The Defense Department also prohibited both federally and privately funded abortions at military facilities. Cronin, "Abortion: The Rate vs. the Debate."

36. National Abortion Rights Action League, 1998 statistics (accesssed on www.naral.org), Washington, D.C.

37. Margaret C. Crosby and Abigail English, "Should Parental Consent to or Notification of an Adolescent's Abortion Be Required by Law? No"; and Everett L. Worthington, "Should Parental Consent . . . ? Yes"; both in *Debating Children's Lives: Current Controversies on Children and Adolescents,* ed. Mary Ann Mason and Eileen Gambrill (Thousand Oaks, Calif.: Sage Publications, 1994), 143 and 133, respectively.

38. Crosby and English, "Should Parental Consent . . . ? No," 143.

39. Court approval by "judicial bypass," the legal remedy to the discriminatory burden such regulations place on girls who can't talk to their families, may even discourage such conversations. Crosby and English, "Should Parental Consent . . . ? No."

40. "Induced Termination of Pregnancy before and after *Roe v. Wade,* Trends in the Mortality and Morbidity of Women," *Journal of the American Medical Association* 268, no. 22 (December 1993): 3238.

41. American Medical Association, Council on Ethical and Judicial

Affairs, "Mandatory Parental Consent to Abortion," *Journal of the American Medical Association* 269, no. 1 (January 6, 1993): 83.

42. Lizette Alvarez, "GOP Bill to Back Parental Consent Abortion Laws," *New York Times,* May 21, 1998, A30. The datum that young women support parental involvement laws was gleaned from a nationwide study of teens and young adult women, but since this fact did not support the political aims of the group that conducted the study, the group's board of directors has chosen not to publicize it.

43. "Woman Is Sentenced for Aid in Abortion," *New York Times,* December 17, 1996.

44. "Debate Continues on Child Custody Protection Act," *Reproductive Freedom News* 7, no. 5 (June 1, 1998): 3–4; "Women's Stories: Becky Bell," National Abortion Rights Action League report, Washington, D.C., undated.

45. Alvarez, "GOP Bill."

46. The bill was reintroduced in 2001. At this writing, it has not been voted on.

47. Tamar Lewin, "Poll of Teenagers: Battle of the Sexes on Roles in Family," *New York Times,* July 11, 1994, A1.

48. Addressing this atavistic social problem, lawmakers in two dozen states have proposed granting money to women who dispose of unwanted infants, as long as the babies are still breathing and the mothers leave them in an authorized location, such as a hospital. Currently, many states prosecute mothers who abandon their newborns. Jacqueline L. Salmon, "For Unwanted Babies, a Safety Net," *Washington Post,* October 20, 2000.

7. The Expurgation of Pleasure

1. Peggy Brick, "Toward a Positive Approach to Adolescent Sexuality," *SIECUS Report* 17 (May–June 1989): 3.

2. *Guidelines for Comprehensive Sexuality Education,* 1.

3. Michelle Fine, "Sexuality, Schooling, and Adolescent Females: The Missing Discourse of Desire," *Harvard Educational Review* 58 (1988): 33.

4. Girls Incorporated, *Will Power/Won't Power: A Sexuality Education Program for Girls Ages 12–14* (Indianapolis: Girls Inc., 1998), V-12.

5. Richard P. Barth, *Reducing the Risk: Building Skills to Prevent Pregnancy, STD, and HIV,* 3d ed. (Santa Cruz, Calif.: ETR Associates, 1996), 89.

6. Tim LaHaye and Beverly LaHaye, *The Act of Marriage: The Beauty of Sexual Love* (Grand Rapids, Mich.: Zondervan, 1976), 289–90.

7. This was the definition given by the majority in Stephanie A. Sanders and June Machover Reinisch's "Would You Say You 'Had Sex' If . . . ?" *Journal of the American Medical Association* 281 (January 20, 1999): 275–77. See also Lisa Remez, "Oral Sex among Adolescents: Is It

Sex or Is It Abstinence?" Alan Guttmacher Institute, Special Report 32, November–December 2000.

8. Mary M. Krueger, "Everyone Is an Exception: Assumptions to Avoid in the Sex Education Classroom," *Family Life Educator* (fall 1993).

9. Cindy Patton, *Fatal Advice: How Safe-Sex Education Went Wrong* (Durham, N.C.: Duke University Press, 1996), 34.

10. The National Survey of Adolescent Males Ages 15 to 19, conducted in 1995 and published in 2000, found that one in ten had experienced anal sex. Tamar Lewin, "Survey Shows Sex Practices of Boys," *New York Times,* December 19, 2000. In one San Francisco survey of seventeen- to nineteen-year-old men who have sex with men, 28 percent had had *unprotected* anal sex, the behavior carrying the highest risk for HIV transmission. U.S. Conference of Mayors, "Safer Sex Relapse: A Contemporary Challenge," *AIDS Information Exchange* 11, no. 4 (1994): 1–8.

11. On the masturbation datum, see Krueger, "Everyone Is an Exception." On the oral sex datum, see Susan Newcomer and J. Richard Udry, "Oral Sex in an Adolescent Population," *Archives of Sexual Behavior* 14 (1985): 41–46. In another survey, of more than two thousand Los Angeles high school "virgins" in 1996, about a third of both boys and girls had masturbated or been masturbated by a heterosexual partner; about a tenth had engaged in fellatio to ejaculation or cunnilingus, with boys and girls more or less equally on the receiving end. Homosexual behavior was rarely reported among these kids, but 1 percent reported heterosexual anal intercourse. Mark A. Schuster, Robert M. Bell, and David E. Kanouse, "The Sexual Practices of Adolescent Virgins: Genital Sexual Activities of High School Students Who Have Never Had Vaginal Intercourse," *American Journal of Public Health* 86 (1996): 1570–76. Remez ("Sex among Adolescents") provides a good review of the scant literature on noncoital adolescent sexual behavior. She also suggests that the incidence and prevalence of fellatio probably far outweigh cunnilingus among teens. Many teens who have had oral sex have not had vaginal intercourse. One of Remez's sources guesses that "for around 25 percent of the kids who have had any kind of intimate sexual activity, that activity is oral sex, not intercourse."

12. Tamar Lewin, "Teen-Agers Alter Sexual Practices, Thinking Risks Will Be Avoided," *New York Times,* April 5, 1997, 8.

13. "Research Critical to Protecting Young People from Disease Blocked by Congress," Advocates for Youth, press release, December 19, 2000.

14. See Thompson, *Going All the Way*; and, e.g., Deborah L. Tolman, "Daring to Desire: Culture and the Bodies of Adolescent Girls," in *Sexual Cultures and the Construction of Adolescent Identities,* ed. Irvine, 250–84.

15. Tamar Lewin, "Sexual Abuse Tied to 1 in 4 Girls in Teens," *New York Times,* October 1, 1997.

16. Lewin, "Sexual Abuse Tied to 1 in 4 Girls."

17. Nancy D. Kellogg, "Unwanted and Illegal Sexual Experiences in Childhood and Adolescence," *Child Abuse and Neglect* 19 (1995): 1457–68.

18. *Not Just Another Thing to Do: Teens Talk about Sex, Regret, and the Influence of Their Parents* (Washington, D.C.: National Campaign to Prevent Teen Pregnancy, 2000), 6–7.

19. "Many Teens Regret Having Sex," National Campaign to Prevent Teen Pregnancy, press release, June 30, 2000.

8. The Facts

1. Adam Phillips, "The Interested Party," *The Beast in the Nursery* (New York: Vintage Books, 1999), 3–36.

2. Janet R. Kahn, "Speaking across Cultures within Your Own Family," in *Sexual Cultures and the Construction of Adolescent Identities,* ed. Irvine, 287.

3. Brent C. Miller, *Family Matters: A Research Synthesis of Family Influences on Adolescent Pregnancy* (Washington, D.C.: National Campaign to Prevent Teen Pregnancy, 1998), 6–12.

4. Diane Carman, in the *Denver Post,* March 2, 1999, posted on the Kaiser Family Foundation Web page.

5. Other good books were *Changing Bodies, Changing Selves,* for teens, by Ruth Bell and members of the Boston Women's Health Book Collective (New York: Vintage Books, 1988); Michael J. Basso, *The Underground Guide to Teenage Sexuality* (Minneapolis: Fairview Press, 1997); and for younger readers, *It's Perfectly Normal: Changing Bodies, Growing Up, Sex, and Sexual Health,* by Robie H. Harris with illustrations by Michael Emberley (Cambridge, Mass.: Candlewick Press, 1994).

6. Go Ask Alice! Columbia University's Health Question & Answer Internet Service, at www.goaskalice.columbia.edu.

7. www.positive.org/JustSayYes.

8. A search for this URL in June 2001 yielded an "Object Not Found" message. However, sites for gay teens are proliferating.

9. *Sex, Etc.* can be accessed on the Internet at www.sxetc.org.

10. David Shpritz, "One Teenager's Search for Sexual Health on the Net," *Journal of Sex Education and Therapy* 22 (1998): 57.

11. Economics and Statistics Administration and National Telecommunications and Information Administration, "Falling through the Net: Toward Digital Inclusion," U.S. Department of Commerce report, Washington, D.C., October 2000, 2–12.

12. See chapter 1 for more discussion of legislated and voluntary Internet filtering.

13. Phillips, "The Interested Party," 14.

14. Stephen Holden, "Hollywood, Sex, and a Sad Estrangement," *New York Times,* May 3, 1998, "Arts & Leisure," 20.

15. Francesca Lia Block, *Weetzie Bat,* in *Dangerous Angels* (New York: HarperCollins, 1998), 29.

16. This insight, of course, must be attributed to the great art critic Leo Steinberg.

17. Journalist Debbie Nathan, ever-vigilant watchdog of cultural absurdity, reminds me that the soundtrack of the 1996 movie *William Shakespeare's Romeo and Juliet* was on the stereo when police arrived at the home of Kip Kinkel to find the dead bodies of his parents. The Springfield, Oregon, boy had just been arrested for the shooting deaths of two of his high school classmates and the wounding of twenty-five others. He is serving a life sentence for murder.

18. William Butler Yeats, "Brown Penny," in *Selected Poems and Two Plays of William Butler Yeats,* ed. M. L. Rosenthal (New York: Macmillan, 1962), 37.

9. What Is Wanting?

1. See, e.g., Barrie Thorne, *Gender Play: Girls and Boys in School* (New Brunswick, N.J.: Rutgers University Press, 1997); and R. W. Connell, *Masculinities: Knowledge, Power, and Social Change* (Los Angeles: University of California Press, 1995).

2. See Michael Reichert, "On Behalf of Boys," *Independent School Magazine* (spring 1997).

3. Males, *Scapegoat Generation,* 46. About 15 percent of tenth-grade students in a longitudinal survey reported fewer experiences of sexual intercourse than they'd claimed in the ninth grade, and of all the kids questioned over the years, two-thirds reported the age at first intercourse "inconsistently." Cheryl S. Alexander et al., "Consistency of Adolescents' Self-Report of Sexual Behavior in a Longitudinal Study," *Journal of Youth and Adolescence* 22 (1993): 455–71.

4. Susan Newcomer and J. Richard Udry, "Adolescents' Honesty in a Survey of Sexual Behavior," *Journal of Adolescent Research* 1, no. 3/4 (1988): 419–23.

5. "Fact Sheet: Dating Violence among Adolescents," Advocates for Youth (accessed at www.advocatesforyouth.org), Washington, D.C., n.d.

6. In *Our Guys,* Bernard Lefkowitz cites another relevant study: "When the psychologist Chris O'Sullivan studied 24 documented cases of alleged gang rape on college campuses from 1981 to 1991, she found that it was the elite group at the colleges that were more likely to be involved. These included football and basketball players and members of prestigious fraternities." Bernard Lefkowitz, *Our Guys* (New York: Vintage Books, 1998), 278–79.

7. A critique of quantitative desire disorders has been mounted by sociologist Janice Irvine, journalist Carol Tavris, sexologist Leonore Tiefer, and some others. Tiefer's sociopolitical perspective is rare in her discipline.

8. Social Security Act, Title V, Section 510 (1997), Maternal and Child Health Bureau, U.S. Department of Health and Human Services.

9. William A. Fisher and Deborah M. Roffman, "Adolescence: A Risky Time," *Independent School* 51 (spring 1992): 26.

10. Deborah Tolman, "Daring to Desire," in *Sexual Cultures and the Construction of Adolescent Identities,* ed. Irvine, 255.

11. Jack Morin, *The Erotic Mind* (New York: Harper Collins, 1995), 83–85.

12. Mary Pipher, *Reviving Ophelia: Saving the Selves of Adolescent Girls* (New York: Ballantine Books, 1994), 208.

13. Pipher, *Reviving Ophelia,* 205–13. These pages contain Lizzie's account, as described here and in the following paragraph.

14. Tolman, "Daring to Desire," 251.

15. This difficulty of putting emotions into words—what one writer called "alyxrythmia"—has been all but naturalized as a masculine trait. (A good example of interpreting everything as biological, even when the description is clearly social, is "Boys Will Be Boys," *Newsweek*'s cover story of May 11, 1998.) But there's plenty of evidence it is completely socialized. Janet R. Kahn interviewed 326 families in 1976 and again in 1983 and found that, across class and race, parents talked less often to their boys about fewer topics related to sexuality and relationships and that fathers talked with their kids far less than mothers. The situation was so serious for boys that she called it "conversational neglect." Kahn, "Speaking across Cultures within Your Own Family."

16. William Pollack, *Real Boys: Rescuing Our Sons from the Myths of Boyhood* (New York: Random House, 1998), 150–51.

17. Pollack, *Real Boys,* 151.

18. Susan E. Hickman and Charleen L. Muehlenhard, "By the Semi-Mystical Appearance of a Condom: How Young Women and Men Communicate Sexual Consent," paper presented at the Annual Meeting of the Society for the Scientific Study of Sex, Houston, Texas, November 1996.

19. Alwyn Cohall, speaking at a Planned Parenthood of New York conference, Adolescent Sexual Health: New Data and Implications for Services and Programs, October, 26, 1998.

20. Kaiser Family Foundation, "National Survey of Teens on Dating, Intimacy, and Sexual Experiences," reported by SIECUS, *SHOP Talk Bulletin* 2 (April 17, 1998).

10. Good Touch

1. Ashley Montagu, *Touching: The Human Significance of the Skin,* 3d ed. (New York: Harper and Row/Perennial, 1986), 33.

2. Stephen J. Suomi, "The Role of Touch in Rhesus Monkey Social Development," in Catherine Caldwell Brown, ed., *The Many Facets of Touch* (n.p.: Johnson & Johnson Baby Products, 1996), 41–50.

3. Montagu, *Touching*, 97–99.

4. Madtrulika Gupta et al., "Perceived Touch Deprivation and Body Image: Some Observations among Eating Disordered and Non-Clinical Subjects," *Journal of Psychosomatic Research* 39 (May 1995): 459–64.

5. The French children were touched more. Author interview, 1999.

6. James W. Prescott, "Body Pleasure and the Origins of Violence," *Futurist* (April 1975): 66.

7. Clellan S. Ford and Frank A. Beach, *Patterns of Sexual Behavior* (New York: Harper/Colophon Books, 1951), 180.

8. Alfred C. Kinsey, Wardell B. Pomeroy, and Clyde E. Martin, *Sexual Behavior in the Human Male* (Philadelphia: W. B. Saunders, 1948), 177. Kinsey also notes observations of infant girls in "masturbatory activity" to what he called orgasm. Alfred C. Kinsey, Wardell B. Pomeroy, Clyde E. Martin, and Paul H. Gebhard, *Sexual Behavior in the Human Female* (Philadelphia: W. B. Saunders, 1953), 141–42.

9. Robin J. Lewis and Louis H. Janda, "The Relationship between Adult Sexual Adjustment and Childhood Experiences Regarding Exposure to Nudity, Sleeping in the Parental Bed, and Parental Attitudes toward Sexuality," *Archives of Sexual Behavior* 17, no. 4 (1988): 349–62; Paul Okami, "Childhood Exposure to Parental Nudity, Parent-Child Co-Sleeping, and 'Primal Scenes': A Review of Clinical Opinion and Empirical Evidence," *Journal of Sex Research* 32, no. 1 (1995): 51–64.

10. Tamar Lewin, "Breast-Feeding: How Old Is Too Old?" *New York Times*, February 18, 2001, "Week in Review."

11. Lewin, "Breast-Feeding."

12. Richard Johnson, unpublished manuscript, March 1998.

13. This has been reported to me by many sex educators, including the veteran Peggy Brick, of Planned Parenthood of Greater Northern New Jersey.

14. Joseph Tobin, ed., *Making a Place for Pleasure in Early Childhood Education* (New Haven: Yale University Press, 1997).

15. "It is unclear whether prevention programs are working or even that they are more beneficial than harmful," concluded N. Dickson Reppucci and Jeffrey J. Haugaard. See their "Prevention of Child Sexual Abuse: Myth or Reality," *American Psychologist* 44 (October 1989): 1266.

16. One study measured a 50 percent rise in fear levels among children who had been subjected to a prevention program that made use of comic-book characters. J. Garbarino, "Children's Response to a Sexual Abuse Prevention Program: A Study of the Spiderman Comic," *Child Abuse and Neglect: The International Journal* 11 (1987): 143–48.

17. Bonnie Trudell and M. Whatley, "School Sexual Abuse Prevention:

Unintended Consequences and Dilemmas," *Child Abuse and Neglect* 12 (1988): 108.

18. Thomas W. Laqueur, "The Social Evil, the Solitary Vice, and Pouring Tea," in *Solitary Pleasures,* ed. Bennett and Rosario, 157.

19. Alice Balint, *The Psychoanalysis of the Nursery* (New York: Routledge and Kegan Paul, 1953), 79.

20. Benjamin Spock, *Baby and Child Care,* rev. ed. (New York: Pocket Books, 1976), 411.

21. John H. Gagnon, "Attitudes and Responses of Parents to Pre-Adolescent Masturbation," *Archives of Sexual Behavior* 14 (1985): 451.

22. *Congressional Record,* 103d Congress, 2d session, 1994, vol. 140, H 9995–10001.

23. Joycelyn Elders, "The Dreaded 'M' Word," in *nerve: Literate Smut,* ed. Genevieve Field and Rufus Griscom (New York: Broadway Books, 1998), 130.

24. William N. Friedrich and Patricia Grambsch, "Child Sexual Behavior Inventory: Normative and Clinical Comparison," *Psychological Assessment* 4 (1992): 303–11.

25. Friedrich and Grambsch, "Child Sexual Behavior Inventory."

26. Robin L. Leavitt and Martha Bauman Power, "Civilizing Bodies: Children in Day Care," in *Making a Place for Pleasure in Early Childhood Education,* ed. Tobin, 39–75.

27. Leavitt and Power, "Civilizing Bodies," 45–46.

28. Peggy Brick, Sue Montford, and Nancy Blume, *Healthy Foundations: The Teacher's Book* (Hackensack, N.J.: Center for Family Life Education/Planned Parenthood of Greater Northern New Jersey, 1993), 2–7.

29. Larry L. Constantine and Floyd M. Martinson, eds., *Children and Sex: New Findings, New Perspectives* (Boston: Little, Brown, 1981), 30.

30. Nancy Blackman, "Pleasure and Touching: Their Significance in the Development of the Preschool Child," paper delivered at the International Symposium on Childhood and Sexuality, Montreal, September 1979.

31. Outercourse was named, but not invented, in the 1970s. Even before the eighteenth century, when travel was slow and distances long, there was "bundling." "The practice allowed a [courting] couple to spend a night together in bed as long as they remained fully clothed or, in some cases, kept a 'bundling board' between them. . . . Parents and youth shared the expectation that sexual intercourse would not take place, but if it did, and pregnancy resulted, the couple would certainly marry." John D'Emilio and Estelle B. Freedman, *Intimate Matters: A History of Sexuality in America* (New York: Harper and Row, 1988), 22.

32. Marty Klein and Riki Robbins, *Let Me Count the Ways: Discovering Great Sex without Intercourse* (New York: Jeremy P. Tarcher/Putnam, 1998), 125.

33. Leonore Tiefer, "Bring Back the Kids' Stuff," in *Sex Is Not a Natural Act*, 71. Note from a detractor who read this chapter: "This strikes me as a crock, remembering instances of petting with strangers. . . ."

34. Tiefer, "Bring Back the Kids' Stuff," 70.

35. Advocates for Youth, "Adolescent Sexual Health in Europe and the U.S." (2001).

36. Klein and Robbins, *Let Me Count the Ways*.

11. Community

1. Patton, *Fatal Advice*, 34. Patton was not the only one to indict abstinence education as a killer. In 1997, the International AIDS Conference proclaimed that the abstinence-only "approach place[d] policy in direct conflict with science and ignore[d] overwhelming evidence that other programs would be effective." In the face of a worldwide health crisis, conferees strongly suggested, teaching "just say no" was worse than a waste of public resources. It was lethal.

2. Half of the forty thousand new HIV infections a year are in people under twenty-five, according to estimates from the Centers for Disease Control and the National Institutes of Health. Bill Alexander, "Adolescent HIV Rates Soar; Government Piddles," *Youth Today* (March/April 1997): 29.

3. They were down 44 percent in the first six months of 1997 compared with 1996. Altman, "AIDS Deaths Drop 48% in New York."

4. Hilts, "AIDS Deaths Continue to Rise in 25–44 Age Group."

5. Including those who inject drugs, the numbers fell from 65 percent in 1981 to 44 percent in 1996. Centers for Disease Control, Atlanta, Ga., March 1996.

6. Interview with Gary Remafedi, director of the University of Minnesota/Minneapolis Youth & AIDS Project, 1998.

7. "Rate of AIDS Has Slowed," *New York Times*, April 25, 1998, A9. African Americans make up half of new HIV infections and 40 percent of full-blown AIDS cases. Doug Ireland, "Silence Kills Blacks," *Nation* (April 20, 1998): 6. Poor neighborhoods, where almost everybody knows somebody with the disease, are being ravaged. In the South Bronx, for instance, AIDS is the leading cause of death in children (interview with GMHC spokesman, 1999).

8. Altman, "Study in 6 Cities Finds HIV in 30% of Young Black Gays."

9. Cherrie B. Boyer and Susan M. Kegeles, "AIDS Risk and Prevention among Adolescents," *Social Science Medicine* 33, no. 1 (1991): 11–23.

10. New York City Health Department, phone interview, April 1999.

11. Barbara Crossette, "In India and Africa, Women's Low Status Worsens Their Risk of AIDS," *New York Times*, February 26, 2001.

12. B. R. Simon Rossner, "New Directions in HIV Prevention," *SIECUS Report* 26 (December 1997/January 1998): 6.

13. Governments of developing countries have won some concessions

from the major pharmaceutical companies, but many observers believe these are too little, too late.

14. The following remarks from people in the Twin Cities came from interviews that I conducted during my visit there in 1998.

15. *District 202 Youth Survey* (Minneapolis, 1997).

16. *District 202 Youth Survey.*

17. Marsha S. Sturdevant and Gary Remafedi, "Special Health Needs of Homosexual Youth," in *Adolescent Medicine: State of the Art Reviews* (Philadelphia: Hanley and Belfus, 1992), 364. The authors cite a study of male prostitutes and other delinquent young men that found that 70 percent of the former group considered themselves gay or bisexual compared with only 4 percent of the latter. D. Boyer, "Male Prostitution and Homosexual Identity," *Journal of Homosexuality* 15 (1989): 151.

18. R. Stall and J. Wiley, "A Comparison of Alcohol and Drug Use Patterns of Homosexual and Heterosexual Men: The San Francisco Men's Health study," *Drug and Alcohol Dependence* 22 (1988): 63–73.

19. "Although there is a significant relationship between substance use and high risk sexual activity, substance use does not cause sexual risk taking," according to a compilation of research by Advocates for Youth. "At-risk teens tend to engage in several inter-related high risk behaviors at once." Marina McNamara, "Adolescent Behavior: II. Socio-Psychological Factors," Advocates for Youth fact sheet, Washington, D.C., September 1997.

20. Studies suggest that as many as 35 percent of young gay males and 30 percent of lesbians have considered or tried suicide. Alan Bell and Martin Weinberg, *Homosexualities* (New York: Simon and Schuster, 1978). As for kids who succeed in self-annihilation, the 1989 U.S. Department of Health and Human Services Task Force on Youth Suicide reported that 30 percent may be gay.

21. Gary Remafedi, Michael Resnick, Robert Blum, and Linda Harris, "Demography of Sexual Orientation in Adolescents," *Pediatrics* 89, no. 4 (April 1992).

22. Patton, *Fatal Advice.*

23. U.S. Conference of Mayors, "Safer Sex Relapse: A Contemporary Challenge," *AIDS Information Exchange* 11, no. 4 (1994): 1–8.

24. Altman, "Study in 6 Cities."

25. D. Boyer, "Male Prostitution and Homosexual Identity," *Journal of Homosexuality* 9 (1984): 105.

26. In one study of New York kids selling sex on the street, only 36 percent of respondents had failed to protect themselves in the last encounter. S. L. Bailey et al., "Substance Use and Risky Sexual Behavior among Homeless and Runaway Youth," *Journal of Adolescent Health* 23 (December 1998): 378–88.

27. Amy Bracken, "STDs Discriminate," *Youth Today* (March 2001): 7–8.

28. *Minnesota's Youth without Homes* (St. Paul: Wilder Research Center, 1997), 5.

29. Ine Vanwesenbeeck, "The Context of Women's Power(lessness) in Heterosexual Interactions," in *New Sexual Agendas,* ed. Lynne Segal (New York: New York University Press, 1997), 173. A 1998 study of homeless youth, however, found that only 36 percent of respondents, who were mostly female, did not use a condom with a casual partner, and the less-well-known a partner was, the more likely they were to use a condom. S. L. Bailey et al., "Substance Use and Risky Sexual Behavior."

30. Author interview, New York, 1999.

31. E. Matinka-Tyndale, "Sexual Scripts and AIDS Prevention: Variations in Adherence to Safer Sex Guidelines in Heterosexual Adolescents," *Journal of Sex Research* 28 (1991): 45–66; S. J. Misovich, J. D. Fisher, and W. A. Fisher, "The Perceived AIDS-Preventive Utility of Knowing One's Partner Well: A Public Health Dictum and Individuals' Risky Sexual Behaviour," *Canadian Journal of Human Sexuality* 5 (1996): 83–90; Linda Feldman, Philippa Holowaty, et al., "A Comparison of the Demographic, Lifestyle, and Sexual Behaviour Characteristics of Virgin and Non-Virgin Adolescents," *Canadian Journal of Human Sexuality* 6, no 3. (fall 1997): 197–209.

32. Carla Willig, "Trust as a Risky Practice," in *New Sexual Agendas,* ed. Segal, 125–35.

33. Graham Hart, "'Yes, but Does It *Work?*' Impediments to Rigorous Evaluations of Gay Men's Health Promotion," in *New Sexual Agendas,* ed. Segal, 119. Gary Remafedi, "Predictors of Unprotected Intercourse among Gay and Bisexual Youth: Knowledge, Beliefs, and Behavior," *Pediatrics* 94, no. 2 (1994): 163.

34. Sarah R. Phillips, "Turning Research into Policy: A Survey on Adolescent Condom Use," *SIECUS Report* (October/November 1995): 10.

35. Willig, "Trust as a Risky Practice," 126.

36. Willig, "Trust as a Risky Practice," 130.

37. Regarding adults who stray, the 1994 University of Chicago "Sex in America" survey put the numbers at 25 percent of married men and 12 percent of married women, but these statistics do not include unmarried committed heterosexual or gay couples and have been considered by others to be extremely conservative. Other studies have found higher incidences. In their extensive 1983 survey, Pepper Schwartz and Philip Blumenstein divided their subjects among married couples, heterosexual cohabitors, and gay and lesbian couples. Their numbers for "nonmonogamy" ranged from 21 percent for wives to 82 percent for gay male cohabitors. Of course, their study was done before widespread awareness of AIDS. Pepper

Schwartz and Philip Blumstein, *American Couples: Money, Work, Sex* (New York: Pocket Books, 1983). Regarding the number of teens who stray, see Susan L. Rosenthal et al., "Heterosexual Romantic Relationships and Sexual Behaviors of Young Adolescent Girls," *Journal of Adolescent Health* 21 (1997): 238–43.

38. Of these, African American teen males report the highest use, at 72 percent, with whites and Hispanics following at 70 percent and 59 percent, respectively. Freya L. Sonenstein and Joseph H. Pleck et al., "Change in Sexual Behavior and Contraception among Adolescent Males: 1988 and 1995," Urban Institute report, Washington, D.C., 1996.

39. Willig, "Trust as a Risky Practice," 130.

40. Jeffrey Weeks, *Invented Moralities: Sexual Values in an Age of Uncertainty* (New York: Columbia University Press, 1995), 42.

Epilogue

1. Jane E. Brody, "A Stitch in Time," *New York Times,* March 21, 1999, "Week in Review," 2.

2. Steve Farkas et al., *Kids These Days: What Americans Really Think about the Next Generation* (New York: Public Agenda, 1997).

3. Children's Defense Fund, Web site, 1999.

4. "The State of the World's Children 2000," United Nations/UNICEF report (accessed at www.unicef.org/sowc00/).

5. "Study Says Welfare Changes Made the Poorest Worse Off," *New York Times,* August 23, 1999; Elizabeth Becker, "Millions Eligible for Food Stamps Aren't Applying," *New York Times,* February 26, 2001.

6. Matt Pacenza, "911, a Food Emergency: Soup Kitchens Are Flooded," *City Limits Weekly* Web site, October 1, 2001.

7. These data come from a small but well-controlled sample. Patrick Boyle, "Does Welfare Reform Hurt Teens?" News Briefs, *Youth Today* (March 2001): 6–7.

8. Children's Defense Fund, Web site, 1999.

9. Most of these children live in homes in which at least one parent has a job. *State of America's Children Yearbook 2001* (Washington, D.C.: Children's Defense Fund, 2001).

10. David G. Gil, "The United States versus Child Abuse," in *The Social Context of Child Abuse and Neglect,* ed. Leroy H. Pelton (New York: Human Sciences Press, 1981), 294.

11. Ethan Bronner, "Long a Leader, U.S. Now Lags in High School Graduate Rate," *New York Times,* November 24, 1998, A1.

12. Children's Defense Fund, Web site, 2001.

13. Forty percent of prison inmates twenty-five and older are illiterate. Marc Maurer, "Young Black Men and the Criminal Justice System: A

Growing National Problem," The Sentencing Project report, Washington, D.C., 1990.

14. At this writing, President George W. Bush and the Republican Party used the September 11 attacks and the ensuing war in Afghanistan to push through an economic "stimulus package" including more tax cuts for the richest individuals and the elimination of the minimum corporate tax. The GOP resisted such Democratic demands as increased, more easily obtained unemployment insurance for people who have lost their jobs since the attacks.

15. Gisela Konopka, "Requirements for Healthy Development of Adolescent Youth," *Adolescence* 8 (1973): 1–26.

Afterword

1. As I write, the Kansas State Senate has voted to cut $3 million from the state university budget unless the school ceases to purchase "obscene" materials used in a popular sexuality education class, such as a slides of naked five- and ten-year-old girls.

Index

Abortion, ix; among Christians, 119; after contraceptive failure, 120; European rates of, 102; health risks of, 123; information sources on, 145; legal vs. illegal, 119, 261n. 10; among low-income teens, 123–24; as a moral good, 120, 126, 262n. 19; regrets about, 121–22; as sex-ed topic, 93, 103, 262nn. 20, 25; teen rates of, 118–19, 261n. 8

"About Your Sexuality" (Unitarian sex-ed program), 14–15

Abstinence education: as child neglect, 109; current emphasis on, xxiv, xxxii, 90–116, 257n. 38; depiction of, as freedom, 107–8; federal government's advocacy of, 91, 97–103, 159, 215, 222, 262n. 25; as ineffective, 93–94, 102, 112–13, 201, 257n. 38; intercourse as emphasis of, 129–33; as lethal, 102, 199–200, 271n. 1; opposition to, 257n. 38; and view of sex as dangerous, 105–16, 159,

199–203, 255n. 28; as a word, 95, 252n. 2

Achilles myth, 172–73

ACLU. *See* American Civil Liberties Union

Act of Marriage, The (LaHaye and LaHaye), 130

ACT-UP, 200, 207

Adebanjo, Toyin, 209

Adolescence (definition), xxix. *See also* Teenagers

Adolescent Family Life Act. *See* AFLA

Adolescent Health Services and Pregnancy Prevention and Care Act, 254n. 17

Adolescents. *See* Teenagers

Adoption, 97, 108, 123

Adults: ambivalence of American, toward children, xxxi–xxxii, 27–29, 219–22; sentencing of children as, xxxii, 88; sex portrayed as only for, 108–10; sexual desire of, for children, xxiii, 20–44. *See also* Parents

Advocates for Youth, 93, 101, 113, 272n. 19

Journalist and independent scholar **Judith Levine** is the author of *My Enemy, My Love: Women, Men, and the Dilemmas of Gender.* Her articles on sex, gender, politics, and psychology have appeared in many national periodicals, including *Harper's,* the *Village Voice, Vogue, My Generation,* and the online magazines salon.com and ncrve.com. She is an active civil libertarian and a founder of the National Writers Union and the feminist guerrilla theater group No More Nice Girls.

Dr. Joycelyn M. Elders is professor emerita of pediatric endocrinology at the University of Arkansas School of Medical Science. She has written many articles for medical research publications based on her studies of growth in children and the treatment of hormone-related illnesses. She served as Surgeon General of the U.S. Public Health Service from 1993 to 1995.